Living and Dying in São Paulo

Living and Dying in São Paulo

Immigrants, Health, and
the Built Environment in Brazil

JEFFREY LESSER

DUKE UNIVERSITY PRESS
Durham and London
2025

Printed in the United States of America on acid-free paper ∞
Project Editor: Ihsan Taylor
Designed by A. Mattson Gallagher
Typeset in Minion Pro and Source Sans 3
by Westchester Publishing Services

Library of Congress Cataloging-in-Publication Data
Names: Lesser, Jeff, author.
Title: Living and dying in São Paulo : immigrants, health, and the built environment
in Brazil / Jeffrey Lesser.
Description: Durham : Duke University Press, 2025. | Includes bibliographical
references and index.
Identifiers: LCCN 2024035214 (print)
LCCN 2024035215 (ebook)
ISBN 9781478030980 (paperback)
ISBN 9781478026723 (hardcover)
ISBN 9781478059936 (ebook)
ISBN 9781478094111 (ebook other)
Subjects: LCSH: Public health—Brazil—São Paulo. | Environmental health—Brazil—
São Paulo. | Social classes—Health aspects—Brazil—São Paulo. | Immigrants—Health
and hygiene—Brazil—São Paulo. | Bom Retiro (São Paulo, Brazil)—Social conditions. |
Bom Retiro (São Paulo, Brazil)—Emigration and immigration—Health aspects.
Classification: LCC RA464.S3 L47 2025 (print) | LCC RA464.S3 (ebook) |
DDC 362.10981/61—dc23/eng/20250121
LC record available at https://lccn.loc.gov/2024035214
LC ebook record available at https://lccn.loc.gov/2024035215

Cover art: "The Plague in S. Paulo." *O Commercio de São Paulo,*
October 28, 1899.

THIS BOOK IS FREELY AVAILABLE IN AN OPEN ACCESS
EDITION THANKS TO THE GENEROUS SUPPORT
OF EMORY UNIVERSITY AND THE ANDREW W. MELLON
FOUNDATION.

Dedicated to the memories of
William Morris Lesser, זײל
Irma Friedlander Lesser, זײל
Michael Shavitt, זײל
Silvana Levi Shavitt, זײל
Warren Dean
Anani Dzidzienyo

CONTENTS

A LONG SET OF ACKNOWLEDGMENTS

This book was conceived during a very boring meeting of department chairs and administrators. Fortunately, I was sitting in the back of the room with the bad kids, including Uriel Kitron, whom readers will meet in the text. As we discussed our mutual research interests in Brazil, we began to think of a project on the relation between immigration and health. It did not take long for us to jointly teach an interdisciplinary seminar on the topic and arrange a grant to bring some students in that class to Brazil.

As the project progressed, and I became more interested in working in teams, the need for funding grew. Many institutions and individuals provided support to this project and what became the Lesser Research Collective (LRC), and all deserve immense thanks. My first major fellowship came from the Institute of Advanced Studies of the University of São Paulo (Instituto de Estudos Avançados, IEA), whose directors, Martin Grossmann, Paulo Saldiva, and Guilherme Ary Plonski, were unfailingly generous. At the IEA, Rafael Borsanelli and Richard Meckien gave me extraordinary support, as did the wonderful staff: Marisa Macedo Gomes Alves, Fátima Moreno, Fernanda Cunha Rezende, Tizuko Sakamoto, Aziz Salem, Raimunda Rodrigues dos Santos, Sandra Sedini, Marlene Signoretti, and João Fernando da Silva. At the IEA I am part of the Intercultural Dialogues (Diálogos Interculturais) research group, coordinated by Sylvia Duarte Dantas and Paulo Daniel Farah, and they and all the members have inspired me in many ways.

The LRC was co-led during most of the research for this book by Dr. Emily Sweetnam Pingel, a policy analyst at the National Center for Immunization and Respiratory Diseases. The team members who conducted research included in this book include Dr. Sara Kauko and Dr. Alexander Cors, along with Bianca Letícia de Almeida, Juliana Casagrande, Jenn Choe, Doris Cikopana, Orlando Guarnier Cardin Farias, Vitória Martins Fontes, Daniella Gonzalez, Sabrina Jin, Beatriz Kalichman, Delphine LaCroix, Julia Chaejin Lee, and Alexandra Caridad Llovet. During the final stages of this project, Cintia Rodrigues de Almeida, Monaliza Caetano dos Santos, Victoria Maza, Luanna Gabrielly Mendes do Nascimento, and Surbhi Shrivastava became interlocutors and improved the book immensely. The wide-ranging research production that emerged from the collective is included in the bibliography.

Over many years, the residents of Bom Retiro have been partners in this project. To those whose homes and workplaces we visited on house calls and whom we have met on the streets, thank you, muito obrigado, muchas gracias, 감사합니, Aguyjevete ndéve, 谢谢, and אדאנק.

The LRC's observations at the Bom Retiro Public Health Clinic began when Dr. Francisco Moreno Carvalho ז״ל, introduced us to Clélia Neves Azevedo, the chief administrator through 2021, and Dr. Fernando Cosentino, who continues to lead Team Green. At the clinic, my thanks go to the physicians, nurses, community health agents, and other health professionals who supported the research and helped make sure that I was in good health. Angélica Souza made everything happen, Sandra Montanari taught me many special Bom Retiro words, and Ana Maria Barreto invited me to her home many times. Team Green members—including Vanessa Wilde Ambrosio, Marcela Borges de Souza, Marina Cândido da Mata, Dany Colin, Leide Dayanne, Muriel Flores, Lene Gonçalves, Tica Porto, Luciana Menjou, Su Ribeiro, and Sheila Vasconcelos—could not have been more supportive. Thank you as well to Evelyn Fabiana Costa, Patricia Debiaze, Sandra Faustino, Barbara Ferreira, Jorge Gutierrez, Sandra Maida, Dafni Paiva, Carol Silva, Patty Torres, Janete Uchoa, and Felipe Lucas Ribeiro da Silva.

A Fulbright Senior Fellowship allowed me to finish the research, and Dr. Luiz Loureiro, Patricia Domenico R. Grijó, Christiane Nagayassu, and Taynara Barros at the Brazilian Fulbright Commission were incredibly supportive, as they have been over many years. My Fulbright host was the State University of São Paulo (Universidade Federal de São Paulo, UNIFESP). I want to thank Dr. Luis Ferla and the members of the History, Maps, and Computers Laboratory (História, Mapas e Computadores, HIMACO) and Pauliceia 2.0 projects—Karine R. Ferreira, Luis Ferla, Gilberto R. de Queiroz,

Nandamudi Vijaykumar, Carlos Noronha, Rodrigo Mariano, Denis Taveira, Gabriel Sansigolo, Orlando Guarnieri, Thomas Rogers, Michael Page, Fernando Atique, Daniela Musa, Janaina Santos, Diego Morais, Cristiane Miyasaka, Cintia Almeida, Luanna Nascimento, Jaine Diniz, and Monaliza Santos. I am especially grateful for the festas de chegada e despedida (welcome and going-away parties) that this group participates in with me several times a year.

Researchers cannot do their work without colleagues at archives, and I want to thank Josianne Oliveira, Elisandra Gasparini, Maria Talib Assad, and Roque Fernandes at the Emílio Ribas Public Health Museum of the Butantan Institute (Museu de Saúde Pública Emílio Ribas do Instituto Butantan) as well as Sergio de Simone, Maria Luisa da Silva, Rodrigo Galvão, and Sandra Pereira. At the São Paulo State Archives (Arquivo Público do Estado de São Paulo), Janaina Yamamoto, Haike Kleber da Silva, and Elzio José da Silva were immensely helpful. The archivists at the São Paulo Municipal Archive (Arquivo Histórico Municipal de São Paulo) and the Aguirra Archive of the Museu Paulista of the University of São Paulo were fundamental in helping me find data, as were Anna Levin at the Ibero-Amerikanisches Institut—Preußischer Kulturbesitz and Dr. Eduardo de Masi and his colleagues in the São Paulo Municipal Ministry of Health.

Three Emory University units funded the students who were part of the LRC: the Global Health Institute, the University Research Council, and the Interdisciplinary Faculty Fellowship Program. A TOME (Toward an Open Monograph Ecosystem) grant from a collaboration of the Association of American Universities, Emory University, and the Andrew W. Mellon Foundation has allowed an open-access version of the book, and my thanks go to Mae Velloso-Lyons, senior program coordinator, and the evaluation committee for Digital Publishing in the Humanities for their support.

Gisela Fosado, editorial director at Duke University Press, has been a constant and encouraging supporter over many years and many books. Her generosity and positive spirit always inspire me. The two anonymous reviewers of the original manuscript provided amazing comments, and I am grateful for their unselfishness in evaluating the book for both its methodological and analytical approaches. At Duke University Press, Alejandra Mejía, Lalitree Darnielle, and A. Mattson Gallagher prepared and designed the monograph, while Ihsan Taylor and Kimberly Miller did heroic work in turning the manuscript into a book.

At Emory, Keith Anthony, Becky Herring, Shinn Ko and her staff, Alexandra Lemos, Phil MacLeod, Xóchtil Marsilli-Vargas, Franzene Minott,

Marissa Nichols and her students, Pablo Palomino, Thomas D. Rogers, Allison Rollins, Karen Stolley, Ana Catarina Teixeira, Leonardo Velloso-Lyons, Katie Wilson, Yanna Yannakakis, and Kelly Yates have encouraged me to be creative and put research, teaching, and academics at the forefront of the university experience.

Doing research outside the United States can be challenging, and History Department chairs James Melton, Kristin Mann, Joe Crespino, and Sharon Strocchia encouraged me to apply for grants and fought for the time I needed to take them. Michael Elliot, Deboleena Roy, Carla Freeman, and Susan Lee supported me as I kept the project rolling despite my own administrative responsibilities.

Jaqueline Wolf and her colleagues in the Department of History at Ohio University inspired me to move forward with the project when I still had not figured out where it was going. The participants in the Toronto Latin America Seminar, organized by Gillian McGillivray, including Peter Beattie, Anne-Emanuelle Birn, Benjamin Bryce, Jerry Dávila, and David Sheinin, improved early paragraphs and pages immensely. Sérgio Costa and his colleagues at the Free University of Berlin, and Benito Schmidt and Ruben Oliven and their colleagues at the Federal University of Rio Grande do Sul, gave me opportunities to present work in progress, while more developed chapters received excellent critiques at the Emory Latin American and Latinx Workshop in 2023, organized by Yanna Yannakakis and Mónica Garcia Blizzard. Members of the National Autonomous University of Mexico's Seminar on the History of Migrations in Mexico (Seminario de Historia de las Migraciones en México), including Daniela Gleizer, Pablo Yankelevich, América Molina del Villar, Irina Córdoba, and Catherine Vézina, provided guidance in making my broader argument. The same was the case at Tel Aviv University, where my thanks go to Leo Corey, Raanan Rein, Miri Shefer-Mossensohn, and Atalia Shragai. Marcos Chor Maio, Gilberto Hochman, and Jaime Benchimol of the Graduate Program in the History of the Sciences and Health at the Oswaldo Cruz Foundation (Programa de Pós-Graduação em História das Ciências e da Saúde da Casa de Oswaldo Cruz) have helped shape this work immensely, as have colleagues at the Maria Sibylla Merian Centre on Conviviality-Inequality in Latin America—including Tomaz Amorim, Sérgio Costa, Jörg Dünne, Roberta Hesse, Barbara Göbel, Susanne Klengel, Anna Levin, Melanie Metzen, Joanna Malgorzata Moszczynska, Marina Falcão Motoki, Marcos Nobre, Barbara Potthast, Joaquim Toledo Jr., Peter W. Schulze, and especially Simone Toji.

One of the pleasures of this project was making presentations around the globe, in Mozambique at the Manhiça Center for Health Research (Centro de Investigação em Saúde de Manhiça) and in Brazil at the Casa do Povo, the Emílio Ribas Hospital, and the UNIFESP School of Medicine in São Paulo. Fabio Valentim and his students at the School of Architecture and Urbanism of the Escola da Cidade helped me think about space in new ways. My special thanks go to Nadya Guimarães Araújo, Sergio Guimarães, Cássio Silveira, Denise Martins, Oziris Simões, and Gildo Magalhães dos Santos Filho for including me in so many different health-related events.

Many of the almost completed chapters of the book were presented in a series of seminars at the University of Zurich, under the auspices of the chair of the Anthropocene, Debjani Bhattacharyya. She and her colleagues and students were remarkably generous with their time. I want to especially thank Martin Dusinberre, Matthieu Leimgruber, Yi-Tang Lin, Moe Omiya, Camille Elisabeth Schneiter, and Leila Girschweiler.

Debjani Bhattacharyya, Alexander Cors, Monaliza Caetano dos Santos, Matthew C. Gutmann, Pablo Palomino, Emily Sweetnam Pingel, Thomas D. Rogers (whose coefficient is the star of chapter 6), Tuli Shragai, Surbhi Shrivastava, Heeju Sohn, and Chris Suh read and commented on the final draft of the manuscript, making this a much better book.

Books start and end with family and friends, and many of both have been mentioned above. Others who have heard way too much about this project include Jung Yun Chi, Laís Miwa Higa, Dária Jaremtchuk, Xochitl Marsilli-Vargas, Denny Tavares, Celso Zilbovicius, Giovani Sacrini, Raanan Rein, Esti Rein, Roberto Lang, Barbara Lang, Roney Cytrynowicz, Monica Cytrynowicz, Patrick Allitt, Samy Katz, Gabriel Londe, and Harold Solomon. The Lessers and Shavitts are a constant throughout all my research. To my growing family, Eliana, Aron and Ana, and Gabi and Sabin, this book could not have happened without your support and love.

An Introduction

Selling a Gun

One day I found a gun. It was hidden in a closet in my deceased in-laws' apartment in São Paulo, a city that has been one of my homes for almost four decades. Why would my spouse's peaceful, law-abiding parents, both refugees from Nazi-era Europe, conceal this weapon? Finding the gun led to a combination of accidents and luck that molded the questions that this book asks about movement, the built environment, and living and dying, whether from disease or violence.[1] The weapon, and my attempts to dispose of it, took me on a journey across geographies, temporalities, and peoples that included immigrants and public health officials, neighborhoods and buildings, illnesses and cures, and life and death.

Getting rid of the revolver, as I explain in more detail below, ended with a long drive in the back of a police car to my research site in Bom Retiro, the central São Paulo city neighborhood that is the geographic focus of this book (map I.1). This district has a long Indigenous and African-descent history but has been popularly stereotyped for more than a century as having primarily immigrant residents. In the late nineteenth century, those newcomers were primarily Catholics from Italy, with other significant populations from Spain and Portugal.[2] In the interwar period, both religion and national origin began to change with the entry of eastern European Jewish and Greek Orthodox immigrants. Korean Christians, primarily Protestant, began settling in the early 1960s. In the 1980s Bolivian

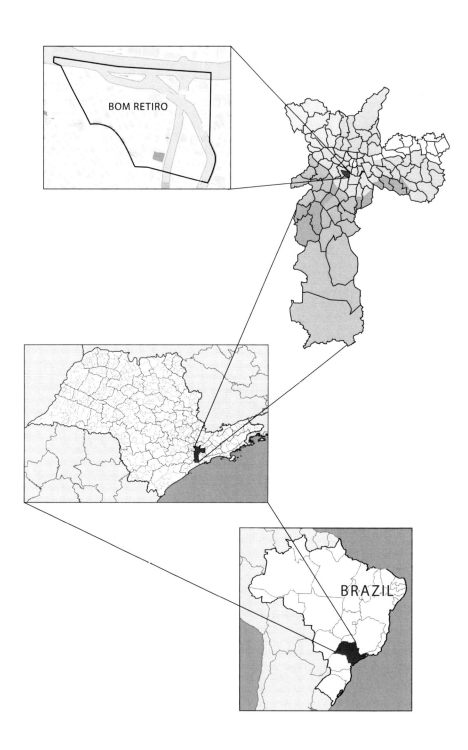

BOM RETIRO

BRAZIL

and Paraguayan newcomers, many of them Protestant Evangelicals, became the labor backbone in unregistered sweatshops/residences, often owned by the descendants of earlier arrivals.[3] More recently, the neighborhood has become home to immigrants from China, Africa, South Asia, and the Caribbean.

Disposing of a gun legally in Brazil in mid-2015 (before Jair Bolsonaro was elected and eased gun-buying and ownership restrictions) had many challenges. Chucking it into the trash was, my family agreed, a terrible idea since gun violence is frequent in Brazil. It was easy to find information about the Brazilian government's weapon buyback program on the federal website, but days of phone calls to the authorities produced brush-offs.[4] Eventually my very determined spouse connected with Inspector Aparecida of the São Paulo Metro Civil Police (Guarda Civil Metropolitana), and she agreed to help me get rid of the gun.

Inspector Aparecida suggested that she, I, and the gun meet at the Sé Metro Station, located in one of the eight districts that make up São Paulo's densely populated and geographically compact historic center. I stuffed the weapon in my backpack along with a Civil Police internet form that provided permission to use public transportation when selling a gun. Buses and metros are how I normally get around São Paulo, but this was the first time I was packing heat. It was scary and exciting.

I got off the metro at Sé station, trying to think of ways to explain the gun if I were searched as I was not entirely confident that my web document would convince the police that I was not a criminal. My paranoia eased when Inspector Aparecida and her two bodyguards appeared, a not-surprising trio since in São Paulo city police generally patrol in pairs or groups.[5] Together we walked to a Civil Police station in the Praça da Sé, the official geographic center and ostensible founding point of São Paulo. A huge Catholic Church looks over the plaza, dominated by a towering statue of the sixteenth-century Padre José de Anchieta, the "Apostle of Brazil," ministering to kneeling Indigenous peoples, although another interpretation regards it as a monument to oppression. In the 1960s the Praça da Sé was the site of some of Brazil's most important political protests, but today it is filled with Evangelical Protestants in the throes of religious fervor, often preaching from churches that are established by placing blue tape on the ground. Businesspeople, increasingly from Africa, sell their wares from tarps with corner cords that can be quickly scooped up to avoid police raids. Many residents of São Paulo without formal housing live on and around the Praça da Sé, where social service organizations provide meals.

We arrived at the police station, located next to the Anchieta statue in a building that once housed an informal hostel for undocumented immigrants. Despite Inspector Aparecida's rank, the officers on duty were dismissive, claiming that they did not have the paperwork at hand to take the gun. They suggested that we try another station, located less than five hundred meters away, in front of the University of São Paulo Law School. Off we went, the inspector, her bodyguards, the gun, and Jeffinho. We found the mobile police unit inside a small converted camper. Remarkably, the van had an internet connection, and the officer on duty agreed to generate the paperwork needed to take the pistol. I patted myself on the back for doing the right thing and prepared to walk the thirty minutes to Bom Retiro, where I had an appointment at the archive of the Emílio Ribas Public Health Museum, which was filled with documents I was eager to read.

As is often the case, I did not really understand what was going on. The policeman told me that I couldn't simply hand over the gun and head off to the archive. Instead, the officer explained that the police had to purchase the gun. That meant paperwork, lots of paperwork. The first forms were straightforward—my personal information and a description of how and where I found the revolver. The second set of documents was about the weapon itself. The name of the manufacturer was stamped on the frame, but the caliber was not. The officer called his colleagues into the tight space as everyone tried to figure out what the gauge was, where the bullets would be inserted, and how the gun worked.

After about twenty minutes of careful analysis, the truth was revealed: the "revolver" that had so terrified me and my family was in fact a starter pistol, which I later learned my father-in-law would fire to begin children's track and field races.[6] When we discovered that the nonlethal revolver had its barrel filled and was not able to fire bullets, I thought it would lead to laughter and me being sent off. Inspector Aparecida saw things differently. If the "gun" had fooled her colleagues, she reckoned, it would fool the public and thus could be used to commit crimes.[7]

The not-so-deadly starter pistol had again become a deadly weapon. It needed to be off the streets, and that could only happen if I sold the gun to the police. The sale needed to be carefully documented since in Brazil and most of Latin America both the population and the political state (i.e., politicians and legislators) largely distrust the latter's agents, such as law enforcement.[8] This distrust is apparent not only when selling weapons. For immigrants, the distrust becomes clear when the Brazilian Federal Police emit a document confirming the approval of immigrant residency, and then, as I learned during my own migration experience, a second document is needed to confirm the legitimacy of the first at border control points staffed by the same Federal Police. The lack of trust also meant that I was not allowed to gift the gun to the police since that might create a scenario where the pistol might be resold or regifted illegally. This should not have been a surprise to me—although it was—given the extensive research on the often-thin lines between lawbreaking and law enforcement.[9]

Systemic distrust meant that the police and I needed to formalize a transaction to prove that I had sold a real gun and that they had bought and then disposed of it. That meant still more paperwork. It took almost two hours to generate the receipt that represented the sale; during that time the officers and I chatted about family, my research, and futebol (soccer). The receipt, the officer explained, was not the end of the process. The gun would only be registered as sold after I went to a Bank of Brazil ATM and entered a special code that would lead me to a special screen for selling guns. By using a unique PIN on this screen, I would receive cash and a receipt that I was required to retain. The officer, quite reasonably thinking that I was a moron for trying to sell a starter pistol in the first place, gave me 1-2-3-4 as my PIN. He wrote it down for me in large numbers on the receipt. He then made me repeat the sequence out loud twice—1-2-3-4, 1-2-3-4—since he may have concluded that I could not read well, and he wanted to ensure that I followed the procedure. I did as I was told and was relieved to be rid of the gun and happy to have the equivalent of about US$25 in extra cash.

With the arms deal concluded, it was time for the inspector to get back to her office at the Civil Police headquarters near Bom Retiro's huge, British-built Luz Railway Station. Since the archive of the Emílio Ribas Public

Health Museum was nearby, Inspector Aparecida offered me a lift, and another adventure began as I was wedged between her bodyguards in the back of the police car. We moved slowly through the traffic-filled streets. Reaching Bom Retiro by car from the Praça da Sé can easily take twice as long as it does on foot. Pedestrians peered into the vehicle to see who had been arrested. Inside the automobile, our conversations were wide-ranging. One officer's mother had recently died, and he ruminated on the relationship between being an officer, a son, and now an orphan of sorts. Inspector Aparecida spoke with great pride about the medical care provided by the Brazilian Unified Health System but criticized the lack of mental health treatment. These dual views are widespread among many sectors of the Brazilian public, who complain about the lack of services, long waits for treatment, and poor facilities.[10] When a different policeman grumbled that Bom Retiro had too many foreigners, the driver rebutted that the problem in Brazil was too many Brazilians.

The flow of the vehicle and the chat show "how geographies, rhythms, politics, economies, cultures, natures, and power relations constitute the everyday urban experience [and become] a powerful means of revealing the rhythms that in large part constitute urban life, inequality, and change."[11] The tale of how I tried to sell the "gun" also underscores my presence in this project. Whether in an archive or in a patient's residence, human interactions and physical spaces influenced how I understood the data I collected.

People and Space

In 1892 a military health official working in the infirmary of Bom Retiro's military barracks called the district "the worst neighborhood in São Paulo."[12] His comment gave the district of less than four square kilometers an oversized place within the imaginary of the city. Size, both geographic and imagined, was on my mind as the police car crept through the city. Inspector Aparecida was late for an appointment, so our first stop was at the headquarters of the Civil Police, one of the institutions that emerged from the nineteenth-century Directorate of Police and Hygiene and the early twentieth-century Police Medical Assistance Unit, both precursors of the contemporary São Paulo Municipal Coroner's Office (Instituto Médico Legal). The contemporary Civil Police building is less than a hundred meters from the Luz Railway Station, where hundreds of thousands of immigrants disembarked in the nineteenth and twentieth centuries after arriving by boat at the port of Santos, about eighty kilometers away. Today the Luz Railway Station is a hub for both the metro and the commuter lines that many in the working classes use to return to their homes on the geographic periphery of São Paulo city.

The Civil Police headquarters is a three-minute walk from what had been a railroad depot. In 1942 that "old and somber building" became the headquarters of the Department of Political and Social Order (DEOPS), a brutal security force created in 1924 that used the building as a location of torture and violence during the military dictatorship (1964–84).[13] These two buildings, and the military barracks mentioned above, are only some of the structural reminders in Bom Retiro of how the state sponsored physical, mental, and symbolic violences. For example, just a mile away from the former DEOPS building was the infamous Tiradentes Prison, in operation from 1852 to 1973.[14] These structures, and what happened to people inside of them, have made Bom Retiro one important location for memories of oppression and resistance.[15] Films like *The Year My Parents Went on Vacation* (*O ano em que meus pais saíram de férias*), nominated by the Brazilian Ministry of Culture for the 2006 Oscar for best foreign film, and Samuel Reibscheid's 1995 short story whose Yiddish/Portuguese title "Plétzale. Marco Zero" (The Jewish quarter, ground zero), for example, use Bom Retiro to explore the harsh years of the dictatorship.[16]

After dropping off the inspector, we made our way to the nearby Rua José Paulino, Bom Retiro's main artery and commercial street, named after a land, bank, and railroad owner who was a philanthropist for health-related causes.[17] When laid out in the late nineteenth century, the thoroughfare's name was the Rua dos Imigrantes (Immigrants Street), but the name was changed to honor José Paulino in 1915, five years after Bom Retiro had been elevated to district status.[18] The new street name was part of an attempt by the city to recognize what the *Correio Paulistano* newspaper, a major journalistic enterprise founded in 1854, called "extraordinarily thrilling" economic growth in the neighborhood.[19] Many businesses were owned and operated by immigrants. Maye Goldstein, an eastern European Jewish immigrant, for example, actively bought, sold, and rented homes and workspaces. The Roman Pharmacy treated many forms of *bad health*, the term I use throughout this book to encompass the broad ways that the public understands physical and mental illnesses. Bad health had many causes, including violence, infectious diseases, falls and collisions, and long hours in small factories like the Italian-American Woodwork and Carpentry Company or large ones like the Germânia Brewery.

Most of the enterprises in Bom Retiro, historically and in the present, connect to the domestic textile industry, where work conditions are often precarious, and workers are often unwell. This makes aspects of life and death in Bom Retiro similar to those in other cities in the Americas with garment districts, such as the Gamarra neighborhood in Lima, Peru, said to have ninety thousand textile workers; and Paterson, New Jersey, United States, once known as America's Silk City.[20] Diana Taylor concluded that the textile industry helped to make Bom Retiro chaotic (like the events related to my arrival in the district above) and often illusionary. She called the district "São Paulo's phantasmagorical world of things" after analyzing a performance that used the streets of the neighborhood as a stage.[21] Those "things," human and not, are in constant movement, and we might think of Bom Retiro and neighborhoods like it as urban ventricular arteries.

In a similar vein, the flows of people and goods indicate that health and immigration are not confined to official geographic contours, or the around forty thousand residents and perhaps twice as many daily workers and shoppers in Bom Retiro. What happens, and happened, in Bom Retiro does not stay in Bom Retiro: it is part of a global dialogue. Former US president Bill Clinton's 1997 speech to Brazilian businesspeople made this clear: "The neighborhoods of São Paulo are a window on the World. . . . The spirit of the Middle East fills Bom Retiro. The rhythms of Africa pervade every quarter. People from everywhere call this place home."[22] As Andrew Britt has noted, Clinton's comments "cast São Paulo's racialized/ethnicized neighborhoods as timeless and essential elements of the city's seemingly distinctive brand of ethnoracial mixture and supposedly harmonious interethnic relations."[23] Britt's comments could also apply to the hipster publication *Time Out*, which named Bom Retiro as among the "coolest" neighborhoods in the world because of its "exhilarating gastronomic scene—thanks to its melting pot of immigrants from Italy, Korea, Greece, Bolivia, Eastern Europe and more."[24]

Rua José Paulino is still lined with clothing- and textile-related shops owned by immigrants and descendants of immigrants, located on the ground floors of two- and three-story buildings. While contemporary textile workers usually, but not always, use electric rather than human-powered sewing machines, their small workspaces are often in the same locations they would have been a century ago.[25] During business hours the street is packed with consumers buying clothing and textile-related products, and salespeople calling pedestrians into their shops to "take a peek." Today the stores are often overseen by Korean immigrant/descendant owners, but fifty years ago the owners might have been eastern European Jews, and a century ago they might have been Christians from the Middle East or southern Europe. Human-pulled and -pushed carts move loads of cloth and accessories, finished clothing, and snacks for purchase, just as they did in the nineteenth century. Police foot patrols are ever present during daylight although they, like everything else, seem to disappear with the arrival of darkness.

If shoppers were to look above the street-level retail and wholesale outlets, which they rarely do, they would see tinted, often barred, windows that keep upper-floor workshop-residences—an imprecise but evocative picture might be painted by the words *tenement-sweatshop*—hidden from public view. Inside, plywood-separated single rooms, often housing entire families, ring workspaces filled with sewing machines and piles of fabric, thread, and buttons. This is yet another way that Bom Retiro fits into a global ecosystem since many of the textile workers are South American immigrants. Most are Bolivians, the largest entering immigrant group following changes in visa rules linked to the 1991 common-market agreement known as Mercosur/Mercosul, along with many Paraguayans, and Peruvians as well.[26] The parts of Rua José Paulino farthest away from the Luz Railway Station have much less street-level commercial activity, and ground-floor retail stores become scarce. The street ends abruptly at the Bom Retiro Public Health Clinic, with the neighboring former São Paulo Central Disinfectory (Desinfectório Central) complex that today houses the archive of the Emílio Ribas Public Health Museum, where I went after selling the "gun." In this part of Bom Retiro, the sound of shopping is replaced by the sound of sewing as the relative quiet allows what is going on in the intimate spaces behind closed doors to become more apparent.

Arrivals

I do not usually arrive in Bom Retiro in the back of a police car. Usually, I take the metro Yellow Line to the Luz neighborhood, named after Nossa Senhora da Luz (Our Lady of Light) in the early seventeenth century. Today a series of long escalators emerges from the platform onto a plaza with small shops offering services to the working classes—butchers, haircutters, clothing sellers—in buildings that had been upper-middle-class residences in the nineteenth century. The upper floors hold short-term rental residences and tenements, many located in buildings with disputed ownership that have been occupied by those in search of housing. To the right of the metro entrance is the impressive Estação da Luz (Luz Railway Station), where police, people without permanent residences, and sex workers of multiple gender

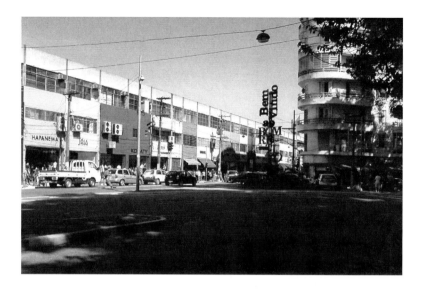

Figure I.1 Entrance to Bom Retiro, showing three-story buildings with retail clothing stores on the ground level and workshop-residences on the upper floors. Source: Paulo Humberto, "Bom Retiro—Região da Estação da Luz—São Paulo," October 24, 2009, Wikimedia Commons, https://commons.wikimedia .org/wiki/File:Bom_Retiro_-_Regiao_da_Esta%C3%A7ao_da_Luz_-_Sao_Paulo _-_panoramio.jpg.

identities seem to watch over the entrances. A beautiful pedestrian bridge traverses the tracks inside the station, and the harsh poverty of the formerly elegant north side of the station is transformed into a wide avenue whose sight line includes the Jardim da Luz (Luz Garden) public park and the Pinacoteca art museum. During my fieldwork at the Bom Retiro Public Health Clinic, I would follow a broken sidewalk around the Jardim da Luz to Rua José Paulino, whose beginning is marked by huge art deco letters spelling "Welcome to Bom Retiro" (figure I.1).

Bom Retiro is a place where people arrive on foot and by motorized transportation, from throughout Brazil and from abroad. Today's immigrants come from different places than those who arrived a century ago. Almost 28 percent of the more than fifty thousand Africans registered with Brazil's Federal Police are from Angola, with another 40 percent from Guinea-Bissau, Cape Verde, Nigeria, Mozambique, or Senegal.[27] There are about a quarter of a million Chinese immigrants and their descendants in São Paulo, overwhelmingly from Taishan, Guandong Province, and Qingtiam, Zhejiang Province, in the People's Republic, and from Taiwan.[28] There are around thirty thousand refugees from Venezuela, Syria, the Democratic Republic of the Congo, and Haiti, as well as a small and growing South Asian immigrant population.[29] Some of these newcomers, unsurprisingly, live and work in Bom Retiro, at times temporarily as they make their way northward to Mexico and then to the United States.[30]

Migration is often a disorienting experience. This was how I felt after selling the "gun" and arriving in Bom Retiro wedged between two armed officers in a police car. My movement through the city that day, while hardly a migratory experience, is a metaphor for the paths that this book takes in its analysis of the connections among immigration, health, and the built environment.[31] I argue that this triangulation explains the mechanisms by which the state and residents engage with and perpetuate everyday practices, spaces, and imaginaries regarding health and migration, all of which occur in periods disaggregated from traditional political periodization.[32] Prior to the mid-nineteenth century, Brazil was marked by a lack of public health policy, but this changed between 1850 and 1910 as the state sought to create health regulations, which would largely be enacted through private enterprise. From 1910 to 1945, the state played an increasing role in public health with many policies emerging from reinterpretations of ones used in the United States.

In 1945 the federal government began to demand state-level financial self-sufficiency in health, leading to large-scale breakdowns as states and municipalities were decreasingly able to fund health care for the broad public. This collapse became increasingly noticeable after 1970 as social inequality, and increasing gaps between rural and urban areas, became the norm. In 1988, with the end of a military dictatorship that had been in power for more than two decades, a new democratic constitution made health a formal right. The result was the creation of the universal and free Unified Health System (Sistema Único de Saúde, SUS), which remains in place today and, legally speaking, is available to any person within Brazilian territory, independent of citizenship status.

Residues

By stressing how people engage with everyday health practices, health spaces, and health imaginaries, I highlight material, political, and social residues that persist even during periods of transformation. We might think of residues as "structures of repetition" that mark permanence based on past activity; "from everything remained a little," as the poet Carlos Drummond de Andrade wrote.[33] This book thus argues that the intractability of the past in the present means that changing public health policies, biomedical advances, and new ideas about multiculturalism may not be as transformative as they first appear.[34]

Residues are "the results or outcome of some already concluded process. They are leftovers. Remnants. In this sense, residues cannot escape their history and provide clues for reconstructing the chemical past."[35] After buildings and roads are destroyed, the rubble that remains indicates "the residues of success and failure," but those solids can be forced together to create building materials such as bricks and prefabricated planks.[36] In Brazil trash is often called a "residue" and frequently provides an income for those who collect it informally, as Carolina Maria de Jesus's widely read 1960 memoir (defined by some scholars as "the poetics of residues") emphasizes.[37] Psychological residues are suspected as the cause of some memory disorders, and even borderlands can create the "emotional residue of an unnatural boundary."[38]

Residues also lead to geographies, and those traces of the past in turn allow me to theorize sites of changing health even while examining forces that impose continuities and thus structures. Some of the structures, like buildings and streets, are *infrastructural*, a term coined by nineteenth-century French engineers for "the substrate of support for rail lines—the structure beneath the structure."[39] Social structures relate to behavior in "health spaces" or with certain types of "health people" as they connect with race, ethnicity, class, gender and/or sexual orientation. Thinking about residues thus highlights the relationship between subjective ideas about diseases and cures and material objects that are supposed to improve health outcomes objectively. Social and cultural residues help to explain long-term gaps in understanding between health providers and patients. They explain why advances in biomedical technologies—such as X-rays and new pharmaceuticals—do not always lead to improved health outcomes in working-class neighborhoods like Bom Retiro.[40]

Global residues are very much part of the Americas. The "living remains [and] lingering legacies" of slavery, immigration, multilingualism and perceived accents, assimilative pressures, and formal and informal industrial development have layered on top of each other for centuries to create what scholars sometimes term *structures*.[41] This book argues that residues both create and are created in the daily lives of people, during visits with medical professionals, during their walks from place to place, and in discussions of everything from gun violence to diseases. Social, discursive, and material residues come to the surface in built environments as distant, yet as similar, as Bom Retiro and Cancer Alley in Louisiana in the United States.[42]

In Bom Retiro and other garment districts around the globe, material residues produced by textile workshops are omnipresent. Piles of cloth remainders and cardboard strips that once held buttons or rhinestones sit on the streets collecting water, and those residues become mosquito breeding grounds each time it rains. The residues of clogged and overflowing sewers do the same. All structure how people walk through the neighborhood, including the routes they choose and the kinds of steps they must take to avoid litter heaps and puddles. Thus, structure(s) and change(s) exist simultaneously, an idea that Gilberto Hochman and Anne-Emanuelle Birn have explored in relation to epidemics.[43] Even toilet facilities engage with residues since, as is the case in much of Latin America, used toilet paper and other waste products (called *resíduos* in Portuguese) are not flushed, to avoid clogging sewers.

I considered using words other than *residues* for this book. *Continuities* seemed more absolute than the sources supported, and I feared that significant gaps in the data (especially for the 1930s and 1940s) might lead readers to ahistorical conclusions. *Sediments* implied a materiality that might exclude cultural dialogues. My use of the word *residues* provides a category that can highlight similarities over time that may be seen in different mediums, ranging from discourses to material objects. My focus on residues does not mean that I reject change over time or cultural and geographic specificities. Yet, as Ajay Gandhi has argued, "residual subjects" emerge when we ask about the constancy of certain types of human activities, for example, the exhibiting of monkeys for a fee by their catchers in Delhi, an activity that was also part of São Paulo's urban landscape in the late nineteenth and early twentieth centuries.[44] Such residues are also apparent in what Diego Armus and Pablo Gómez call the "gray zones of medicine," and using historical and contemporary data allows me to analyze why biomedical change and health-related stasis frequently coexist.[45]

One of the recurring images, across class lines, of Bom Retiro was as sick, foreign, and industrial, a picture that emerged from observable migration patterns and labor and living conditions. Scholars of the Americas will recognize these patterns and the stereotypes that arose from them as typical of geographies where much of the labor took place in large formal factories (called *fábricas* in Portuguese) and smaller workshops (called *oficinas*). The English-language academic literature sometimes refers to oficinas as *sweatshops*, but I avoid that term since it implies a sharp distinction between workplace and residence. In central São Paulo city, workspaces were and are frequently residential spaces as well, just as in many garment districts.[46] In Bom Retiro these working/living areas were often located in cortiços (literally "beehives" but often translated in English as "tenements"), high-density housing where environmental health is precarious and where entire families live in single rooms and share bathroom and cooking facilities with others. To emphasize the overlap between work and residential space, I use the term *oficina-residência* (workshop-residence) to distinguish these spaces from those that are strictly for labor or for residence. Oficina-residências, like urban and suburban slums, are places where race and space merge symbolically and experientially.[47] While labor/living conditions in Bom Retiro's oficina-residências are harsh, I do not use terms related to enslavement since doing so would diminish the real conditions of slavery in Brazil. Furthermore, contemporary immigrant workers, while in often-abusive labor regimes, often participate in circular migratory patterns linked to economic cycles and overwhelmingly have access to schools and health care.[48]

Spaces

This book focuses on individual cases (human, structural, and environmental) and what they teach us about continuities broadly in urban working-class districts with many immigrants and their descendants, as is the case of Bom Retiro.[49] By asking about how living and dying over time relate to space (at the level of the home, the workplace, the street, the block, the neighborhood, and the city), I aim to create counterpoints to the homogenizing aspects of state-produced data.[50] This spatial focus allows me to better see how the state and its representatives flatten cultural differences, making responses to diseases and cures often surprisingly similar over time. It brings to light why diverse immigrant communities, despite differing historical and cultural trajectories, often generate similar antagonistic responses to policies such as state-imposed prevention and eradication programs.

Bad health in Bom Retiro is not limited to disease; it also results from noise, abuse, precarious infrastructure, bites from nonhuman animals (as small as a scorpion and as large as a dog), crime, and violence. By connecting everyday experiences of bad health with language and cultural activities, material structures like buildings and streets, and social structures like race, class, or citizenship, I read geographies and the people who inhabit them through the lens of health. My lens, to be sure, is not limited to discourses about cures during public health crises or the public-awareness work of health care workers. I am also interested in how the population and representatives of public health negotiate actions within spaces. For the public, these negotiations often demand creativity as they "live" health processes and state projects related to disease prevention and cures.

Movement inflects every chapter of this book. Health professionals today, as in the past, move throughout Bom Retiro on foot to bring health care to packed oficina-residências and enforce health policies. Brazilian residents of Bom Retiro, often Black, were frequently displaced occupationally and residentially by immigrants and their descendants. Some then migrated to other parts of the city or to other countries, creating new racially tinged residential and labor spaces for new arrivals.[51]

Movement plays a role in how residents remember the neighborhood. When journalist Marcos Faerman spoke with older residents of Bom Retiro in the 1980s, he found that they often used inaccurate global chronologies to suggest that their own self-defined ethnic group had arrived in an un-populated place but was then expelled once others entered. "Among some old Italians, there was the feeling that they had lost Bom Retiro. Among some old Jews, the feeling remained that the best of Bom Retiro is dead. Some old Italians resent the 1930s [claiming that it] was around this time that prostitutes were dumped on three of its most important streets. Italian families fled the neighborhood. The Jews brought money from Europe to buy their houses. Was it so?"[52]

Teresinha Bernardo's oral histories with two former residents of Bom Retiro—Dona Nidia, described as a "White Woman," and Sr. Raul, described as a "Black Man"—show the connection between racial ideas and migratory processes:[53]

> Dona Nidia: "It was a very happy neighborhood, with three cinemas and two dance halls. It was a neighborhood where everyone was friends, but it began to change when the Jews arrived, and we started to leave."

> Sr. Raul: "Mr. Stacchini preferred Italians like himself. It was 1927 and I remember it like it was today. I put up with all those years of the onslaught of Italians because I was basically brought up in the store (Stacchini Shoemakers). In 1927 Italians rained down on Bom Retiro and Blacks left, there were no more jobs for Blacks as shoemakers or tailors. Even today, I won't set foot in Bom Retiro."

Dona Nidia and Sr. Raul both express what Emily Sweetnam Pingel calls a "racialized geography" where each new immigrant group is "not quite part of the neighborhood, rather they are passing through."[54] Pingel's 2019 conversation with Maria, a self-identified Afro-Brazilian woman and longtime resident of Bom Retiro, makes the point clear:

> Today you have an immense quantity of Koreans. So, you have the Koreans, the Jews, who are traditional, the Bolivians. Today you have Paraguayans arriving, Angolans. So, it's a very mixed neighborhood. But—those who are *truly* from the neighborhood know each other . . . so you can go to the corner fruit stand and the owner knows you'll pay at the end of the month. But when a new foreigner arrives, we all know, look, this foreigner is new. And that has happened really quickly . . . and since it is a commercial neighborhood, people come in to work. They come to work and then they leave, but we stay. So, we know who is actually from the neighborhood.[55]

My own experiences with residents and ex-residents of Bom Retiro reflect those described above. In 2006, when *The Year My Parents Went on Vacation* was released, I participated in many formal and informal conversations because of the film's geographic setting in Bom Retiro and its themes of political resistance, marriage between Jewish and non-Jewish Brazilians, and intergenerational conflicts between immigrants and their Brazilian-born children. I interpreted the film as a love letter to an *imagined* Bom Retiro with its portrayal of close relations between those of different immigrant backgrounds, and between whites and Blacks, despite normalized racism. Yet some former residents of the neighborhood whom I knew were less enthusiastic. They did not "remember" the film's rendering of affective relationships across ethnic, racial, and religious backgrounds since their own memories were of ethnoreligious segregation by choice.

I had not thought about the conversations regarding *The Year My Parents Went on Vacation* for many years, but that changed in 2020, right before the COVID-19 pandemic. I was asked to discuss the relationship between immigration and health at the Casa do Povo (the People's House), a Bom Retiro political-social organization founded after World War II by progressive Jewish Brazilians and Jewish immigrants from eastern Europe. The participants were mostly Jewish Brazilians who had been brought up in the

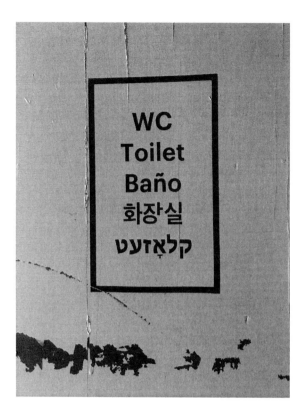

Figure I.2 Multilingual sign (Portuguese, English, Spanish, Korean, Yiddish) for bathroom facilities at the Casa do Povo, Bom Retiro. Source: Photograph by Raphael Schapira, October 14, 2022. Used by permission.

district but had migrated to upper-middle-class São Paulo neighborhoods. A few in the audience had never lived in Bom Retiro but felt a deep connection because of stories told by their parents and grandparents. There were also current residents, some multigenerational and others recent arrivals of Korean and Andean descent.[56] The nonresidents were dismissive of my claims that Bom Retiro had long been multiethnic, despite my attempts to use statistics and the Casa do Povo's own multilingual signage (see figure I.2). Instead, they presented an idyllic view of a single-ethnicity past. Current residents disagreed, speaking about Bom Retiro as a multicultural neighborhood suffering from long-term health challenges and racism. All attendees thought that I was wrong about the significant Afro-Brazilian presence in the neighborhood, an attitude that I discuss in more detail in chapter 2.

I do not believe the divergences between me and the audience were related only to self-identification. Indeed, one common aspect of ethnic identities across the globe is the in-group imaginary tales that often exclude everyday multiethnic experiences.[57] Such recollections often conflict with academic research, but I have tried to take remembered experiences seriously, even when they challenge my arguments. Taking memory seriously, however, does not diminish the importance of the historical documents and contemporary observations that I analyze. All reflect assumptions by state representatives, by the press, by health care providers, and by residents and nonresidents that immigrants are exotic and dangerous and thus exacerbate long-term health inequalities despite medical advances over time. These attitudes bubble to the surface in topics like nutrition, chemical dependency, epidemics, sexual health, eugenics, middle-class values, border control, international collaboration, and population politics, where residues help to structure contemporary relationships.

Starting in the nineteenth century, urban districts around the globe linked to immigrants and working-class industrial labor became health battlegrounds.[58] Many of these spaces were in city centers that those in the dominant classes considered geographically marginal. This is also the case today. In 2019 a tour guide who works for a company focused on university study-abroad programs in São Paulo told me he would be fired if he suggested a Bom Retiro walking tour. When I asked him why, he talked about fears of the neighborhood's residents—as working class, as nonwhite, as immigrants. Places like Bom Retiro, then, are often targets of state and popular focus even as inhabitants are marginalized in relation to health, access to rights, and public policy.

There are many working-class neighborhoods where immigrant labor specializes in the production of garments and textiles, and enduring and connective legacies appear when we view small spaces as global. Bom Retiro in São Paulo is also Praça Onze in Rio de Janeiro and Novo Hamburgo in Rio Grande do Sul, both in Brazil. It is the Lower East Side in New York City and the Flats in Cleveland in the United States, Once in Buenos Aires in Argentina, the Ward in Toronto in Canada, and South Tel Aviv in Israel.[59] While each is distinct (obviously!), the differences do not prevent us from pondering similarities, be they in social structures, discourses and actions about health, or cultural repertoires that revolve around and move within the built environment.[60] Indeed, looking for similarities across place and time creates questions that do not appear, or might be discarded, when the focus is difference. Shlomo Shmulevitsh's 1912 Mentshn-Fresser ("People Devourer") may have been inspired by the 1889 "Russian" flu or the "sequence of epidemics of the early twentieth century—TB, polio, cholera, and influenza."[61] While the ballad was written in the Russian Empire, it would make as much sense to immigrants then as it would to those living in Bom Retiro today:

> A terrible plague is spreading
> around the world
> With the blazing speed
> of a great fire
> Human minds are helpless,
> wisdom is without use
> No remedy can be found for . . .
> a bacillus
> Microbes, bacilli, what do you want?
> Whose will do you serve?
> You devour your victims without mercy
> You take aim at blossoming life
> You bathe in our tears
> You suck the marrow from our bones
> You poison our innards.

Remembering that geographic centers are often health peripheries helps to understand how maps of São Paulo and other cities frequently and falsely represent space as continuous and organized.[62] The flatness of maps, with their often proportionally erroneous lines and symbols representing streets, hides flooded roads, broken sidewalks, garbage piles, and roaming and flying nonhuman animals.[63] Maps, then, are residues of the intentional ignorance and self-deception of bureaucrats and represent a spatial "double articulation," to play with Doreen Massey's argument about how geographic space and cultural place do not always overlap.[64]

Maps of São Paulo city, starting in the mid-nineteenth century and continuing into the 1950s, consistently show Bom Retiro (located in the northern central quadrant) as a largely empty periphery to the rest of the central city.[65] The 1890 map (figures I.3a and I.3b), for example, shows that going more than a few blocks into the neighborhood meant entering emptiness, in effect going off the grid since the streets had not yet been mapped.[66] Artur Saboia's 1929 map (figures I.4a and I.4b) uses a different approach, giving Bom Retiro a larger footprint but ending abruptly at the edge, suggesting that São Paulo did not exist outside of the map. As late as 1951, maps represented Bom Retiro as a frontier space, with urban organization and all that came with it stopping suddenly.[67]

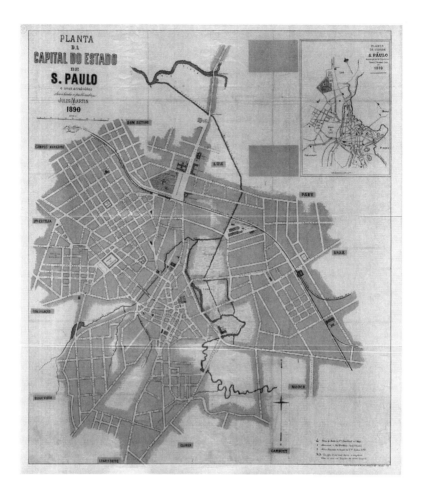

Methods Leading to Questions

This book reflects the many approaches that I use to generate and analyze data. Like many in the humanities, I spent most of my career thinking of myself as a solitary researcher even while acknowledging the help of archivists, librarians, and students. For this project, however, I worked with three interconnected teams whose data, ideas, and conclusions influence every sentence of this book. Those who read endnotes will notice that the research is informed by disciplines including history, cultural studies, public health, anthropology, geography, and sociology. In some of these areas of knowledge, publications include multiple authors, indicating a different kind of academic production than that typical of the humanities, where single-authored publications dominate.

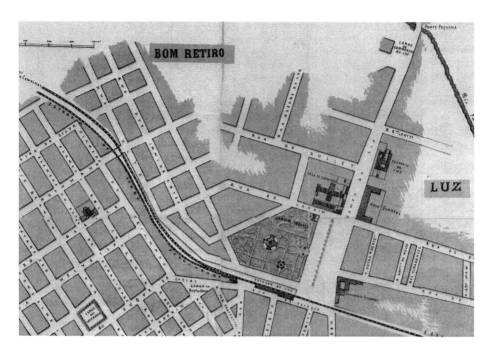

Figures I.3a & I.3b 1890 map of São Paulo and detail view showing Bom Retiro as largely an "empty" space. Source: Jules Martin, "Planta da Capital do Estado de S. Paulo e seus arrabaldes desenhada e publicada por Jules Martin em 1890," *Informativo—Arquivo Histórico Municipal* 4, no. 20 (September–October 2008), http://www.arquiamigos.org.br/info/info20/img/1890-download.jpg.

I used a variety of historical and contemporary sources, including archives, observation, oral histories, cartography, digital map creation, photographic exhibits, and participation in city-sponsored health programs. Much of the material was found in the archives of the Emílio Ribas Public Health Museum, situated in the building that had been São Paulo's Central Disinfectory, and the archival and historical space became an actor in the interpretation of some of the documents.[68] I have tried to provide readers with a sense of the dilemmas we faced in analyzing data by sometimes providing multiple conclusions. I used the Pauliceia 2.0 Historical Geographic Information Systems Platform to link quantitative data (e.g., demography, infrastructure planning, health outcomes, and socioenvironmental challenges) to the built environment, especially in order to see continuities in spatial patterns over time.[69] I often matched the quantitative data with blueprints, architects' notes, street notes, and press reports to map contemporary human flows through and around the buildings, which I then compared

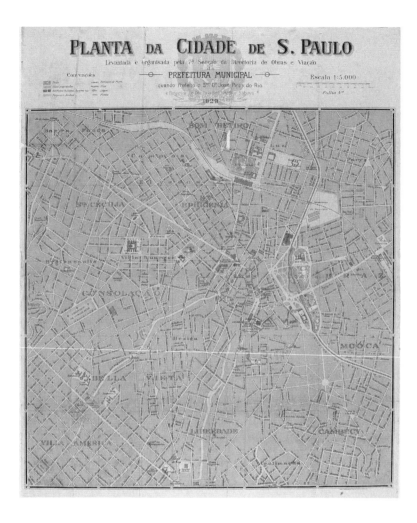

with photographs and etchings from earlier periods. My own observations and oral histories emerged from multiple years embedded in a primary care team at the Bom Retiro Public Health Clinic.[70]

By examining the interplay between people's lives and what those lives tell us about broader structural determinants over time, this book engages with multiple national academic literatures that are not always in conversation with each other. For example, historians of Latin America who study immigrants often focus on single groups, and in previous publications I have sometimes taken this approach. Such a focus tends to generate data that emphasizes closed ethnic communities with little national or multiethnic interaction. Scholars of immigration, whether based in Brazil or the United

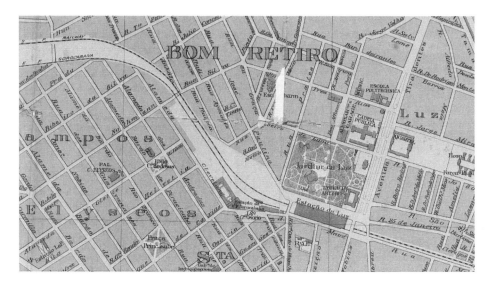

Figure I.4a & I.4b 1929 map of São Paulo and a detail view showing Bom Retiro as an urban neighborhood. Source: Artur Saboia, "Planta da Cidade de S. Paulo (1929)," Coleção João Baptista de Campos Aguirra—7ª Seção da Directoria de Obras e Viação—Prefeitura de São Paulo—Seção Cartográfica da Companhia Litográfica Ipiranga (São Paulo e Rio de Janeiro), Museu Paulista, https://upload.wikimedia .org/wikipedia/commons/b/ba/Planta_da_Cidade_de_S._Paulo_-_1%2C_Acervo _do_Museu_Paulista_da_USP.jpg.

States, often examine how immigration intersects with broad socioeconomic and health issues but rarely via comparisons with other countries.[71] Scholars who study health buildings like hospitals will, I hope, find my focus on urban materiality like sidewalks and sewer systems of use. Epidemiologists and medical anthropologists who prioritize contemporary data will see that the residues of the past are always reflected in the present. While this specific study ends with the publication of this book, the processes that link health, immigration, and the built environment in working-class neighborhoods like Bom Retiro continue.

Teams

Much of the research and analysis included in this book was generated by three multidisciplinary, multinational teams whose members often interacted with each other. One Brazilian partner was the Family Health Strategy "Team Green" (Equipe Verde), led by Dr. Fernando Cosentino at the

Unidade Básica de Saúde (UBS; primary health care clinic) Bom Retiro, the district's Sistema Único de Saúde (SUS; Brazilian Unified Health System) health clinic (in this book referred to as the Bom Retiro Public Health Clinic [BRPHC]). The importance of UBSs cannot be overstated since they provide basic and family health care to over 70 percent of Brazil's population, and some services to almost everyone, including those with private health insurance plans. Press coverage of health in Brazil often takes place with a reporter stationed inside of or in front of a UBS, and there is even a multi-season television series that focuses on the work of a fictional clinic in an underprivileged São Paulo neighborhood.[72] Public health clinics serve coverage areas determined at the municipal level, and Bom Retiro, in sector 16 (map I.2), is spatially central rather than peripheral to the city of São Paulo.[73]

The BRPHC's coverage area has five subsections, each defined by a color name and each comprising more than four thousand patients.[74] I joined Team Green in 2015 because its territory in the western portion of Bom Retiro (highlighted in map I.3) included the areas that held a mid-nineteenth-century immigrant hostel; the Ministry of Health's late nineteenth-century Central Disinfectory, a municipal institution that included infectious disease research, policy creation, and enforcement; and multiple twentieth-century health institutions, like a leprosy treatment center and a sexual health clinic that operated when the city sanctioned prostitution in the 1940s.

Team Green's patients were diverse, and when Emily Sweetnam Pingel conducted research in the BRPHC in 2019, she found that about 38 percent were immigrants while the others listed their country of origin as Brazil. The racial categories, sometimes expressed by the patient and sometimes judged without asking by the health care provider, were listed as white (about 47 percent), Brown (about 34 percent), Black (about 4 percent), Yellow (1.5 percent; note that this is a formal racial category in the Brazilian census and is used in many official records), and Indigenous (a small number). Among non-Brazilians, the largest numbers came from South America (Bolivia, Paraguay, and Peru) with the next-largest group from Asia (overwhelmingly Korean, with some Chinese).[75]

Like all the Family Health Strategy teams at the BRPHC, Team Green includes a physician, a nurse, one or two nurse technicians, and five or six community health workers (CHWs).[76] At the BRPHC the community health workers are almost all women, a change from the past, when state-employed public health workers were overwhelmingly male. Each CHW covers a microregion within the subsection and is expected to visit patients at home once a month. This system emphasizes the relationship of geography to

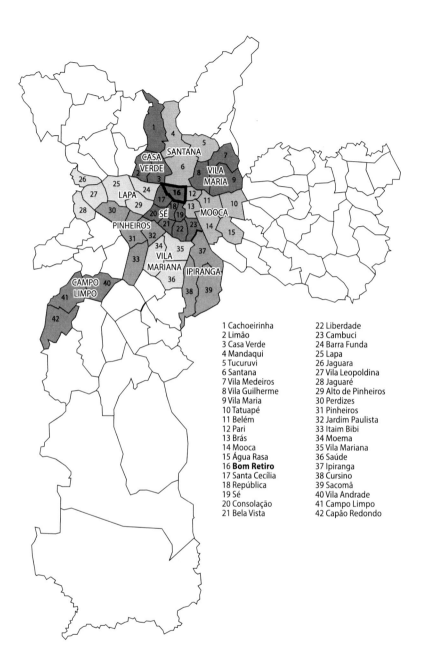

1 Cachoeirinha
2 Limão
3 Casa Verde
4 Mandaqui
5 Tucuruvi
6 Santana
7 Vila Medeiros
8 Vila Guilherme
9 Vila Maria
10 Tatuapé
11 Belém
12 Pari
13 Brás
14 Mooca
15 Água Rasa
16 **Bom Retiro**
17 Santa Cecília
18 República
19 Sé
20 Consolação
21 Bela Vista

22 Liberdade
23 Cambuci
24 Barra Funda
25 Lapa
26 Jaguara
27 Vila Leopoldina
28 Jaguaré
29 Alto de Pinheiros
30 Perdizes
31 Pinheiros
32 Jardim Paulista
33 Itaim Bibi
34 Moema
35 Vila Mariana
36 Saúde
37 Ipiranga
38 Cursino
39 Sacomã
40 Vila Andrade
41 Campo Limpo
42 Capão Redondo

Map I.2 A map based on information from the São Paulo Municipal Secretary of Health showing central health coverage areas by district. Bom Retiro is in the northern part of the city, within the larger Sé district. Source: Prefeitura de São Paulo, Secretaria de Saúde, http://smul.prefeitura.sp.gov.br/historico_demografico /img/mapas/1992.jpg.

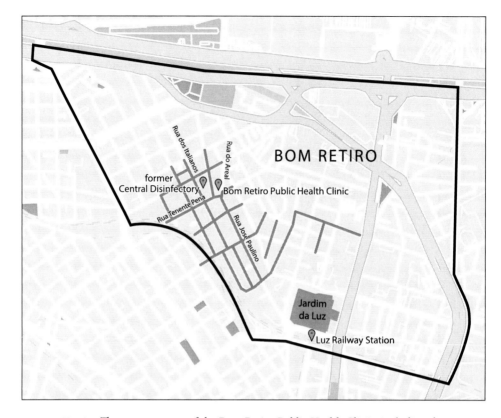

Map I.3 The coverage area of the Bom Retiro Public Health Clinic, including the northern boundary created by the Tietê River. Note the Jardim da Luz (Luz Garden) in the southern part. Team Green's coverage area is in the western part of the neighborhood and includes what had been the Central Disinfectory. Source: Dr. Fernando Costa de Carvalho Cosentino, Unidade Básica de Saúde Dr. Octávio Augusto Rodovalho, Bom Retiro, June 2, 2021.

health and emerges from one that originated with home visits by Brazilian female nurses in the early twentieth century, a time when male physicians often refused to make house calls to those in the lower classes.[77] In all of Brazil, those registered with the Unified Health System, including me, have access to routine visits at the health post. Since some health care barriers common in the United States, like lack of insurance, are largely absent in Brazil, the personal relations that Emily Sweetnam Pingel has defined as "who and what one "knows" about health care are critical. Health workers had and have an oversized presence in Bom Retiro, as was made clear both by the historical documentation and by the data I collected during the five years I worked with Team Green.

Another Brazilian partner for this project was composed of researchers at the Federal University of São Paulo's (UNIFESP) History, Maps, and Computers laboratory, directed by Luis Ferla. The laboratory connected to Pauliceia 2.0, a multiyear historical-mapping project funded by São Paulo state that included UNIFESP, the São Paulo State Archives, the Brazilian National Institute for Space Research (Instituto Nacional de Pesquisas Espaciais, INPE), and Emory University.[78] The third team was the Lesser Research Collective, known by its members as Team Lesser/Equipe Lesser.[79] This group of Emory and Federal University of São Paulo undergraduate, MA, and PhD students of diverse citizenships did not act as traditional research assistants. Rather, each team member conducted an individual research project, focused on some aspects of health, immigration, and space in Bom Retiro, that connected with all others. These projects included a sociological study of obstetric violence and the reproduction of health inequities; historical, epidemiological, and neuroscientific examinations of maternal health; a project on Hansen's disease; an investigation of Korean church-organized community health systems; and a comparative project on health among Chinese, Korean, and Bolivian immigrants in Bom Retiro.

Team Lesser shared data generated across disciplines and methods, leading to often-unanticipated questions.[80] Perhaps the most challenging was how our research might directly influence the lives of both health care workers and residents in Bom Retiro. One answer came in 2016 when Dr. Sara Kauko created a photographic exhibit showing daily life in Bom Retiro within the BRPHC. Another response came in 2018 when Team Lesser participated in a Ministry of Health project to map socioenvironmental challenges to health in the neighborhood. One finding of the 2018 study was that areas around textile-workshop residences had high incidences of mosquito-borne diseases like dengue. The initial response of some health care workers was that a lack of personal hygiene was common among the Bolivians and Paraguayans who lived and worked in these spaces. Using other types of data, Team Lesser was able to demonstrate to health care professionals that the workshop-residences were in locations that had been flood prone since the nineteenth century. Standing water, the state's highly inconsistent collection of litter, and resulting mosquito-borne illnesses had a long history unrelated to national origins.

Living and Dying in São Paulo argues that time and space are critical to understanding health. My interest in migration and other forms of human movement means I ask about globalized ideas about the construction, function, and perception of health spaces, broadly construed. I analyze the relationship between dense urban spaces (such as streets, homes, sewers, buildings, and sidewalks) and health outcomes in working-class neighborhoods.[81] I want to understand how and why disease, epidemics, cures, accidents, and crime have intersected with the histories of migration and spatial development, and how immigrants and their descendants have produced alternatives, ranging from homeopathic medicine to protests, to state-imposed health programs such as vaccinations or the use of chemical sprays to kill mosquitoes.

The organization of this book is itself a methodological argument, and each of the chapters creates residues that influence what follows. The words on the real or virtual page, including the observational postscripts that end each chapter, seed ideas about immigration, health, and the built environment that I hope create a visible final structure. The historical and contemporary data are, of course, mediated in various ways. For example, the voices of immigrants often emerge through documents written by public health specialists and government bureaucrats, and many of my observations began with context provided by health care workers, not patients. Within each chapter there are shifts, at times abrupt, between past and present. Readers will notice that the discussions overall do not range equitably over the decades. Some years or months or even days receive much more coverage than others because of how historical data linked to health come to the surface. When writing about the past within chapters, I use traditional chronologies to show how laws create institutions that generate residues even after legislation is revised or institutions are shut.

Chapter 1, "Naming a Death," dissects how life and death are negotiated when immigrants and state representatives hold competing ideas about good and bad health. It is followed by "Bom Retiro Is the World?," a spatial analysis within a broader context of immigration, anti-Blackness, health concerns, and urbanization in the Americas. Chapter 3, "Bad Health in a Good Retreat," focuses on material structures, including buildings and streets, and asks why certain types of health incidents occur repeatedly over time. Chapter 4, "Enforcing Health," scrutinizes the São Paulo Medical Police, an organization that was dismantled in 1940 but whose residues are apparent in the contemporary activities of São Paulo's Civil Police, the coroner's office, and the municipal Health Surveillance Office. Chapter 5, "A Building Block of Health," opens amid Brazil's 2016 Zika outbreak when I spent two months with a municipal health surveillance team investigating complaints of mosquito-filled standing water. It then shows how one building, the Central Disinfectory, came to embody the hygienist state. Finally, "Unliving Rats and Undead Immigrants" analyzes how health crises led to the targeting of immigrants and how immigrants in turn reacted.

A POSTSCRIPT

There are many ways to arrive in Bom Retiro. In addition to three metro stations on two different lines, there are buses, and the neighborhood is a relatively easy walk from many other central parts of the city. The experience of entering the neighborhood and walking to Bom Retiro Public Health Clinic from the Tiradentes Metro Station, however, is completely different from the stroll from the Luz Metro Station that I described earlier in this chapter. Exiting at Tiradentes Metro Station, you take a short escalator to the Praça Colonel Fernando Prestes flanked by the Military Police Command Barracks, the Municipal Archives, a public elementary school, city offices, and the socially progressive Institute Dom Bosco and its associated church. From there you walk down Rua Três Rios, with residential buildings as tall as ten stories, shops, hip coffeehouses, restaurants with signs in Portuguese and Korean, Jewish communal and religious organizations, and impressive structures built in the nineteenth century and linked with education and health, like Brazil's first School of Dentistry.

Many visitors go to Rua Três Rios for the "cool" Bom Retiro of K-pop and K-coffee. They see ascendant immigrants and their descendants, and upper-middle-class and middle-class residents who own commercial and residential properties. My own first experience in the neighborhood was one of unseeing, to use a term perhaps coined by China Miéville.[82] It was the mid-1980s, and I was conducting research on images of Jews in Brazil. As I walked the streets, I focused on finding Jewish life while ignoring everything else. At the time I participated in several social movements, and in one of them I met "Jacob," a medical student who would soon leave Brazil for Israel. Decades later, as I began research for this book, a friend told me that Jacob was a physician at the Bom Retiro Public Health Clinic (readers will meet Dr. Jacob in chapter 3). He and I renewed our acquaintance as we walked through the district, and a new Bom Retiro appeared. This one did not look like the one I had known decades earlier, nor the one that visitors hailed as they drank fancy coffee and ate "ethnic" foods in relatively expensive restaurants. For the first time I saw many Bom Retiros, not a single Bom Retiro.

1

Naming a Death

The revolver that killed Amelia Marini with a shot through the heart in Bom Retiro in 1913, unlike the twenty-first-century starter pistol we met in the introduction, had real bullets. She was one of the many newcomers who died violently in central São Paulo each year. Born in Italy, Amelia Marini, as she was called by the influential *Correio Paulistano* newspaper, was one of the millions of immigrants who arrived in Brazil in the four decades starting in 1880. Recorded in the police records as Amelia Marino, she had first migrated to Argentina and then remigrated to Brazil in 1909 as a seventeen-year-old after being abandoned by her husband.

While weapons and resulting deaths were not recognized by many representatives of the state as a public health problem, for the immigrant working classes gun violence was a frequent cause of bad health as the population of São Paulo exploded starting in the late nineteenth century (see figure 1.1). Indeed, Amelia Marini was just one of the almost four hundred deaths, many of them violent, among Bom Retiro's roughly thirty thousand residents in 1913.[1] Marini was classified by the police as a domestic worker, and she lived in one of the cortiços that dominated São Paulo's working-class residential landscape. Her cramped residence was at the Rua dos Italianos, 37, less than a block from the rail line and just two blocks from the Central Disinfectory, an imposing municipal building that since 1893 had housed São Paulo city's most important health research, policy, and enforcement

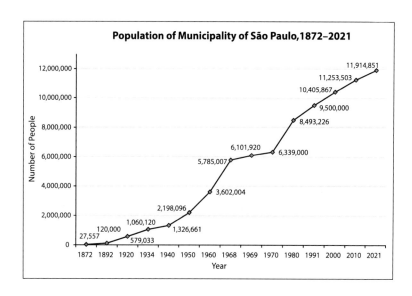

Population of Municipality of São Paulo, 1872–2021

Figure 1.1 Sources: Império do Brasil, "Quadro geral da população livre considerada em relação aos sexos, estados civis raça, religião, nacionalidades e grão de instrucção," in *Recenseamento do Brazil em 1872*, vol. 12 (Rio de Janeiro: Typ. G. Leuzinger, 1874), https://biblioteca.ibge.gov.br/visualizacao/monografias /GEBIS%20-%20RJ/Recenseamento_do_Brazil_1872/Imperio%20do%20Brazil%20 1872.pdf; Ministério da Agricultura, Indústria e Commércio, Directoria Geral de Estatística, *Recenseamento do Brazil—realizado em 1 de setembro de 1920*, vol. 4, pt. 4 (Rio de Janeiro: Typ. Da Estatística, 1922); Cidade de São Paulo, "Dados demográficos dos distritos pertencentes às Subprefeituras," https://www.prefeitura .sp.gov.br/cidade/secretarias/subprefeituras/subprefeituras/dados_demograficos /index.php?p=12758; Instituto Brasileiro de Geografia e Estatística, *Censo Demográfico 2010*, accessed June 28, 2024, https://censo2010.ibge.gov.br/sinopse/index .php?uf=35&dados=4; and Instituto Brasileiro de Geografia e Estatística, *Censo Demográfico, Séries Historicas, População residentes, 1872-2010*, https://www.ibge .gov.br/estatisticas/sociais/populacao/2098-np-censo-demografico/9662-censo -demografico-2010.html?edicao=9673&t=series-historicas. Prepared by Surbhi Shrivastava, Lesser Research Collective, 2023.

units. Marini could not miss the large building as she left her residence each day since the tall, block-encompassing physical structure dominated Bom Retiro spatially and visually, reminding the public that the state could "see" them and was ready to aggressively intervene in their private health lives.

The two different ways Marini's surname was spelled, and the known and unknown stories of her life and death, are important. The physicians at the São Paulo Medical Police, inaugurated in 1911 as a unit of the Secretary of Justice and Public Safety, would not agree with me. They recorded Marini's demise by filling in a form with perfunctory information about her nationality, age, residence, and race. They treated her death as just one more example of the explosive link among health, immigration, and working-class life.[2] The word SUICIDE was stamped in large letters across the medical incident report, relieving law enforcement of the need to investigate the case.

The *Correio Paulistano* represented the state's oligarchs, who demanded European immigrants for their plantations, to the less than 30 percent of São Paulo's population that was literate.[3] It told a different story about Amelia Marini. The headline shouted "Suicide or Crime? An unhappy girl, abandoned by her husband, goes to live in the company of a Syrian dentist—a shot in the heart—the police, suspecting a crime, open a rigorous investigation—being heard by the authority, the dentist declares he believes in a suicide, because the lover was extremely nervous."[4] The article itself told of an honorable, but naive, Italian young woman making good even though life had treated her badly.

After arriving in Bom Retiro, Amelia Marini had met another immigrant, this time an apparently upwardly mobile one from Syria.[5] Alexandre Naban was a dentistry student at the School of Pharmacy, Dentistry, and Obstetrics, another important health building in Bom Retiro, inaugurated in 1905 (today the Oswald de Andrade Cultural Center, located at Rua Três Rios 363). After receiving his license, he opened a practice in a São Paulo neighborhood associated with Middle Eastern immigrants (on Rua Florencia de Abreu). In love and with his income apparently secured, Naban suggested that the couple live together but in separate rooms, perhaps because they were not formally married. It appears that Marini agreed, and the dentist rented two vacant rooms in the cortiço on the Rua dos Italianos, "surrounding her with relative comforts and offering her a chance to rest" from her exhausting work as a domestic laborer.

The *Correio Paulistano* report on Marini's death was filled with stereotypes of immigrants as challenges to medical and moral health. The article told of an honorable immigrant woman (at the time Italian women were often associated with promiscuity; see chapter 2) and portrayed Naban as an exploitative Middle Easterner.[6] The building where they lived was presented as a physical representation of Marini's honor and a contrast to stereotypes linking immigrants to a lack of hygiene: "The cortiço (where she lived), unlike so many others in São Paulo where filth rules supreme, is made up of four or five poor residences, but clean and relatively comfortable." The suggestion that the dead woman's home was healthier than other cortiços deemphasized that she was unmarried, had a child, and lived "in a matrimonial state" even while reminding readers that immigrants created "bad health" through their living conditions.[7]

About eighteen months after Marini and Naban became a couple, little Alberto was born. The *Correio Paulistano* suggested that the birth triggered tension over whether the union should become formal and full-time. It was the crying of this "strong and well-treated" child that led the owner of the cortiço, Diogo Baroni, to ask Carmella Cicca, an Italian immigrant neighbor, to check on Marini on that late November evening. It was then that Marini was found dead, with Naban's revolver and a spent cartridge by her side.[8]

Intertwined Pasts and Presents

Bom Retiro is filled with the residues of Amelia Marini's death, from its causes to its repercussions. The neighborhood still has a high index of daily violence (including suicides and attempts) and health issues that lead to state interventions and popular cures. Broken sidewalks remain lined with informal factories, flooding is common, and garbage is piled on the streets. Bom Retiro remains today, as it was throughout the twentieth century, a geography that is "poor, full of cortiços, without any comfort, not even paving, with little water, almost useless, without hygiene."[9] Residents continue to be stigmatized by geography, residential type, and citizenship status, and the district's public schools continue to educate the children of working-class immigrants and nonwhite nonimmigrants, just as they did a century ago.[10] The contemporary Rua dos Italianos is still filled with precarious, cramped, and poorly ventilated residences and textile workshops. The most imposing building on the Rua dos Italianos in the late nineteenth century was the city's nerve center for epidemic control—the Central Disinfectory— and it is still owned and used by the Municipal Ministry of Health.

Amelia Marini's multiple migrations, her relationship and child with another immigrant, and her life and death in Bom Retiro form a global story. For many in the interconnected Brazilian dominant classes— landowners, politicians, bureaucrats, and media owners—immigrants like Marini were part of their attempt to remake Brazil racially and economically following the abolition of slavery in 1888.[11] To attract "white" immigrants, São Paulo's leaders had to challenge a widespread belief in Europe that settling in Brazil was dangerous and often fatal. As Brazil transitioned from empire to republic, politicians enacted new health policies that they believed would convince immigrants to choose Brazil and prevent them from bringing new diseases into what they believed was an already "sick" country.[12]

Brazil became a republic on November 15, 1889, during an outbreak of yellow fever. Sanitation and the elimination of epidemics were top national priorities, both to encourage foreign investment and to keep the working classes at work.[13] Health policy was placed under state, not federal, control, and in 1890 São Paulo state's new Sanitary Service received 46 percent of the state budget, a huge jump from the 1 percent that the previous imperial government had directed toward health.[14] With this investment, São Paulo state's official public health infrastructure, including hospitals and medical educational institutions, became the most sophisticated in Brazil.[15] Much of the state funding was targeted to Santos, the port city where immigrants arrived, and São Paulo, the city where almost all newcomers went first after leaving the docks. While the percentage of state funds directed toward public health decreased over the decades, it remained between 10 and 20 percent through 1920.[16] Under the leadership of Emílio Ribas, a physician and São Paulo's leading public health specialist, bureaucrats regulated medical professions and championed scientific approaches to assessing infectious disease through health institutions, starting with the Bacteriological Institute in 1892.[17]

Bom Retiro's immigrant population and industrial labor structures made the district a target of health officials, just like similar neighborhoods throughout the globe, ranging from Buenos Aires to Bombay.[18] Two of the city's important late nineteenth-century health buildings were placed in the neighborhood, the Central Disinfectory and the nearby and fascinatingly inclusive School of Pharmacy, Dentistry, and Obstetrics.[19] These buildings, although with different uses, continue to be among the largest in the district. Two other types of buildings made up the built environment in Bom Retiro. At the end of the nineteenth century, the neighborhood had among the highest percentage of cortiços in the city and the highest numbers of factories, including of ceramics, beer, and textiles.[20] Both types of structures were largely filled with immigrant workers and their descendants.

State political leaders promulgated São Paulo's 1894 Sanitary Code. The 520 articles dealt with everything from "standards for the hygienic construction of housing and public buildings—schools, jails, hospitals—and private ones—factories, workshops, shops, butchers, and markets. The law defined measures for the prevention and treatment of epidemics and infectious diseases. It determined vaccination and revaccination, created lists of notifiable diseases, and set penalties for non-compliance with the law. In addition, it legislated on the work of women and minors in factories and workshops."[21]

The new health regulations and infrastructure came as technological advances in oceanic transportation shortened the time it took people, diseases, and ideas to come to Brazil from the rest of the world. Long-term Black residents were pushed out of central neighborhoods as the numbers of immigrants, who politicians and their allies in the media proposed would "whiten" Brazil with European Christians, skyrocketed. The newcomers often went to rural plantations, where they replaced ex-slaves, but many settled in the city of São Paulo, where they became industrial laborers. Some of these new urbanites were emigrants from the same places as those going to the countryside, like Italians, Spaniards, and Portuguese. Others came from places (like the Middle East or Asia) or from populations (non-Christians) that Brazil's opinion makers had not considered.

Bom Retiro was and is a stand-in for industrial neighborhoods around the globe where immigrants and their descendants make up a noticeable percentage of the population.[22] In the late nineteenth century, the largest contingent of foreign-born residents in Bom Retiro and São Paulo came from Italy; Brazil received over 800,000 Italian immigrants between 1880 and 1920.[23] Prior to World War I, most were Venetians and Tuscans. One Italian visitor in 1908 wrote, "The most outstanding characteristic of the city is its Italianness. We hear more Italian in São Paulo than in Turin, Milan, or Naples, because . . . in São Paulo all the dialects come together under the influence of the Venetians and Tuscans, who are in the majority, and the natives adopt Italian as their official language."[24]

Nineteenth-century health officials and politicians throughout the Americas linked specific types of labor, geography, and nationality to poor health outcomes and a lack of modernity among the working classes, both immigrant and native.[25] In São Paulo working-class immigrants often lived in central neighborhoods near rivers that, beginning in the mid-nineteenth century, powered factories that in turn created sewage and bad health. These districts were often low-lying, making changes to the built environment, like building canals and paving streets, complex and often unsuccessful because of minimal state investment and technological challenges.

The lack of modernization terrified some authorities, one of whom noted in 1892 that residents of the central city were getting ill "in their homes, or on the streets of the city . . . which are hotbeds of disease."[26] Jacob Penteado was one of those residents. He lived in Bom Retiro as a child and would go on to become a well-known editor, translator, postal service employee, and chronicler of city life. He remembered how the district's population was targeted for its bad health even as it suffered from "almost nonexistent health measures, like medical clinics, health education, and prophylactic measures."[27] Common illnesses were tuberculosis, syphilis, smallpox, typhoid fever, the bubonic plague, and mosquito-borne and other diseases linked to standing water and poor waste removal. Bad health also included child abuse and poisoning (both accidental and otherwise). Fights between residents, workplace accidents, and collisions between pedestrians and vehicles like horse-drawn carriages, human-pulled carts, horse-drawn trolleys, and motorized vehicles were significant aspects of daily life.[28] Moral "diseases" such as worker activism, real and perceived suicide, sex work, and masturbation among school-age children, on whom "reprimands, punishment, and even expulsion, had little effect," also worried those in the middle and upper classes as they peered into Bom Retiro via the lens of newspaper reports that highlighted violence in police actions and workers' movements.[29]

In Bom Retiro "old" diseases have endured until the present, including tuberculosis, typhoid, alcoholism, and cholera.[30] "New" diseases often have residues of past ones since flooding from the Tamanduateí and Tietê Rivers continues to be part of everyday life and make *Aedes aegypti*–borne illnesses chronically relevant.[31] Resident complaints, whether via the government, the press, or public actions, have generally been ignored as public health workers and policymakers focus on immigrant culture as the primary cause of disease, just as they did in the nineteenth century.

Crowded Spaces

In 1890 Aluísio Azevedo (1857–1913), a journalist, diplomat, and novelist, published his influential novel *O cortiço* (the 1926 English translation was entitled *A Brazilian Tenement*), in which he described the housing type as follows:

> Today a few meters of land, tomorrow a few more, step by step the vender acquired the considerable field lying between his frontage and the quarry at the base of the hill. And as fast as a new patch of ground became his it was promptly covered by a twin sister of the original structure made possible by the involuntary contributions of the neighborhood. All were for rent, and as fast as new huts arose there appeared new tenants to occupy them. . . . [Nothing] delayed

the progress of the tenement, whose compact sections reared their heads, one after another, like a line of soldiers in close formation. . . . The completed structure enclosed an open rectangular space toward which all of the houses faced, and which was the common front yard of all the ninety-five cramped dwellings.[32]

Azevedo's description of cortiços emerged from his experiences in nineteenth-century Rio de Janeiro. Yet even today politicians and public health specialists point to poor housing in districts like Bom Retiro as a primary cause of bad health, often using language similar to Azevedo's.

The São Paulo municipality currently defines *cortiços* as "multifamily residences, built out of one or more buildings on the same urban lot, subdivided into various units that are rented, sublet, or used by third parties."[33] The seemingly neutral words hide the impact of social class on health outcomes. For example, Brazil's renowned "good" contemporary national health system with its long history of successful vaccination campaigns sits together with the bad health created by difficulties with access to basic water, sanitation, and hygiene services. In the past, the truly wealthy looked for care abroad, but most of São Paulo's well-off used private clinics and hospitals located in the affluent neighborhoods where they lived, as remains true today. In the nineteenth and early twentieth centuries, private health spaces in São Paulo were often directed by well-known immigrant physicians and nurses, who were hailed by the same dominant classes that believed foreigners were disease vectors. Between 1872 and 1932, a little over 9 percent of doctors registered with the São Paulo state Sanitary Service were foreign born and trained, overwhelmingly Italian, and the clinic names often emphasized their European origins.[34]

In places like Bom Retiro, there were also immigrant health care workers. These physicians, nurses, and midwives were frequently less well trained than their upper-class counterparts, received low fees, and did not have access to the newest medical technologies.[35] Immigrant health thus often revolved around popular treatments that emerged out of premigratory experiences and connected to existing Brazilian formulations. Cures ranged from prayers, to the use of herbs, to the wearing of amulets that linked Catholicism with African religious rituals present in Brazil such as the figa (an amulet in the shape of a fist with crossed thumb and forefinger) or the use of colored beads signifying connections to African deities.[36] For serious illnesses, many of those living in Bom Retiro went (and still go) to the Santa Casa de Misericórdia, a Catholic philanthropic institution that managed health for the city's nonelites. The Santa Casa also managed death, from picking up cadavers to providing caskets to burying people.[37]

The 1894 Sanitary Code, modeled after the French one, reflected widespread anxieties among the dominant classes that working-class immigrants and nonwhites were prone to becoming disease vectors. Health policies and actions linked race, class, nationality, and geographic residence and focused on contagious diseases and improvement of the built work and residential environment. The code was poorly enforced, frequently modified, and subject to intense criticism across class lines. Even so, public health officers promoted drops in overall mortality rates, including in deaths resulting from nontransmittable and transmittable disease, in the city of São Paulo from 10.6 percent in 1894 to 4.2 percent in 1899, a level that remained stable until the global H1N1 influenza epidemic of 1918.[38] These officials hailed the city's "splendid position" vis-à-vis natality and mortality, especially in comparison with other global cities.[39] By focusing on mortality, nationally prominent public health leaders and politicians simultaneously promoted São Paulo as "the most forward-looking and advanced in Brazil" while blaming working-class immigrants and their neighborhoods and housing for the infectious diseases that continued to spread through the city.[40] Public health officials used the same approach to explain a rise in child mortality rates, despite the state Sanitary Service's programs for expectant mothers.[41] Public health officials correctly noted that the urban population was growing rapidly because of immigrant entry but then tended to treat adult and child mortality and morbidity as cultural, rather than structural, issues.[42]

Bom Retiro Takes Shape

Bom Retiro did not exist as a named place when Brazil declared itself an empire and became independent of Portugal in 1822. At the time, São Paulo city had fewer than ten thousand inhabitants, and at least 25 percent were enslaved. Even so, residents were keenly aware of the geographic importance of the hill that rose out of the floodplains (*várzeas*) of the Tamanduateí and Tietê Rivers. The upward-sloping land was attractive to the wealthy, who believed—as did, for example, the British, who founded the summer capital of Shimla to avoid Calcutta's rivers—that its altitude made people less prone to sickness. By the middle of the nineteenth century, the area that would become Bom Retiro was ringed by eight huge slave-built rural estates, often called *chácaras*, partially built on land that had been an Indigenous market. With Portuguese colonization these Indigenous spaces were deeded to a small, landed elite connected to the empire. Joaquim Egídio de Sousa Aranha (1821–93), the coffee baron, banker, and politician known by his title the Marquês de Três Rios, was one of those landowners.[43] His enormous Chácara Bom Retiro (Bom Retiro Estate) was larger than the historic center of São Paulo city through much of the nineteenth century.[44]

Healthy life on the hill changed over the course of the nineteenth century. Bom Retiro's first industries, ceramic factories that took advantage of the mud along the floodplains, began to increase the population density and environmental pollution. Owners began to sell their chácaras to land investors, many of them immigrants, who then subdivided the lots for rent or repurchase, usually by other immigrants.[45] Each year during the late nineteenth and early twentieth centuries, the numbers of factories grew and along with them came workers. River straightening, railroad tracks, and new zoning codes remade Bom Retiro into a working-class neighborhood that those with money and power often glossed as a "foreign" space.[46] The changes to the built environment also created new boundaries. To this day Bom Retiro is filled with streets that abruptly end in unpassable viaducts, which makes entering and leaving the neighborhood a challenge. The streets that do provide entries and exits funnel people toward the parts of the neighborhood with large law enforcement buildings and military barracks (today near Luz Railway Station and the Tiradentes Metro Station).

The marking of Bom Retiro as foreign was far from neutral; it had (and has) a direct impact on health policies and outcomes. Some in the dominant classes, for example, believed foreigners would improve the country by de-Africanizing the population and implanting "modern" labor ideas. Others believed foreigners brought diseases and dangerous ideas like socialism and anarchism. Bom Retiro became and remains a "foreign" space because of unmodern "residences . . . interspersed with small shops, diverse workshops, and, as is characteristic of this area, locations for illicit rendezvous and suspicious-looking dwellings."[47]

The connection of foreignness to danger continues to this day, but I do not think that the Marquês de Três Rios would have imagined Bom Retiro in those ways as he traveled to his weekend estate in the mid-nineteenth century. Like many powerful men at the time, the three-time president of the Province of São Paulo expected to be recognized; he is reputed to have enjoyed traveling through Bom Retiro and down Rua Três Rios by public streetcar rather than in his private carriage because when others embarked, they would doff their hats to him with a respectful "Good day, Mister Marquês!"[48] Mister Marquês would be shocked to walk down the "cool" paved Rua Três Rios today, with its self-identified Jewish cultural centers, Korean coffeehouses and supermarkets, and informal textile factories staffed largely with Andean laborers. To be fair, it would be equally hard for contemporary residents of Bom Retiro to imagine that their crowded streets, homes, and workplaces had been a rural retreat at the confluence of two rivers.

In the late nineteenth century, planners began to reorganize São Paulo's city center from six colonial-era parishes into twenty-one districts, with Bom Retiro receiving the official designation in 1910. A decade later, the 1920 Brazilian census provided the first complex demographic glimpse of the district, whose population of 29,804 ranked tenth of twenty-one, representing a little over 5 percent of the population of the central city. The political reorganization of the city center continued throughout the twentieth century. Today Bom Retiro is one of the eight districts within the center-city Sé subprefecture, one of the thirty-two subprefectures that make up the municipality of São Paulo. The center city has more than 460,000 inhabitants, but Bom Retiro's approximately thirty streets have less than 10 percent of them.[49] While sources vary greatly in their population estimates, in part because immigrants are often reticent to engage with census takers, all agree that around 1970 there was negative growth in the district. Middle-class residents, often the children of immigrants who had attended university, were moving out of what they saw as an increasingly dangerous and disease-filled neighborhood to upper-middle-class parts of the city. This led to a population low of 26,678 in 2000 (figure 1.2). In the twenty-first century, those figures began to trend upward in all central city districts, and the official figure for Bom Retiro's 2021 population was 39,202.[50]

Working-class immigrants were not the first foreigners in Bom Retiro. Much of the transformation from a healthy "Good Retreat" to an unhealthy urban neighborhood was led by central Europeans, whom Warren Dean has defined as an "immigrant bourgeoise." These newcomers had a higher-than-average tolerance for risk and took advantage of an "environment of almost perfect laissez faire" to build urban industries in the economic spaces often ignored by native-born, plantation-based oligarchs prior to World War I.[51] The male immigrant bourgeoise frequently married Brazilian women, some of them the daughters of rural oligarchs and others of well-off immigrant parents. This dynamic was clear into the twentieth century when annual reports published by São Paulo health authorities included tables for "marriages by nationality." In 1912, for example, there were 254 marriages of Brazilian men to foreign women and 658 marriages of foreign men with Brazilian women.[52]

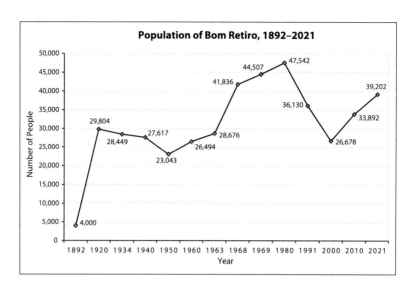

Figure 1.2 Sources: Henrique Raffard, *Alguns dias na Paulicéia* (São Paulo: Academia Paulista de Letras, 1977), 109; Cidade de São Paulo, "Dados demográficos dos distritos pertencentes às Subprefeituras," https://www.prefeitura.sp.gov.br/cidade/secretarias/subprefeituras/subprefeituras/dados_demograficos/index.php?p=12758; Liziane Peres Mangili, *Bom Retiro, bairro central de São Paulo: Transformações e permanências, 1930–1954* (São Paulo: Alameda, 2011), 69–70; Decio Amadio, "Desenho urbano e bairros centrais de São Paulo: Um estudo sobre a formação e transformação do Brás, Bom Retiro e Pari" (PhD diss., University of São Paulo, 2005), 5; United Nations, *Population Growth and Policies in Mega-Cities: São Paulo* (New York: United Nations, 1993), 3; Seade, "O Perfil dos Municípios Paulistas, Bom Retiro," accessed June 28, 2024, https://perfil.seade.gov.br/; and Hilário Dertônio, *O bairro do Bom Retiro* (São Paulo: Prefeitura Municipal, Secretaria de Educação e Cultura, Departamento de Cultura, 1971), 19. Prepared by Surbhi Shrivastava, Lesser Research Collective, 2023.

As the landed and titled lost influence and wealth over the course of the nineteenth century, they began to sell their properties to immigrant entrepreneurs/land speculators. The new owners modified land tenure patterns in Bom Retiro by subdividing the former estates and building roads. They then resold the plots to relatively well-off investors who built collective housing or structures for factories. The progression from estate to large lot to subdivision meant that the working class could only afford to rent. If immigrant dreams of "fazer á America" (making it in America) included land- or homeownership, they were rarely fulfilled in Bom Retiro. Whether the housing was called *tenements* in North America or *vecindades, conventillos,* or *inquilinatos* in South America, renting and crowding marked working-class urban geographies.[53]

The creation of urban Bom Retiro emerged largely from land subdivision by four immigrant landowners who came to Brazil in the mid-nineteenth century: Alsatian-born Manfred Meyer, US-born Charles Dimmit Dulley, and German-born Frederico Glette and Victor Nothmann. The latter pair purchased the Visconde de Mauá's chácara and transformed it into the district of Campos Elísios and one small part of contemporary Bom Retiro.[54] More important for our story were Meyer and Dulley. Meyer was an agent for the French consulate in São Paulo, and in 1859 he opened the Meyer Brick Yard and began purchasing similar industries in the region. Soon he was the primary producer of bricks, tiles, and other construction products in the city. In 1859 he married Elvira Isabel de Souza Queiroz, the daughter of a rural landowner, and the couple acquired the enormous lot owned by the coffee baron and politician Antônio da Silva Prado, which today makes up part of the Bom Retiro and Barra Funda districts.[55] Less than a decade later, the couple generated additional funds for purchasing land by selling some of their ceramic factories. They sold one to João Ribeiro da Silva, a cement importer who had learned a new technique for producing artificial stones that would spur the construction of private homes in the central part of São Paulo.[56]

By 1870 Meyer and Queiroz were focused on land acquisition, subdivision, and sales although they would continue to own ceramic factories into the 1880s.[57] They soon owned three large estates located between the rail lines (completed in 1861) and the várzeas of the Tietê and Tamanduateí Rivers, including some of what had been the Marquês de Três Rios's Chácara Bom Retiro. Between 1881 and 1892, the Meyers were involved in more than half of the land and home sales in Bom Retiro (forty-two as a seller and one as a buyer), spurred by municipal tax incentives intended to encourage industrialization and its associated immigration and population growth.[58] Many of the Meyers' land sales were to the city and state governments, including the lot that would become the geographic nexus of public health and immigration with the city's first immigrant hostel in 1881 and the Central Disinfectory in 1893. The Meyers also were pioneers in the controversial technique of donating land to the municipality to construct streets along which they would then sell lots, sometimes even before the streets were built.[59]

Charles Dimmit Dulley, a native of Pittsburgh, Pennsylvania, United States, was also a primary land buyer and seller in Bom Retiro. He arrived in São Paulo as a twenty-two-year-old in 1861 and worked as a tunnel construction engineer for the São Paulo Railway Company, known colloquially as "the English." Like many in the immigrant bourgeoisie, Dulley largely socialized with expatriates, in his case from the United States, the United Kingdom, and Germany. Two were Harriet Matilde Rudge and her spouse, Henry Fox, an English watchmaker responsible for the public-facing clock at São Paulo's central Cathedral da Sé. Rudge and Fox had multiple Brazilian-born daughters, and Dulley married Ana Luiza Fox in December 1866, around the same time that he left his job to become a construction magnate hired on a large-scale contract basis by the railroad.[60] Charles's ever-growing income and Ana Luiza's commercial connections and Brazilian citizenship meant land purchases were relatively straightforward.[61]

Those individual purchases soon became the Chácara Dulley, a center for expatriate social life.[62] Charles Dimmit Dulley died in 1878, but it was only at the end of the century that plans began to subdivide the land and integrate it into the growing urban environment largely created by Manfred Meyer. Likely led by Charles and Ana Luiza's son, Charles John Dulley, himself trained as an engineer in England, the land was sold off in large plots, one of which became the School of Pharmacy, Dentistry, and Obstetrics in 1905. In 1907 the Society of Saint Francis de Sales (also known as the Salesians of Don Bosco) purchased a large plot where the Santa Inês boarding school opened in 1911.[63]

Immigrants and Urban Expansion

Amelia Marini was just one of the about five million immigrants from Europe, Asia, the Middle East, and the Americas who settled in Brazil before 1950, most following the 1888 abolition of slavery and rapid industrialization (see figures 1.3 and 1.4). Her story reminds us that while immigration is often studied quantitatively, immigrants have names, healthy and sick lives, and deaths. The overwhelming majority arrived by ship at the port city of Santos, where many trudged off the docks to board a train for the British-built Estação da Luz (Luz Railway Station). Construction for the "Grand Victorian Train Station," located at the southwestern edge of Bom Retiro, began in 1861 and was finished six years later. That many immigrants passed through the Luz Railway Station, and thus Bom Retiro, on their way to São Paulo state's plantations has two important ramifications for our story. First, the neighborhood carries a symbolic weight as the central hub for immigration. In this sense it is like Ellis Island or Angel Island in the United States

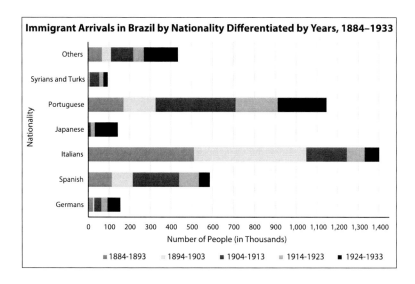

Figure 1.3 Source: Instituto Brasileiro de Geografia e Estatística, Centro de Documentação e Disseminação de Informações, "Apêndice: Estatísticas de 500 anos de povoamento," in *Brasil: 500 anos de povoamento* (Rio de Janeiro: IBGE, 2000), 226. Prepared by Surbhi Shrivastava, Lesser Research Collective, 2023.

although neither location had a resident immigrant population as did Bom Retiro. Second, the immigrants transiting through the Luz Railway Station often carried diseases. Thus, yellow fever outbreaks and public health actions throughout the state between 1889 and 1896 followed the rail lines.[64]

Not all immigrants, however, went to plantations. Many stayed in São Paulo city or remigrated back after disappointing rural experiences. These newcomers often settled in what Jacob Penteado called the immigrant industrial working-class "neighborhoods that start with 'B': Bom Retiro, Brás, Belenzinho, Bexiga, and Barra Funda."[65] Penteado himself was born in Sorocaba (an industrial city about one hundred kilometers from São Paulo city) in 1900, migrated as a child to Buenos Aires, and then returned to Brazil as a seven-year-old, settling first in Bom Retiro and then in Belenzinho.

Immigrants were critical to Brazil's industrialization, and São Paulo's transformation into a city of factories meant laborers needed to be housed, fed, and kept healthy enough to work (see figures 1.5 and 1.6).[66] In 1893 the census showed that 55 percent of the city's population had been born outside of Brazil, and in 1920 that number was still high, at 35 percent.[67] Newcomers made up more than half the patients at São Paulo's Santa Casa de Misericór-

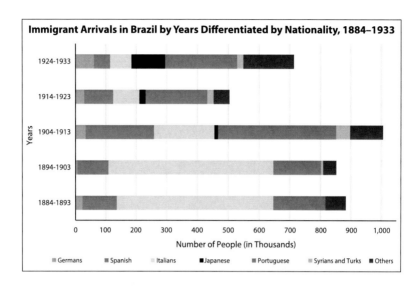

Figure 1.4 Source: Instituto Brasileiro de Geografia e Estatística, Centro de Documentação e Disseminação de Informações, "Apêndice: Estatísticas de 500 anos de povoamento," in *Brasil: 500 anos de povoamento* (Rio de Janeiro: IBGE, 2000), 226. Prepared by Surbhi Shrivastava, Lesser Research Collective, 2023.

dia hospital, and one director, who earlier in his career had worked at São Paulo's Hospedaria dos Imigrantes (Immigrant Hostel and Reception Center), complained in 1901, "Rapid growth based on immigration causes inconveniences, serious inconveniences, at least from the pathological point of view."[68] These concerns were personified at Luz Railway Station, where immigrants were met by representatives of the São Paulo Ministry of Health for disease screening and treatment and were subject to having their luggage chemically disinfected.[69]

São Paulo city's demographic explosion began in the late nineteenth century, and today the metropolitan population exceeds twelve million, and Grande São Paulo has more than twenty million residents. The small city with an economy centered on coffee before 1880 became a frenzied, industrial, and often-unplanned urban madhouse soon thereafter. The influx of people, money, and institutions meant new ideas about space. Soon São Paulo's leaders, like so many around the Americas, were redesigning the city cartographically and topographically as part of what they believed would be a transition from a colonial to a European-like metropolis.

Changes to the built environment were accompanied by new discourses on improvement and modernization. Residents of working-class

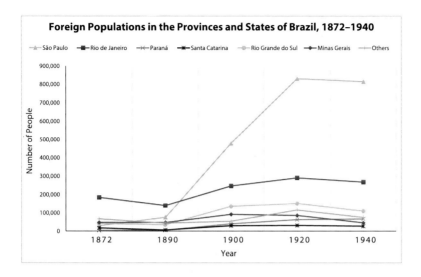

Figure 1.5 Sources: Instituto Brasileiro de Geografia e Estatística, *Censo Demográfico, Séries Historicas, População residentes, 1872-2010*, https://www.ibg .gov.br/estatisticas/sociais/populacao/2098-np-censo-demografico/9662-censo -demografico-2010.html?edicao=9673&t=series-historicas.; and Maria Stella Levy, "O papel da migração internacional na evolução da população brasileira (1872 a 1972)," *Revista de Saúde Pública* 8, suppl. (June 1974): 49–90, https://doi .org/10.1590/S0034-89101974000500003. Prepared by Surbhi Shrivastava, Lesser Research Collective, 2023.

neighborhoods, however, often complained that they did not see the benefits. For example, electric streetlights were first installed in São Paulo in 1905 and within a decade were the rule in most upper-middle-class neighborhoods of the city.[70] In Bom Retiro, however, gas streetlamps were in use until 1937, the latest in the city.[71] The lyrics of the waltz "Lampião de Gás" (Gaslight) suggest how past inequities can become nostalgic pleasures in the present: "My São Paulo, calm and serene. It was small, but really grand. Now it has grown up, but everything died. Gaslight, what yearnings I have for you."[72]

Immigrant Labor Geographies

The processes leading individuals and groups to immigrate involved complex social, family, economic, and geographic networks. In Bom Retiro these networks were initially visible through monied immigrants like Meyer and Dulley. This changed around 1880 as immigrants from Italy, Portugal,

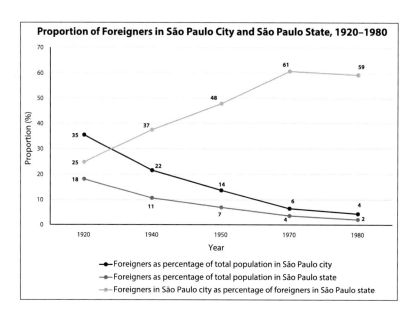

Figure 1.6 Sources: Instituto Brasileiro de Geografia e Estatística, *Censo Demográfico, Séries Historicas, População residentes, 1872-2010*, https://www.ibge.gov.br/estatisticas/sociais/populacao/2098-np-censo-demografico/9662-censo-demografico-2010.html?edicao=9673&t=series-historicas.; and Maria Stella Levy, "O papel da migração internacional na evolução da população brasileira (1872 a 1972)," *Revista de Saúde Pública* 8, suppl. (June 1974): 49–90, https://www.scielo.br/j/rsp/a/gSZkx3b5kCrf8TkWjGRxmfx/?format=pdf&lang=pt. Prepared by Surbhi Shrivastava, Lesser Research Collective, 2023.

and Spain settled and began to bring new ideas about clothing usage, food consumption, language, and political activities. Racism was another kind of network, and many immigrants learned that their success could be hastened by pushing long-term residents of African descent out of the city center. Health was a particularly visible kind of network since factory work was dangerous and laborers could rarely afford private health care, a topic I explore in chapter 4. Even so, officials saw immigrant self-care, for example, the use of popular Brazilian cures to replace those actually or mythically used premigration, as unmodern. Residues of nineteenth-century prejudices about southern Europeans among health care professionals and businesspeople are also found in descriptions of twenty-first-century Andeans. One example is the continued use of the word *indolent* by factory owners who seek ever-faster production and by health care workers who are disappointed when immigrants do not comport themselves like middle-class Brazilians.

Factory owners used networks to employ immigrant workers. Yet the expanding numbers of large and small factories did not just add to Bom Retiro's population but also helped to sicken them. Access to rivers created energy for factories that in turn generated huge amounts of industrial waste. The effluence flowing into the Tamanduateí and Tietê Rivers created "putrid mud deposits" along the floodplains, while the associated flies and mosquitoes generated "powerful and growing infection outbreaks."[73] The pollution and disease, however, did not stop children from playing, swimming, and fishing in rivers.[74]

Since industrial legislation went largely unenforced, factories were a persistent generator of bad health in Bom Retiro. Accidents were common in the district's "incalculable number of small shoemaking and woodworking factories . . . foundries, clothing and hat factories, and home workshops that produced food, drinks and chemicals such as soap and candles."[75] Chimneys and smoke created a visual landscape in São Paulo that made Bom Retiro seem much larger than its measured space. Jorge Americano, a politician and former president of the University of São Paulo, remembered looking out at the neighborhood in the late nineteenth century: "There were thirty or forty chimneys, spewing black coke smoke like in England (there was still no electricity in São Paulo). The Paulistas spoke of it proudly, 'Brazilian Manchester!'"[76] The human and material global networks that came together in Bom Retiro, sometimes called the "São Paulo Model," created an industrial central city marked by packed housing and factories open twenty-four hours per day.[77]

Many of these processes were at play in the 1885 opening of the Anhaia and Company textile factory (Fábrica de Tecidos de Anhaia e Cia), the first large-scale one in Bom Retiro.[78] The business was owned by Luís Antônio Anhaia, a large landowner and city councilperson from Itú, at the time an area of plantations, including of cotton, about a hundred kilometers from São Paulo city. Anhaia's Bom Retiro factory took advantage of a location next to the railroad tracks to move textiles quickly. By the turn of the century, the factory employed 350 workers working in two twelve-hour shifts and producing more than twelve thousand meters of textile products, along with the associated waste, each day.[79] To maintain these production metrics, the company enforced social and labor compliance. In response, in late 1902 female loom workers began a strike (just one of many) following poor treatment from a floor manager and the firing of a seventeen-year-old seamstress after three years of service.[80] Each of these strikes resulted in police intervention and violence, further intertwining labor and health issues.

State repression did not stop worker activism, and Bom Retiro's streets were often taken over by immigrant workers.[81] When requests to use indoor spaces for strike meetings in other parts of the city were denied, Bom Retiro's open fields were often used.[82] The intersection of Rua dos Imigrantes, Rua do Areal, and Rua Tenente Pena became a prime location for public protests, often sponsored by *A Lanterna* and later by *A Plebe*, two anarchist newspapers edited by Edgard Frederico Leuenroth.[83] The meetings made the intersection one of great symbolic value. In 1913 a speech by Antonio Soares dos Santos of the People's League against High Prices was "stupidly interrupted" by an opponent who tried to drag him from the improvised stage to the local police station. The crowd was on the side of dos Santos, and Leuenroth himself returned dos Santos to the stage to finish his speech.[84] In 1917 strikers in Bom Retiro "formed barricades [against] the unaware and militarized defenders of the State and Capitalism, the principal cause of their own misfortune and the misfortune of those who are their brothers in suffering."[85]

The intersection's residual symbolic power was also used by the state. In 1925 the São Paulo municipality decided to create model health posts focused on prenatal and postnatal care, early childhood health, nutrition, venereal diseases, and tuberculosis. Only three were opened in the city, one at that same intersection in Bom Retiro, named after Geraldo de Paulo Souza, a physician and founder of the University of São Paulo's School of Public Health.[86] Today the Bom Retiro Public Health Clinic sits at the intersection, continuing to show the importance of specific spaces to state conceptions of health.

Public health authorities often portrayed working-class neighborhoods in the Americas as unhealthy, unruly, and violent and thus needing state interventions that linked health and policing.[87] Brazil was no different, and as Paulo César Garcez Marins has argued, "Turmoil and disorder were words easily and widely applied to the dynamics of Republican capital cities, to the occupation of houses, and to the increasingly numerous and unstable inhabitants. The emerging elites believed they had a duty to rid the country of what they considered 'backwardness' that they attributed to the country's colonial and imperial past, and that was visible in the apparent confusion in urban spaces, populated with crowded and noisy streets, overcrowded housing, and epidemics that spread rapidly through the neighborhoods, continuously ravaging the great coastal capitals."[88]

Government officials' prejudices against foreign laborers often intertwined with racism against nonwhites, a category that included in different moments southern European Catholics and eastern European Jews.[89] These same politicians and those allied to them often blamed workers for the environmental deterioration typical of unregulated and rapid industrial expansion. In Bom Retiro diseases came with the regular flooding of the Tietê and Tamanduateí Rivers, whose waters entered homes, streets, and factories. In 1872, 1887, and again in 1929, São Paulo was hit by heavy rains that necessitated the removal of families from Bom Retiro's cortiços and disrupted public transportation in and out of the neighborhood.[90] Each incident led to government investigations and angry public responses but flooding and related health issues continue into the present.[91]

One of those investigations was led by Luiz Bianchi Betoldi, an Italian immigrant from Lombard, who moved to São Paulo in 1872. He was an engineer, a property owner in central São Paulo, and a recruiter of Italian workers for Bom Retiro's factories. He was an employee of the city's Public Works Department, and his 1887 report on the flooding and consequent malaria explosion, was depressing. Without major structural changes, he noted, "Sadly, by my observations from the last flood, it will be impossible to prevent a recurrence, even with a less significant inundation."[92] Betoldi argued, without much success, that municipal leaders should take more responsibility for "the street" by placing litter collection containers, with scheduled pickup times, in front of cortiços.[93] Another engineer employed by the city, Theodoro Sampaio, did a similar study half a decade after Betoldi's and reached the same conclusions, noting that little had changed in the five-year span.[94]

Bom Retiro's health challenges, and the different anxieties they produced for residents and city leaders, made the district a focus of municipal health actions. It also made the neighborhood a laboratory for future health policies when the new São Paulo state Sanitary Service was inaugurated in 1890. Even so, the image of bad health has continued to the present, worsening during epidemics. Henrique Raffard, son of the Swiss consul in Rio de Janeiro, visited the rapidly expanding neighborhood in 1886 and again in 1890, noting that the built environment was not conducive to good health: "It is a pity that the subdividing of Bom Retiro was not done better to prevent rainwater from pooling in some places, and there could also have been better organization in the alignment of some buildings."[95] In 1901 Antonio Francisco Bandeira Jr. produced a microscopic look at São Paulo's industrial growth, cataloging individual streets by their factories and stores. His visits to Bom Retiro connected the built environment to bad health: "The houses are filthy, the streets, almost in their entirety, are unpaved, there is a lack of water for the most necessary tasks and a shortage of electricity and sewers."[96]

The view of Bom Retiro as dirty, flood prone, and sick was so widespread that newspaper readers only needed to see the name of a street in the neighborhood to jump to negative conclusions. As Valéria Guimarães argues, an article telling the story of someone who lived in Bom Retiro instantly conjured up a place that was "industrial and proletarian, a lowland plain of the Tietê River, subject to frequent floods. It had one of the highest rates of epidemics in São Paulo. Its wells were unhealthy, and its residential plots, narrow and long, five or six meters in front, were lined up in small houses where many families lived."[97] These images help to explain why the *Correio Paulistano* emphasized the cleanliness and order in Amelia Marini's home.

For most residents of Bom Retiro, flooding brought hardships as they walked for blocks, barefoot, to get clean water, even in the more well-off parts of the neighborhood.[98] Protecting nonhuman animals, cleaning mud-filled houses, and rushing for vaccines to prevent new waterborne and mosquito-borne illnesses was the norm.[99] These harsh realities continue in Bom Retiro, but memories often hide this: Dona Alice was born in the interior of the 96,000-square-mile state of São Paulo, and her family migrated the 175 kilometers from their hometown to Bom Retiro when she was three years old. Her conversation with Ecléa Bosi as part of an oral history project with older residents of São Paulo includes this nostalgic recollection that connects flooding with immigration and the homeland where she had never been: "When it rained a lot, lower Bom Retiro became the Brazilian Venice. The flood dominated everything. All the families had a boat, and at night they strolled in the flooded streets, with lights on the boats, singing and serenading. For us, the youngsters, it was a joy when the Tietê overflowed."[100]

Flooding, sewer problems, and a lack of potable water were so severe that the city's first Department of Water and Sewers was placed in Bom Retiro.[101] The district began to receive sewers in 1894, but early twentieth-century studies showed that São Paulo's working-class neighborhoods suffered from untreated water because of infrastructural malfunctions and uneven water distribution.[102] Within Bom Retiro, the distribution of clean water and sewers was also unequal because the northern parts of the neighborhood were most prone to flooding. Even so, some of Bom Retiro's cost-of-living protests prior to World War I included the complaint that sewers in the neighborhood were increasing rental costs and thus pricing out the working class.[103]

Bad health in Bom Retiro was not generated only by flooding and poor sewers. Litter, because it moved through the neighborhood due to water and poor removal programs, was and is a particular issue.[104] In the nineteenth century, like today, trash from residences, factories, and the city's rivers overflowed onto streets in low-lying neighborhoods with each significant rainfall. Household waste was often deposited in vacant lots or directly outside of homes, since São Paulo's first trash incinerator only opened in 1913. The material residues of family life were eaten by cows or dogs or picked up in carts by those without formal employment to be sold as fertilizer, or more recently for recycling.[105] In the 1890s there were regular complaints about litter thrown into holes next to public wells, which "may be infected by the liquid infiltrations."[106] In the mid-1980s Bom Retiro was described this way in the *Jornal da Tarde* newspaper: "25,109 residents, five hundred thousand people running through the streets daily, sixty-eight tons of litter every day."[107] Other observers linked real negative health outcomes in the neighborhood to culture rather than structure such as working conditions, overcrowding, and meager social services, often describing industrial working-class districts in the language of disease. Indeed, poor sanitary conditions in homes and in Bom Retiro were often blamed on immigrant workers rather than on environmental pollution from rivers and factories.[108]

Flooding and poor waste removal were a dangerous combination. Mosquito-borne diseases were thus part of everyday life for residents of Bom Retiro, and insect repellants with names like Terror to Mosquitoes became part of the commercial landscape.[109] Public health officials often blamed the residents, but neighborhood dwellers saw the state as the problem. Water-based complaints became a regular part of the reporting of the *Correio Paulistano*; this 1912 notice was typical:

> *Gripes and Complaints*
>
> *The residents of Rua General Flores, in the stretch between Rua Sólon and Rua Jaraguá, write to us requesting our intervention with the municipal government, to remove the existing water drain, which floods frequently, closer to the Tietê River.*
>
> *The waters coming from Rua Guarany, and the surrounding areas, flow into there (to Rua General Flores), putting the health of its residents at serious risk, since across the street a veritable stream has formed that breeds mosquitoes and can produce dangerous fevers.*[110]

Almost a century later, the complaints from residents are similar as flooding and standing water continue to make Bom Retiro one of the central neighborhoods with the highest incidences of dengue.[111] The Good Retreat of rural leisure was transformed into a place of Bad Health.

Illuminating the Darkness

While the historical past may not be part of the overt day-to-day consciousness of the living, the contemporary built environment includes residues of the past and connects to lived experiences. One way that happens for those residing in, working in, or passing through Bom Retiro is the presence of São Paulo's first botanical garden, opened in 1798 (figure 1.7). Renovated and reopened to the public in 1825 as the Jardim da Luz (Luz Garden), the space emphasized to "slaves, immigrants, workers, and others not in the elite" that strolling outside was a health privilege.[112] In 1890 the Jardim da Luz became the center point of a series of new streets linking Bom Retiro to other parts of the central city.[113] A decade later, local aristocrats financed the municipal School of Arts and Crafts to educate specialized industrial workers (the building today is the Pinacoteca do Estado de São Paulo art museum).

In recognition of the role of immigrants in Bom Retiro, a bronze and granite monument to the Italian revolutionary Giuseppe Garibaldi was inaugurated in the Jardim da Luz in 1910. Garibaldi was connected to Brazilian politics through his involvement in the 1836 revolt in the southern Brazilian state of Rio Grande do Sul. In São Paulo, children played the "Garibaldi game," which involved tricking a participant to hold his hands to help a hobbling "Garibaldi" (who, among his other war injuries, was once shot in the ankle) mount a "horse" with his feces-covered boots.[114] Adult immigrant "Garibaldinos" also played in public as they celebrated Italy's unification by marching through Bom Retiro playing Italian patriotic marches each September 20, starting in the early 1900s.[115]

In the later decades of the twentieth century, popular impressions of the Jardim da Luz became connected to sex work, crime, and homelessness, leading the city to lock the gates of ornate fencing at nightfall. A heightened police presence expelled those living in the park with the stated intent of returning the space to people of all generations, classes, and national origins. Today the Jardim is no longer technically in Bom Retiro, a district whose official size has ranged from two and a half to four square kilometers, but virtually no one knows that. Elder exercise classes sponsored by the Bom Retiro Public Health Clinic take place in the park, as do activities that were common in the nineteenth century such as taking family pictures or purchasing musical serenades by the song.

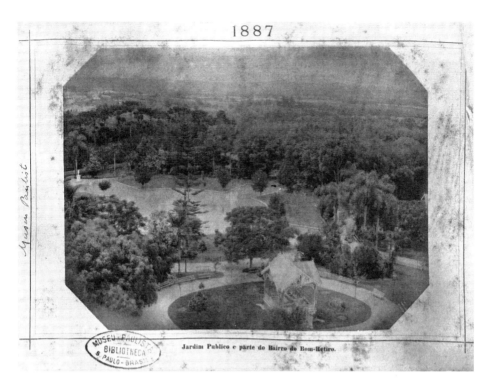

1887

Jardim Publico e parte do Bairro do Bom-Retiro.

Figure 1.7 An 1887 photograph of the Jardim da Luz (Luz Garden) with a caption emphasizing that it is part of Bom Retiro. Source: Militão Augusto de Azevedo, "Jardim Público e Parte do Bairro do Bom Retiro," São Paulo, 1887, Fundo Museu Paulista, Página 57 do Álbum Comparativo da Cidade de São Paulo USP, https://commons.wikimedia.org/wiki/File:Milit%C3%A3o_A._de_Azevedo_-_%C3%81lbum_Comparativo,_57_-_Acervo_do_Museu_Paulista_da_USP.jpg.

The distinct borders of the Jardim da Luz, within the much less clear neighborhood frontiers, connect the past to the present. The east side is home to the impressive Pinacoteca art museum, mostly visited on school field trips and by adult members of the dominant classes. To the west and north of the park, and visible from the Pinacoteca's floor-to-ceiling windows, are Bom Retiro's two- and three-story mixed residential, commercial, and industrial buildings. The southern exit of the Jardim da Luz is less than twenty meters from the entrance to the British-built Luz Railway Station.[116] The physical contours of the park have created long-term conflict over ground-level access. In the nineteenth century, there were disputes over safe pedestrian crossings over the already existing railroad tracks while more recently there are issues over the expulsion each night of everyone in the park.[117]

Today the Luz Railway Station, Jardim da Luz, and the railroad tracks represent an insurgent urban planning since Bom Retiro's informal borders include places no longer officially in the district. This geographic sense is relatively new. As I showed in the introduction, nineteenth-century maps showed the area north of the botanical garden as empty, although these spaces had been occupied long before the arrival of the Portuguese. Cartography visually reinforced colonization by showing lands as unpopulated and thus available for occupation. These maps justified, with sometimes erroneous streets, the deeding of chácaras to the imperial elite and the later sales to land developers whose subdivisions became part of the city's growth. Representing Bom Retiro as empty, even when it was densely populated at the end of the nineteenth century, allowed politicians to withhold services.

"Emptiness" was rapidly transformed by developers into an urban neighborhood. As rural estates became urban lots, Bom Retiro became a space filled with factories and the workers needed to keep them running.[118] By 1890 city leaders increasingly sought to link Bom Retiro to other parts of the city with roads, hoping this would spur more industrial output and growth.[119] In 1900 the district became the second location in São Paulo city to have a tram line to get factory workers to and from the district.[120] The changes further increased the lack of demarcation between geographies of work and nonwork. Growing numbers of factories and commercial services sprang up near residences/small workshops, making industrial pollution a typical part of life and death in Bom Retiro.

This chapter has made three arguments. The first shows what we can learn when we analyze individual lives in our studies of overarching topics like immigration, health, and geography. The life and death of Amelia Marini helps to illustrate how violence and nationality connect to health for immigrants and state officials, from legislators to law enforcement officials. The second argument is that the transformation of Bom Retiro from a rural weekend retreat for the wealthy into an urban industrial district filled with working-class immigrants created residues related to labor oppression, repression, and the othering of Blacks and immigrants by the dominant classes. Finally, I have argued that the state used mapping both to justify its creation of working-class neighborhoods and then to classify those same neighborhoods as not deserving infrastructural benefits. Bom Retiro is thus part of a series of concentric spatial circles including the city of São Paulo, Brazil, the Americas, and the globe. Part of what makes Bom Retiro global, as I argue in the next chapter, is how it is seen from the outside, as a "foreign neighborhood," linked to immigration, health, labor, and racism.

A POSTSCRIPT

Bom Retiro is at the center of a contemporary memory and political dispute in São Paulo that relates to immigration, naming, and geography. While there was little outcry in the mid-1980s when the Ponte Pequena Metro Station was renamed Armênia Metro Station—to acknowledge that immigrant group's historical presence—that changed in 2018 when São Paulo's governor, Márcio Luiz França Gomes, changed the name of the Liberdade Metro Station to Japão-Liberdade Metro Station. The connection between Japan and the Brazilian neighborhood of Liberdade was a surprise to many since most residents of the neighborhood have never been of Japanese descent. Afro-Brazilian activists correctly read the change as an example of how immigration is used to disappear São Paulo's African presence. They insisted on recognition of Liberdade's historical importance for enslaved Africans' struggle for freedom, represented in the built environment with the Church of the Holy Cross of the Souls of the Hanged on the site of the former Portuguese central whipping post.[121] Nikkei activists were equally vociferous in their opposition, noting that they were Brazilian, not Japanese. In 2020 a member of the Legislative Assembly, José Américo (of the Worker's Party, or PT), proposed adding África to the official name of the metro station. In 2023 the plaza's name was modified to Japão-Liberdade-África, continuing a long discursive tradition of denominating Brazilianness with the names of distant geographic spaces.[122]

Conflicts over place-names and national identity also take place in Bom Retiro. In 2017 São Paulo's mayor, João Doria, in collaboration with the Korean consul general and the directors of Korean multinationals, sought to rename Bom Retiro as Little Seoul.[123] "Bom Retiro Is the World" became an opposition rallying phrase, and the Little Seoul proposal was shelved following protests from neighborhood residents who were not of Korean descent. In 2021 the Korean consulate renewed the idea, this time proposing that the district be called Korea Town (in English!) as part of the government's "Hallyu" (Korean Wave) not-so-soft-power project, which has included everything from providing the boy band BTS with diplomatic passports to promoting Korean-made products via programs shown on streaming platforms. The Korean consul argued that the name change would bring foreign investment and tourism to Bom Retiro, and many Korean immigrant and Korean-descent business owners supported the idea. They contended that neighborhood economic growth would follow a new image of modern, hip, and healthy Koreanness rather than that of working-class and disease-ridden immigrants from Paraguay or Bolivia working in semihidden *oficina-residências*.

One evening in October 2021, I attended an anti–Korea Town naming event that, as had been the case four years earlier, used the banner "Bom Retiro Is the World." It was sponsored by the Bom Retiro political-social organization the Casa do Povo (the People's House), founded in 1946 by left-wing and progressive Jewish Brazilians and Jewish immigrants from eastern Europe.[124] The Casa do Povo occupies a large building (a former theater) on the "cool" Rua Três Rios, although when I visited to interview activists in the 1980s, the structure was mostly deserted (these oral histories were not a great success because my surname, which comes from my father's central European Jewish parents and not my mother's working-class Russian ones, led the elderly men to be suspicious of my motives).[125] In the 2000s the Casa do Povo reinvented itself as a promotor of multiethnic Bom Retiro, and thus the Korea Town proposal was particularly irksome.[126] The 2021 rally included a series of short lectures about the multicultural history of the neighborhood and a samba jam session. During the public comments, an older resident suggested that the Corinthians soccer team, founded in the early twentieth century by immigrants in Bom Retiro, was evidence of the multicultural nature of the neighborhood.[127] He brought the house down by leading the audience in a rousing version of the team chant, which includes lyrics suggesting that the British founders of the team created "the most Brazilian club."[128]

2

Bom Retiro Is the World?

Pedro [Álvares] Cabral invented Brazil
Yes sir! He had to go to Africa to fetch slaves but then got lost on his way there.
. . .
Well, what was he thinking? That the ocean never ends?
Naturally, he was bound to find land anyway, but since he was lost and had no
idea where he was, he ended up in Brazil, where he found the savages, the Bom
Retiro neighborhood, the cute Italian girls, as well as my grandpa, who was a
public service old timer . . .
Pedro Cabral loved the party, and so did I.

Juó Bananére (Johnny the Banana Seller), "A invençó do Brasile"

Juó Bananére was fed up with complaints about Bom Retiro's immigrant
population. He insisted that Pedro Cabral (ca. 1468–1520), the Portuguese
colonizer who "invented" Brazil, had come ashore in 1500 to find a fully
formed Bom Retiro. If this were true, the neighborhood and its residents
were central to the national origin story. Bananére was also not buying that
Bom Retiro had only thirty thousand residents since it was "the biggest district of São Paulo, the most beautiful and the one I most admire."[1]

Bananére, the pseudonym of journalist and civil engineer Alexandre
Ribeiro Marcondes Machado (1892–1933), used "macaronic Portuguese" to
chronicle the dialect and culture of Bom Retiro's Italian immigrants, often

in Oswald de Andrade's humorous magazine *O Pirralho* (The brat). Paulo Menotti del Picchia also thought about immigrants, but his modernist poetry was not as funny as Bananére's. In "Tower of Babel," Menotti del Picchia connected country of origin with a variety of physical and political traits:

> Jovial Italians,
> Leopard-eyed Hungarians,
> Caboclos from the Tietê River, dragging the redneck,
> Ukrainian Bolsheviks,
> Polish supporters of Wrangel [a White Russian exile in the 1920s]
> Yellow Japanese like dwarf gnomes carved in amber
> Among the foremen's pests,
> The creaking of the scaffolding,
> The metallic grating
> of steel beams and sounding hammers,
> in São Paulo's free sky,
> made the confusion of languages,
> without disturbing the rigorous geometry
> of the cyclopean skyscraper![2]

In the early twentieth century, many policymakers were less enthusiastic than poets about immigrants, often presenting them as both problems and saviors. Newcomers moving through São Paulo's first major immigrant reception center, opened in Bom Retiro in 1882, became healthy components of political projects (i.e., last week five hundred strong immigrants arrived) and sick ones whose disease would infect the national body.[3] A century later, when city officials began to publicize Bom Retiro as a place where a person could take a trip "abroad" without leaving the city, the duality continued, placing a significant price on those tagged as foreign. The long-term construction of Bom Retiro as a place of radical segregation between different immigrant groups meant cultural opinion makers in the press, in food blogs, and in the municipal tourist office encouraged stereotyping and prejudice, perhaps unintentionally.

The promotion of Bom Retiro as a space where different "foreign" people lived in closed communities reinforced racist ideas about the danger and sickness of the neighborhood and its residents. The visibility of the people and the place reinforced a fear among São Paulo's dominant classes that real and imagined moral and biomedical sicknesses in Bom Retiro were poised to spread to more monied parts of the city.[4] Bom Retiro's different ethnic communities are deeply connected to each other. Yet when Brazil's National Historic and Artistic Heritage Institute (Instituto do Patrimônio Histórico e Artístico Nacional, IPHAN) began to focus on Bom Retiro in the early twenty-first century, they focused on segregation: "Bom Retiro, Bó Ritiro of the Italians, the 'small shtetl' of the Jews, the neighborhood of Korean signs, of English football, of Armenian church bells, of the South American identity of Bolivians, of the 'Acropolis' of the Greeks, of the northeastern-ers, of the merchants and wholesale buyers, of coffee and the railroad that made São Paulo a metropolis—Bom Retiro is a world map embedded in the city of São Paulo."[5] São Paulo's Secretariat of Culture and Secretariat of Education took a similar approach when they co-produced "Bom Retiro Is the World," a twenty-five-minute video that posits that "Bom Retiro was a Good Retreat for people from all over the world: Portuguese, Italians, Jews, Greeks, Syrians, Koreans, and Bolivians. By welcoming people from all over the world, Bom Retiro ended up being a very Brazilian neighborhood, where there is disorder and organization, wealth and poverty, western gods and eastern gods. On the streets of this neighborhood, you can find all kinds of people . . . Brazilians and foreigners, and Brazilian-foreigners."[6]

The seemingly positive casting in "Bom Retiro Is the World" is embedded with other, less favorable stereotypes. A segment about Emanuel, a Jewish Brazilian who goes to pray once a week, describes him as "breaking down barriers" by marrying "a Japanese" (i.e., a Brazilian of Japanese descent, not an immigrant from Japan) since "most Jews marry among themselves." Yet in 2006 most Jewish Brazilians, like most Jews in the Americas, rarely attended religious services, and well over 50 percent married non-Jewish Brazilians. The film is available on YouTube, and the posted comments continued to appear through 2024. Those remarks fit into patterns that I discussed earlier, with memories of the good old days and "yearnings" for "my Bom Retiro." The posts ranged from spatial memories of specific streets and buildings to ones like "my father owns the Greek restaurant" and "an Italian took care of me." One comment even referenced the often-ignored relations between ethnic groups in the 1960s and 1970s, commenting on "my Greek, Italian, Jewish, Northeastern Brazilian, and Portuguese neighbors," most of whom were undoubtedly Brazilians.

The depictions of Bom Retiro as a neighborhood where "the world" shares a single space suggest a geography of closed communities with distinct and visible ethnic markers such as clothing, facial hair, public habits such as smok-ing, and birth rates. Jorge Americano's early twentieth-century list of "The People That We Saw" typecasts many of the working-class immigrants in

Bom Retiro: "Portuguese with giant mustaches . . . Spaniards with jackets and sideburns, one eye green and the other hollow . . . Italians from Calabria, with odd quirks, smoking huge pipes . . . those rare Jews with blue eyes, one eye on each side of their pointy nose. . . . White teeth gleaming in naive black faces . . . Syrians with the hair below the back of their necks and vulture-winged eyebrows over immense noses."[7] Jacob Penteado's memories of Bom Retiro also described ethnicity in absolutes, claiming that immigrants from one country disappeared as others took their place. In his vision Bom Retiro was "an Italian stronghold" in the early 1900s, but eastern European immigrants made it a "a real ghetto, a Jewish city," starting in the 1920s.[8]

While immigration from places as distant from each other as Greece and Korea increased over the course of the twentieth century (see figure 2.1), Catholic Italians and Jewish eastern Europeans remained the focal point for many outside the neighborhood. The journalist Marcos Faerman concentrated on the two groups in a series of articles for the *Jornal da Tarde* in 1981, using the word *community* to suggest closed and unchanging populations. Part 1, "Remembering the Good Old Days," focused on "Italian Bom Retiro," while part 2, presumably describing less good days in the present, was entitled "The Neighborhood of Szmul, Isaac, Jacob, Bagels, Herring, [and] Ten Synagogues," which had become "the Neighborhood of the Jews."[9] While Bom Retiro never had a majority of foreign-born residents, the neighborhood, like so many in the Americas, was and is glossed in the popular imagination as one of immigrants. This makes the human/spatial markings in articles like Faerman's complex. The motifs suggest that residents, including the majority who are citizens, are not fully Brazilian and that globality is negative. At the same time, Brazil's past, present, and future appear to lie in its multiculturality, making globality a positive.

These dualities often appear when I conduct oral histories. While I do not attach the word *community* to specific groups or neighborhoods, my subjects usually do, even when presented with evidence showing that multiple ethnic groups lived next to each other, went to school together, and participated jointly in class-based political movements.[10] Indeed, people often tell their own stories as ones in which their community is unique, more hardworking, more successful, and/or more victimized than others. Exceptionality and its link to neighborhoods can be also seen in the cartoon in figure 2.2, rife with stereotypes, published in the widely distributed *Folha da Manhã* and drawn by Belmonte, one of Brazil's most famous caricaturists. The title of the cartoon, "Dize-me em que rua andas e eu te direi que és," is a São Paulo insider/outsider twist on the Spanish intellectual José Ortega y Gasset's

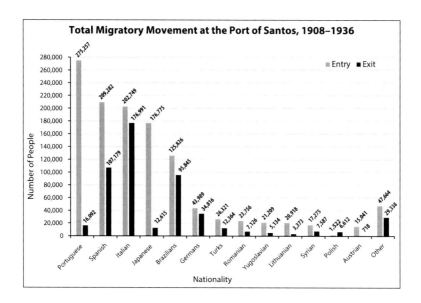

Figure 2.1 Sources: Instituto Brasileiro de Geografia e Estatística, *Censo Demográfico, Séries Historicas, População residentes, 1872-2010,* https://www.ibge .gov.br/estatisticas/sociais/populacao/2098-np-censo-demografico/9662-censo -demografico-2010.html?edicao=9673&t=series-historicas; Maria Stella Levy, "O papel da migração internacional na evolução da população brasileira (1872 a 1972)," *Revista de Saúde Pública* 8, suppl. (June 1974): 49–90, https://www.scielo .br/j/rsp/a/gSZkx3b5kCrf8TkWjGRxmfx/?format=pdf&lang ; and Jeffrey Lesser, *Immigration, Ethnicity and National Identity in Brazil* (New York: Cambridge University Press, 2013), 78. Note: Some Brazilians are included since legislation at the time classified all those who purchased tourist-class passages as immigrants.

comment "Dime el paisaje en que vives y te diré quién eres" (Tell me the landscape in which you live and I will tell you who you are).[11] From one perspective, the title of the caricatures of Arabs, Japanese, Afro-Brazilians, Portuguese, Italians, and Jews reads, "Tell me the street on which you live and I will tell you who you are," suggesting that ethnicity organically dominates the urban body (i.e., neighborhoods). Another reading is "Tell me on which street you are walking, and I will tell you who you are," suggesting that even visitors are transformed biologically, one might even say infected, by entering ethnic territory.

The cartoon focuses on physical otherness by emphasizing that male immigrants were easily distinguishable in the public sphere by their facial hair, clothes, and large noses, images not unlike Jorge Americano's descriptions

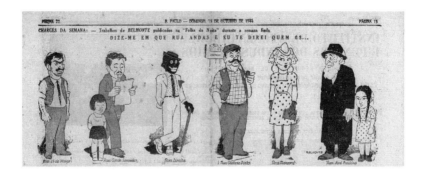

Figure 2.2 Belmonte cartoon, "Tell me the street on which you live, and I will tell you who you are." Source: *Folha da Manhã*, October 15, 1944, 15.

above. The center city streets would be instantly recognizable, even today, since the neighborhood geographies all are linked to specific groups: Arabs (Rua 25 de Março in São Bento), Japanese (Rua Conde de Sarzedas in Liberdade), Afro-Brazilians (Rua Direita in Sé), Portuguese (Rua Caetano Pinto in Brás), Italians (Rua Marconi in República), and Jews (Rua José Paulino in Bom Retiro).[12] Eastern European Jews and Japanese are shown multigenerationally, highlighting a concern expressed by some politicians and intellectuals in the interwar era that these two immigrant groups would produce large families and thus change the racial composition of Brazil for the worse.[13]

Discourses about the single-group globality of Bom Retiro often contrasted a healthy and economically productive "world" with a "Brazil" of sickness and danger. This bifurcation was starkly presented on a single page of São Paulo's *Diário Popular* in 1997 when a glowing article on Bom Retiro's "cultural mixture" included an insert focusing on how neighborhood economic growth was hindered by nonimmigrant drug trafficking and prostitution.[14] In the thirty years that I have been conducting research in Brazil, I have frequently heard Bom Retiro defined in binaries by health care workers, neighborhood activists, and immigrant and immigrant-descent residents: healthy/sick, them/us, ascension/decline, Brazilian/foreign. These complex expressions of human and geographic identities often appear in my conversations, and I am reminded that Bom Retiro was never a closed geographic space inhabited by only one group.[15] Yet for the immigrant laboring classes who spent twelve-hour-plus days doing repetitive work in factories or workshops, the world of Bom Retiro is a very small, enclosed space. The different views, occurring simultaneously, help to understand why the neighborhood and so many like it are defined as unchanging in otherness even if the immigrants—Portuguese, Italian, eastern European, Korean, Bolivian, Chinese, Bangladeshi—have changed over time.

Othered Geographies

Spaces denominated as foreign are typical of cities. They might be called Chinatown or Little Italy or Pequena África. Sometimes "foreignness" is so established that a nonnational term can create a geographic/ethnic image, such as with the Lower East Side in New York, Buford Highway in Atlanta, Liberdade in São Paulo, or Once in Buenos Aires. In Brazil and elsewhere, the designation of a space as foreign includes geography (within and outside of the nation) and identity (us and them).[16] Brazilian-born majorities in geographic spaces like Bom Retiro have never prevented popular and state denominations of the neighborhood as foreign (see figure 2.3). Many Brazilians are described as Arab, Japanese, or German even though their immigrant ancestors arrived generations prior.[17]

When we disaggregate the classification of "foreign" from citizenship, Bom Retiro fits roughly within what John Logan, Wenquan Zhang, and Richard Alba have termed an "immigrant enclave." In their model "ethnic neighborhoods in central cities serve relatively impoverished new arrivals as a potential base for eventual spatial assimilation with the white majority. . . . [S]egregated settlement can result from group preferences even when spatial assimilation is otherwise feasible. In some cases, however, living in ethnic neighborhoods is unrelated to economic constraints, indicating a positive preference for such areas."[18] While Bom Retiro has been home to different immigrant groups, the demographic realities show that the "enclave" is heterogeneous and transnational.

Since state documents sometimes categorized the children and grandchildren of immigrants as foreign, it is no surprise that others did as well. The Austrian American writer and diplomat Ernst von Hesse-Wartegg (1851–1918) spent three extended periods in Brazil in the first decades of the twentieth century. His 1915 German-language *Zwischen Anden und Amazonas* (Between the Andes and the Amazon) described São Paulo this way: "[It] is not a Brazilian city of 450,000 inhabitants, but an Italian city of approximately 100,000, a Portuguese city of perhaps 40,000, a Spanish city of equal size, and a small German city [Kleinstadt] of about 10,000 inhabitants, with few of its advantages and many of its disadvantages. There are some 5,000 Syrians, who alone have three newspapers printed in Arabic characters, Russians, Japanese, Turkish, Poles, Scandinavians, English, and

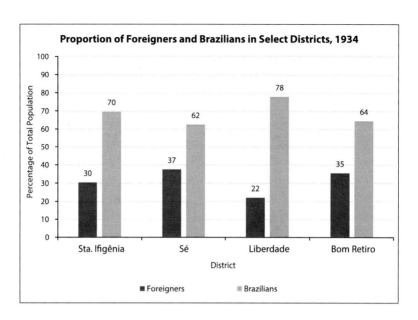

Proportion of Foreigners and Brazilians in Select Districts, 1934

Percentage of Total Population

	Sta. Ifigênia	Sé	Liberdade	Bom Retiro
Foreigners	30	37	22	35
Brazilians	70	62	78	64

District

■ Foreigners   ■ Brazilians

Figure 2.3 Source: Oscar Egídio de Araújo, "Enquistamentos étnicos," *Revista do Arquivo Municipal* 65 (March 1940): 235.

Americans in unknown numbers for lack of reliable statistics. The rest, probably a third of the total, must have been Brazilians."[19] Four decades later, Hesse-Wartegg's words were repeated, almost verbatim, by Pasquale Petrone, the Italian-born chair of the University of São Paulo's Geography Department and president of the Association of Brazilian Geographers. His article on turn-of-the-century São Paulo continues to be widely cited.[20]

Brazilian-born intellectuals took a similar approach to foreign-born ones in understanding how immigration, ethnicity, and space connected. Guilherme de Almeida, a poet and cultural critic, was a member of Brazil's prestigious Academy of Letters. In 1929 he wrote a series of eight articles on his "impressions of our diverse foreign neighborhoods" for *O Estado de S. Paulo*. At the time, his acknowledgment of the importance of immigrants was progressive, but his racially charged satirical language used many of the dominant racist tropes in circulation then and now. Each essay suggested that immigrants segregated themselves from national society to engage in nefarious social, cultural, and economic practices.[21] He termed Bom Retiro "the Ghetto" because of its growing eastern European Jewish population, conjuring up an image of poverty and otherness that non-Jews often associated with eastern European shtetls. Almeida saw the immigrant inhabitants of

Bom Retiro as somehow less than completely human, not unlike the depictions in the World War II–era Belmonte cartoon discussed above: "I found myself face to face with the first face [I saw] in the São Paulo ghetto. Face? Beard: beard and nose. The first Jew."[22]

The presentation of foreignness as genetic was emphasized by statistics, for example, in the 1907 annual demographic-health report by the São Paulo State Health Service (Serviço Sanitário do Estado de São Paulo) emphasizing high birth rates among immigrants.[23] Almost five decades later, the historian Richard Morse marked São Paulo by ethnicities, calling out Bom Retiro as a "foreign bairro."[24] In 1958, Aroldo de Azevedo, in an official publication from the Association of Brazilian Geographers, did the same—marking neighborhoods as had Belmonte in 1944 (figure 2.2) while arguing for what might be called *ethnic democracy*:

> From the ethnic point of view, the *marks* are very visible: Syrian-Lebanese and Armenians concentrated at Rua 25 de Março and surrounding; Japanese in the blocks around Rua Conde Sarzedas; Jews from west-central Europe in Bom Retiro; Italians in Brás, Mooca, and Bela Vista; Black [people] in Barra Funda, Casa Verde, and also Bela Vista; foreigners of varied provenance disseminated in many "Garden City neighborhoods" and all of them coexisting, in the most complete harmony, with those that pride themselves in descending from old colonial stock or of proceeding from other corners of the State of São Paulo and other regions of the country.[25]

Despite the focus on difference, statistics generated by federal, state, and municipal authorities suggest that Bom Retiro was average in almost every single category.[26] The census of 1920 showed the neighborhood's population was about 35.22 percent foreign born, eighth among the sixteen center-city districts, with most newcomers coming from Italy, Spain, Portugal, and Turquia Asiatica, today's Syria and Lebanon. This percentage continued through the mid-1930s when the foreign population was almost exactly at the city's 35.44 percent average, a surprisingly low number given the neighborhood's reputation as foreign. Bom Retiro is like much of the city of São Paulo in other ways as well. Its class structure fits in broadly with that of the city, with the rest of urban Brazil, and with many urban working-class districts in the Americas.[27]

In the early twenty-first century, Bom Retiro remains an average São Paulo center-city district. In 2000 the working-age population was sixth among the ten center-city districts, and its income of about R$1,520 per month was fifth.[28] Information from 2018 and 2019 shows that 20 percent of residents were under fifteen years old (just slightly higher than in the municipality and the state), while older residents over sixty (often immigrants or their children) made up 14 percent, slightly lower than in the city as a whole and slightly higher than in the state.[29] The ratio of men to women was 94.49 to 100, again slightly higher than in the city as a whole and slightly lower than in the state. Fifty-nine percent of Bom Retiro's residents were literate. In terms of natality, Bom Retiro looks like São Paulo although mortality rates for those between fifteen and thirty-four and for those over sixty years old were lower than in the city and the state (2016 figures). Finally, in terms of income, Bom Retiro is a poor place, like most of Brazil. In 2010 the percentage of people earning little or nothing in the district was almost twice as high as that in São Paulo city and state. The per capita monthly income in 2010 was 933 reais per month, around 10 percent less than the citywide average and about 10 percent higher than in the state.[30]

In some respects, Bom Retiro's population is poorer than those in many other center-city neighborhoods. In 2010 more than 39 percent of Bom Retiro's residents remained unconnected to the city sewer system, and a 2018 São Paulo municipal study found Bom Retiro to have the largest number of cortiços of any central district.[31] The constancy of housing types in Bom Retiro is related to high population density and large numbers of oficina-residências, whose workers seek to avoid motorized transportation because of its relatively high cost. Not surprisingly, Bom Retiro had the lowest average travel time between residence and workplace in the city in 2010. High rates of unemployment and underemployment have marked Bom Retiro since the late nineteenth century. In 2010, of the ninety-six districts in São Paulo, Bom Retiro had the ninth-highest index of heads of households without income while ranking fifty-six in terms of heads of households making more than twenty times the minimum monthly salary.[32]

Available statistics suggest that since the end of the nineteenth century, the neighborhood has sat in the middle of others in São Paulo city in terms of health.[33] When I analyzed early twentieth-century figures produced by São Paulo's Sanitary Service for twenty-five central city neighborhoods, Bom Retiro's disease incidence and prevalence, morbidity, and mortality were average. The total number of deaths from common diseases ranged over time, with Bom Retiro sometimes sixth in deaths, sometimes nineteenth. In other words, the neighborhood was never the healthiest and never the unhealthiest in the city. The situation is similar today. Age-adjusted statistics place Bom Retiro in the middle of the central districts in terms of social inclusion/exclusion, a municipal designation that includes health outcomes.[34]

Afro-Diasporic Bom Retiro

Embedded in the concept of immigrant or foreign spaces in the Americas is the (in)visibilization of nonimmigrants, especially those of African descent. What some scholars and activists term *whitewashing* occurs in diverse socioeconomic, ethnic, and racial geographies, including in Bom Retiro.[35] The reality of both the Black and nonwhite citizenry residing, working, and socializing in the same geographic spaces as immigrants and their descendants links to the ebbs and flows of health hierarchies in Bom Retiro and Brazil more broadly.[36] For many politicians and large landowners in the nineteenth century, immigrants both brought sickness *and* represented the potential for racial improvement vis-à-vis the African-descended population.[37] From the establishment of the Brazilian republic, an official policy, termed *whitening*, sought to subsidize "white" immigrants while prohibiting the entry of those deemed nonwhite. Whitening policies financially incentivized millions of Europeans to emigrate to Brazil, and soon after they were followed by non-Europeans, notably from Japan and the Middle East. At the same time, many potential immigrants, and politicians in nations of emigration, believed Brazil was a dangerously unhealthy location precisely because of the Black population. Thus, as Guilherme Leite Gonçalves and Sérgio Costa show, racism was part of how capitalism and industrialization linked to national identity in Brazil.[38] Places like Bom Retiro, with both long-term Black populations and immigrants, became a focus of state concerns about bad health.

In 1893 those of African descent made up almost 13 percent of the population of the district that at the time included Bom Retiro.[39] Between 1911 and 1915, Fábio Dantas Rocha estimates that Blacks made up almost 16 percent of the population in Bom Retiro, with Italians at 51 percent and Portuguese at 23 percent. Rocha derived these figures from analysis of documents from the Medical Police, a dataset that is the focus of chapter 4, "Enforcing Health."[40] For 1916 to 1920, the percentage of Blacks in Bom Retiro rose to almost 27 percent, with Italians at 48 percent and Portuguese at 16 percent. From 1921 to 1925, Rocha finds that Bom Retiro's population was almost 36 percent Black, 34 percent Italian, and 18 percent Portuguese. From 1926 to 1930, the population was 40 percent Black and 24 percent Italian and, for the first time, had a large percentage of whites who were not Italian,

Spanish, or Portuguese: 26 percent, an indication of the growing number of Brazilian-born children of immigrants in the neighborhood.

Population percentages generated from Medical Police reports overcount nonwhites since state authorities targeted people of color and immigrants in both law enforcement and public health actions. The numbers do suggest that in the broad categories of Black, white, and immigrant, Bom Retiro sits in the middle of the twenty-three central districts that appear in that document set, a position affirmed in oral histories.[41] The 2010 census shows that Bom Retiro has not changed that much demographically, with nearly half of Bom Retiro's residents identifying as nonwhite, a category encompassing self-declared Black and Brown Brazilians (in the 16–35 percent range) and immigrants from Asia and the Andes.[42] In 2020, Bom Retiro ranked fifty-eighth of ninety-six neighborhoods in São Paulo in terms of average monthly salary (R$2,693, about US$500) for those with formal employment (the statistics do not reflect the high numbers of residents with informal employment in the district).[43] The class and race statistics for Bom Retiro mirror those in Brazil overall, emphasizing that the foreign or immigrant denomination is not demographically accurate. Bom Retiro's Afro-Brazilian population is rarely discussed in academic work, which is often focused on immigration and a related assumption that the district does not have a significant Afro-Brazilian population.[44]

The invisibilization of Afro-Brazilian people in geographic spaces denominated as foreign should not come as a surprise. The abolition of slavery in 1888 led many formerly enslaved peoples to seek industrial jobs in São Paulo, where they often settled in the precarious housing of central districts, including Bom Retiro. Over time many were forcibly relocated to outlying parts of the expanding city, often following state-sponsored housing demolitions and the building of roadways.[45] By the twentieth century, nonwhite Brazilians also began internally migrating to São Paulo. Some settled in Bom Retiro, mainly those from the poverty- and drought-stricken northeastern region, where in the seventeenth century Brazil's first enslaved Africans had labored on sugar plantations.[46] Historian Kim Butler has shown that claims that São Paulo state was uniquely white were discursive, not factual, a position echoed by historian Barbara Weinstein.[47] Fábio Dantas Rocha separated Brazilians by race and non-Brazilians by national origin and found that São Paulo often had higher numbers of Afro-Brazilian residents than of any single immigrant group. Butler found that the numbers of Afro-Brazilian live births in the state were comparatively high in both 1925 and 1929, and of the thirteen districts in the central city, Bom Retiro had 5.6 percent of the total in 1925 and 4.9 percent of the total in 1929—the fifth highest in both cases.[48]

Immigrants themselves were often eager to whiten the neighborhoods where they lived. One way they did this was through school choices. The first Italian school in São Paulo, Bom Retiro's Scuola Sempre Avanti Savoia! (the name, used by many Italian schools, references a war cry in favor of a royal Italian family), was founded in 1887 by immigrants who did not want to send their daughters to the municipal school, opened just a few years earlier.[49] Maintaining their language and culture intersected with prejudice, since avoiding public schools meant minimizing interactions with Black and Brown Brazilians. While Jacob Penteado remembered many students and educators of color at the Marechal Deodoro Public School in the early twentieth century, this changed over the decades.[50] Samuel Harman Lowrie's 1938 analysis showed that Bom Retiro's school had among the lowest percentages of Black and Brown children in São Paulo.[51] A more recent study by Marcia Luiza Pires de Araújo shows that in 1938, 7 percent of the children at the Marechal Deodoro Public School, opened in 1907 as the Bom Retiro Joint Schools (Escolas Reunidas do Bom Retiro) and located at the Rua dos Italianos, 78 and 80 (moving two years later to number 405), across the street from the Central Disinfectory, were registered as "pardo" (Brown) or "preto" (Black).[52]

Agronomist and economist Decio Zylbersztajn grew up in 1950s and 1960s Bom Retiro, and his novel, O filho de Osum (Osum's son; Osum, or Oxum, is a Yoruba deity widely celebrated in Brazil), is filled with Black Brazilians, Jewish immigrants, and Jewish Brazilians in constant, although not always pacific, relations.[53] Generally, however, Bom Retiro's ethnic geography of immigrants, Black Brazilians, Brown Brazilians, and white Brazilians goes undiscussed. For example, most of the doorkeepers, apartment building superintendents, and domestic workers in Bom Retiro are Nordestinos, a term that connects race and class and, like foreignness, extends for generations after the physical migration.[54] These jobs represent a very different ethnoracial geography from that of the largely Andean and Paraguayan immigrants and their descendants, who are linked to textile production, or Korean immigrants and their descendants, who are linked to store and factory ownership.[55] Yet another racialized space is the Zumbi dos Palmares University, founded in 2003 with the "primary mission of the inclusion of Black and/or low-income people in higher education, enabling the integration of Blacks and non-Blacks in an environment favorable to the discussion of social diversity, national and international contexts."[56]

Bom Retiro, despite its reputation as a foreign space, was an important part of twentieth-century Afro-Brazilian mobilization. The neighborhood was the home of the first Afro-Brazilian newspaper in São Paulo, *O Menelick*, founded in 1915 within a broader expansion of the Black press in the Americas.[57] Edited by the poet, accountant, and former foundry worker Deocleciano Nascimento, the paper was named after the ostensible first emperor of Ethiopia, Menelik I, son of King Solomon and Makeda, the Queen of Sheba.[58] The newspaper's office, at Rua da Graça, 207, was less than two blocks from the Sinagoga Kehilat Israel, erected in 1913 by Bessarabian Jews as São Paulo's first synagogue. In 1916 Nascimento moved the newspaper from his home to a building on the Rua do Areal, the tiny street that today houses the Bom Retiro Health Clinic and that, as I show in chapter 4, was often associated with Afro-Brazilians and illness. Articles in *O Menelick* show a vibrant Afro-Brazilian cultural presence in Bom Retiro, with dance clubs and beauty contests.[59] Even so, as Paulina Alberto has argued, *O Menelick* and other Afro-Brazilian newspapers in São Paulo often "evince a consciousness of being watched and judged."[60]

Relations between Black people and immigrants were part of daily life in both rural and urban Brazil. Newcomers separated themselves from the Afro-Brazilians who worked and lived alongside them to create whiteness. Many immigrants refused to marry Afro-Brazilians as one way of reinforcing the color line, and police records are filled with cases of immigrant-on-Black violence.[61] Racism worked to the advantage of many immigrants, whose Black neighbors were "banished from the wage labor systems and craft work because of competition from 'white Europeans' [and] observed with anxiety and resentment the almost magical transitions in the fates of former neighbors who had lived with them in the basements and in the tenements."[62]

José Benedito Correia Leite (1900–1989) founded the Afro-Brazilian newspaper *O Clarim da Alvorada* in 1924. In his memoir he speaks of cultural markers, such as "cheap clothes and walk(ing) with sandals or barefoot" that made Black people living in the "periphery [of] Barra Funda, Bixiga, Liberdade, Bom Retiro and Brás" aware of their difference from immigrants. As a child, Correia Leite lived and worked in the home of an Italian family in Bixiga, a central São Paulo neighborhood that, like Bom Retiro, was associated with immigrants despite its Black Brazilian presence. Leite remembers that his connection to immigrant culture sometimes meant that he was "de-Blackened" with the phrase "he is not very Black."[63]

Bom Retiro's racialized geographies had a direct relation to bad health, including both health outcome and ethnic violence. Jorge Americano, who would become rector of the University of São Paulo, was in a youth gang whose "wars" used both physical violence, from clubs to stone throwing, and discursive violence through mocking chants. He recounted his memories of space and immigrant/nonimmigrant relations in Bom Retiro in "Challenges and Wars between Boys":

> Jaime (I don't know who he heard from) brought the news that the boys from Bom Retiro had declared war on us and were going to attack us. Jaime was 8 years old, and I was 13.
>
> We, who lived in Campos Elísios, were "good people," and those from Bom Retiro were not.
>
> I didn't really believe it, but "the careful die of old age." Jaime believed it. My friends didn't really believe it, but Jaime did.
>
> We entered the arms race.
>
> I don't know about the Bom Retiro side, but on ours, we manufactured weapons. They were sticks with wax tips, to hit the head, stick, and pull out hair. And sticks with nails, to beat and pierce the head. There were sharp knives. Stones. Elastic slingshots.
>
> No one knew how the rumors started or ended. But the war did not come.[64]

In the mid-1940s, the sociologist Florestan Fernandes studied the discourses of inclusion and exclusion among Bom Retiro's children's gangs, focusing on mockery. His spatial focus led him to conclude that for children, unlike their parents, nationality (i.e., immigrants, Brazilians of immigrant descent, Brazilians of nonimmigrant descent) was less important than geography (i.e., what street you lived on). Like today, streets were not formally segregated although they did have concentrations of specific ethnic and racial groups, making gangs ethnic and multiethnic at the same time. As a result, the mocking chants often used ethnic language that might not match perfectly with membership. For example, gangs that included Jews might mock other groups for their Jewishness.[65]

Building Heights and Their Discontents

In São Paulo, residential verticalization, both higher-altitude neighborhoods and tall buildings, is statistically linked to better health outcomes.[66] Towering structures, however, do not dominate Bom Retiro and other working-class neighborhoods in São Paulo, for multiple reasons.[67] In Bom Retiro the nineteenth-century buildings that housed the Central Disinfectory and the School of Dentistry continue to be among the biggest in the neighborhood. Both have huge footprints, and their height was intended to reinforce the state's role in enforcing health. Furthermore, the neighborhood is filled with warehouses that, like the health structures, sit on large plots that had been factories. The well-cared-for Corinthians Fan Club Headquarters is one of those structures, but so are many plots that are abandoned or in some cases (as I learned during a series of visits with health surveillance workers) owned by well-off individuals who have been diagnosed with obsessive-compulsive spectrum hoarding disorder. Finally, a series of zoning restrictions in the 1970s sought to convert the area to institutional use, with a low population density.[68] As a result, most Bom Retiro streets are dominated by low buildings (of three stories or less).

Jung Yun Chi has divided Bom Retiro into three geographic sectors that show the microsegregation—based on class, labor, building usage, and ethnicity/race—typical of immigrant-populated working-class neighborhoods in the Americas.[69] Sector 1 has at its center Rua José Paulino (the former Rua dos Imigrantes), lined with two- and three-story buildings that house both retail textile outlets and oficina-residências where workers labor and reside. It has about 1,700 commercial establishments and produces more than 50 percent of all the women's clothes in Brazil. Residents of Sector 1 in the past were Brazilians of African descent or immigrants from southern Europe and today tend to be Bolivians, Paraguayans, or nonwhite Brazilians. This part of Bom Retiro through the 1930s was filled with small alleyways that ended in brick walls, sometimes under the train lines, intended by politicians to make leaving the neighborhood a challenge.[70]

Bom Retiro's few upper-middle-class apartment buildings of more than three stories are in the small Sector 2 (figure 2.4). This is the part of the neighborhood farthest away from and above the floodplains. Paving came first to this part of the neighborhood, limiting noise (from hooves and metal-wheeled vehicles) and improving traffic flow by replacing the often mud-filled gravel-and-stone byways. It is where the Marquês de Três Rios liked to stroll in the early twentieth century and was the target of developers, who denominated it "upper Bom Retiro" after World War II.[71] Residential buildings in Sector 2 were built to code and were among the first to have guest bathrooms, as residential spaces became important for entertaining among the middle classes. When I went on home visits to these buildings with the Bom Retiro Public Health Clinic team, many exterior doorways had either a mezuzah (a small case containing verses from the Jewish Bible)

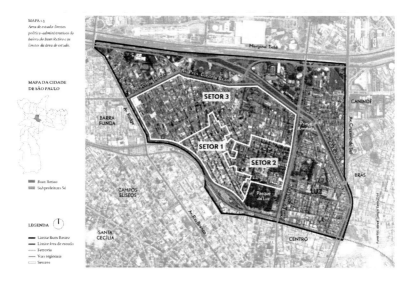

Figure 2.4 The three geographic ethnic/labor/class sectors of Bom Retiro. Source: Jung Yun Chi, "O Bom Retiro dos coreanos: Descrição de um enclave étnico," MA thesis, Universidade de São Paulo, 2016, 39. Used by permission of Jung Yun Chi.

or a discoloration where one had been removed, often by new owners who were Korean immigrants and/or their descendants. A discussion of the ethnic changes and mixing within single buildings appears in a 1990 series of essays about Bom Retiro, which Cremilda Medina called a "Jewish City" of the past. Journalist Marcos Seil Kim used the metaphor of three rivers (as in the "cool" Rua Três Rios) to suggest that the neighborhood is typically Brazilian (coisas do Brasil) because its immigrant and immigrant-descent residents, like the rivers, are "together, yet separate."[72]

Sector 3 is the largest and poorest sector of Bom Retiro and includes the precarious Moinho Favela along the rail lines, named after a mill with its own train platform.[73] Among the buildings are the former Central Disinfectory (today the Emílio Ribas Public Health Museum and a Ministry of Health warehouse), the Marechal Deodoro Public School (still in operation) and private schools, many religious institutions, and the Bom Retiro Public Health Clinic. In the nineteenth and early twentieth centuries, most of the residences were wooden cortiços, but by the 1930s these gave way to two- and three-story brick or concrete structures, many of which remained cortiços. Later in the century, a few multistory apartment buildings for the middle class were erected, but today they often contain oficina-residências.

The Lesser Research Collective analyzed the height of residential buildings in Sectors 2 and 3, where most residents of Bom Retiro live. We sought to determine if there might be a correlation between building heights and the poor state services and much worse health outcomes in Sector 3. Not surprisingly, Sector 2 had many more tall buildings with multiroom single-family apartments than Sector 3 (map 2.1). Buildings in Sector 2 tended to have internal systems where trash bags were collected by the service staff and placed in large dumpsters. Buildings in Sector 3, on the other hand, were filled with oficina-residências, and residents/workers placed waste on the street in inexpensive bags. Since pickups were irregular, these bags were often ripped open by both humans (for food and resale materials) and nonhumans (for food and breeding space). These same bags, and street litter in general, became reservoirs for standing water after rainfall, leading to mosquito breeding and the long-term differential health impacts discussed in the following chapters. Indeed, street litter is a primary dengue breeding ground in São Paulo and most of urban Brazil.[74]

Litter is a material residue that leads to real sickness and creates stereotypes connecting class, race, and ethnicity to sickness. While state trash collection in Bom Retiro is spotty, informal trash separation and collection has been the norm since the nineteenth century. Informal trash collectors often did/do their work at night, to avoid the judgmental gaze of the public, since, as Marta Pimenta Velloso notes, "the people who work or live off garbage—collectors, resellers, and even sanitary engineers—are stigmatized by society . . . (just as are) spaces for the treatment and final destinations—dumps, deposits, treated landfills, recycling plants and sewage treatment stations."[75] Bom Retiro's residents have complained about the problem of street litter for 150 years, often pressing their case in the press because of government inaction.

Historical associations of sickness, immigrants, and trash are sometimes repeated by contemporary health care professionals. In June 2018 Team Lesser participated in a São Paulo Ministry of Health project to identify socioenvironmental risks in Bom Retiro, with the goal of better focusing health actions. The initial charting was done with a huge map laid on a giant table in which colored stickers represented different challenges, including water based (for example, open sewers or severe flooding), atmospheric (for example, air pollution), social (wooden building construction inside or outside, street dwellers, cortiços), residual (for example, garbage on the street), and zoosanitary (for example, bugs and mosquitoes) (figure 2.5).

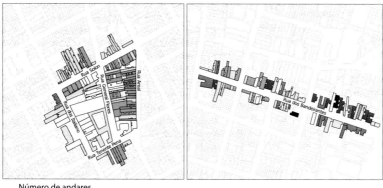

Altura dos prédios no quarteirão de estudo e na rua dos Bandeirantes definida a partir dos números de andares.

Número de andares
☐ Terreo
☐ 1 andar
▨ de 2 a 4 andares
▨ de 5 a 7 andares
■ de 8 a 11 andares
■ de 12 a 17 andares

Map 2.1 Comparison of building heights by stories in Bom Retiro around the Public Health Clinic (and encompassing the former Central Disinfectory) and the upper-middle-class part of the neighborhood closer to the Tiradentes Metro Station. The data was gathered by street-level observation and plotted using geographic information system techniques. Source: Prepared by Delphine LaCroix and Juliana Casagrande, Lesser Research Collective, 2017.

If the mapping had taken place in the late nineteenth- and early twentieth-century Bom Retiro, the socioenvironmental risks and their most common locations would have been similar because of continuities in flooding sites, lack of infrastructure, and class. For example, zoonotic vulnerabilities linked to flooding, which increases mosquito-borne diseases, are more present in Sector 3 than in Sector 2, just as they were in the past. Conversations among health care professionals about sickness and geography might also be similarly tinged with racial and class assumptions. I was told, multiple times, something like "of course this location has litter—mosquitoes—poor work conditions—sewage problems—etc. because there are Bolivian/Paraguayan oficina-residências there." In this case, the spatial and racial residues were more than just theoretical; they had a direct impact on all aspects of health.

This chapter places the demographic and material history of Bom Retiro within a broader context of immigration, health concerns, and urbanization

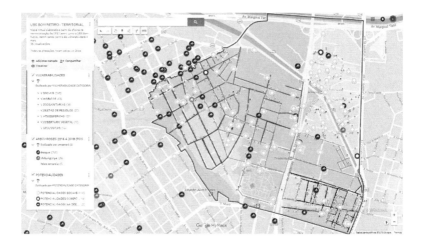

Figure 2.5 Locations of socioenvironmental risks in Bom Retiro, 2018. The hybrid map was constructed by health professionals at the Bom Retiro Public Health Clinic and Team Lesser. Source: Cidade de São Paulo sus/pavs/psp, "Relatório Diagnóstico Socioambiental," Unidade Básica de Saúde Bom Retiro—Supervisão Técnica de Saúde—Santa Cecilia (2018).

in the Americas. It challenges the concept of Bom Retiro as an immigrant or foreign neighborhood by demonstrating the long-term multiethnicity of the district. I also analyze how the negation of Blackness was part of a wider political and cultural strategy to whiten Brazil, a process imagined as leading to a healthier population. Legislation thus prohibited the entry of nonwhites and placed Brazil within a racialized global labor market. Despite the belief in immigrant racial transformation among many racist politicians, educators, and health officials, the geographies that emerged in dense urban working-class neighborhoods were judged as insalubrious. In other words, many people promoting whitening through immigration simultaneously believed that most newcomers were not fulfilling their racial health obligations. Immigrants were rarely judged as victims of the health geographies that emerged from the natural environment, notably the presence of rivers and related flooding, and from the built environment of factories and cortiços, which often turned climatic occurrences and industrial output into health crises. By the late nineteenth century, public health officials and their allies usually judged immigrants as the perpetrators of bad health and glossed Bom Retiro, like so many working-class neighborhoods in the Americas, as sick.

It was March 2016, and I did not know that Paris Fashion Week had just ended, or even that it existed. Even if I had, I would not have understood why Bom Retiro's main shopping street was filled with luxury cars whose drivers were opening the doors for elegantly dressed passengers. What I learned was that a small group of Bom Retiro clothing makers mainly sold to an upper- and upper-middle-class clientele, unlike most shop owners, whose wholesale and retail establishments focused on volume. These exclusive shops regularly sent designers to global fashion shows, where they took photos and made drawings of the newest designs and emailed them to Bom Retiro. Designers quickly produced mockups, and fittings took place on the following day. The clothing would eventually include a logo and a brand name.

Years later, a friend who owns an upscale clothing factory/store recounted how they see the process. Multiple times each year, the owners of chic establishments in Bom Retiro, often Korean or of Korean descent, travel to Europe to see the new seasonal designs. Going to boutiques and taking photographs is awkward and often leads to being asked, or forced, to leave the establishment. As a result, Bom Retiro's traveling fashion bosses now go to department stores—the Zara chain in Spain is a favorite—whose floor plans and clothing designs are social media friendly. In these stores taking photos of clothing is common. The images are then WhatsApped to each factory's clothing designers, who then put their mark on the new collections. In other words, while the originals are the same, each Bom Retiro factory/store creates a unique version that only they sell.

Seasonal hemispheric differences mean that summer fashions in Europe today are appropriate for Brazil in the future. The clientele knows the dates when the different seasonal collections will be launched in Bom Retiro, and they reserve their visits well in advance. My friend's customers tend to be well-off white women in their fifties and sixties, often from smaller cities in the interior of São Paulo and neighboring states. For these patrons, European-inspired fashions are important class markers, and they tend to patronize only one store, working with individual salespeople, whom they treat as employees in their personal boutiques. In Bom Retiro, buying Brazilian-created global clothing is not unlike eating Brazilian-created global food since both allow those with some money to feel cosmopolitan and international without ever leaving the country.

3

Bad Health in a Good Retreat

The late-night shooting on the Rua dos Italianos left five people injured. Paschoal Tura, a thirty-nine-year-old Italian immigrant and small business owner, had invited some neighbors to his residence for a drink in August 1914. The group comprised immigrants and Brazilians, unsurprising since about 35 percent of the city's residents were foreign born.[1] All had work the next day, ranging from shoemaker to factory worker, but that did not stop them from drinking late into Sunday night. Soon "they drank too much beer, becoming so excited that they began insulting and provoking each other."[2]

Jeronymo Barbelia, one of Tura's neighbors, was one of the revelers. Once intoxicated, he became abusive, and sometime after midnight the other partyers decided it was time for him to leave. Barbelia, however, did not go home after being thrown out of Tura's house. He waited for the others, and as they left, he pulled out a straight blade, challenging each one to a fight. After being ignored or perhaps laughed off, Barbelia grabbed a shotgun and fired twice, injuring each of the five as the small shot scattered. Barbelia then fled while the others were taken or went to the Medical Police clinic, although the documents do not explain how they got there.

The *Correio Paulistano* reported the shootout on the Rua dos Italianos in a moralist tone like the one it used in in describing Amelia Marini's death a year earlier. The headline, "Shotgun Fired—the Consequences of Alcohol," led into an article connecting working-class status and Bom Retiro's cortiços to immigration, liquor, and gun violence. The Medical Police documentation provides different perspectives than the newspaper reports. Each victim had their own one-page report, and all show that health professionals called law enforcement officers.[3] While the documents do not say what happened after the group was treated, they do teach us much about immigrant lives in São Paulo. The Barbelia and Tura families lived next to each other on the Rua dos Italianos, in numbers 175 to 205, a numbering pattern that indicates a series of cortiços that later in the century might be replaced with single buildings with multiple entrances. All the victims were judged by the attending physicians to be white. The youngest victim, Paschoal's sixteen-year-old son, Leonardo, was not badly injured. He worked as a shoemaker in 1914, but like many children of immigrants, he moved up the social ladder, becoming the player-owner of the Turano FC soccer club in 1923.[4]

In the long history of the Americas, the press, police, politicians, and public health workers have connected immigrants to violence, criminality, poor sanitary and labor conditions, and sickness. In the process, broad cultural ideas have emerged, linking bad health to geographic locations, often specific neighborhoods.[5] In the late nineteenth and early twentieth centuries, politicians targeted southern and eastern European immigrants and nonwhites, and the places they lived, as "the city of São Paulo began to divide between 'the side over there,' the territory of working immigrants . . . and 'the side over here,' seen as the richest part and closest to sophisticated shops and services . . . and currently recognized as the expanded center of the city of São Paulo."[6] This distinction continues to be the case, and health outcomes "over there" are consistently worse than those "over here."[7]

Sick Immigrants in Unhealthy Housing

There is a great irony in the history of real and imagined immigrant health in Brazil. Sojourners and their home-country governments were as concerned about the bad health of Brazilians as Brazilian policymakers were about the bad health of newcomers. Indeed, emigration to Brazil was halted at various moments by European governments because of health issues. In 1886 the Italian Ministry of the Interior issued a memorandum opposing emigration to Brazil, and especially to the province of São Paulo, deemed the "most unhealthy and inhospitable in the empire."[8] Three years later, as Brazil became a republic, the Italian government went further, prohibiting emigration to Brazil for almost two years because of yellow fever outbreaks in ports like

Santos and Rio de Janeiro. Some Italian politicians alleged that remigration to Italy resulted from "the ferocity of epidemic outbreaks among immigrants in São Paulo."[9] The 1902 Prinetti Decree prohibited emigrants from accepting passages subsidized by the state of São Paulo, and two decades later, even the São Paulo Italian-language newspaper *Fanfulla* came out against Italian entry because of local poor health and labor conditions.[10]

Despite the anxieties on both sides of the Atlantic, people and disease did travel oceanically. Health policies often connected to immigration, for example, when authorities in Brazil traced an 1893 cholera epidemic that left fifty-three dead to ships that had stopped in Genoa and Marseilles, two cities amid their own outbreaks. Ports were closed around Brazil, leading to a drop in immigrant entry and anger from rural landowners and urban factory owners. As a result, health officials developed a plan to build a quarantine center between the port of Santos and the city of São Paulo. The location was São Bernardo do Campo, at the time a town of about 2,500 residents surrounded by fazendas worked largely by Italian immigrants. Since preventing ships from leaving Europe was impossible, and landowners demanded labor, public health officials proposed to quarantine immigrants with scarlet fever, cholera, yellow fever, or smallpox, all diseases that had the potential to spread rapidly.[11] The buildings that would house newcomers were to be constructed out of fragile materials and then burned down to prevent disease spread. The test structure, however, collapsed on itself, scuttling the plan.

Bom Retiro was often the focus of health and immigration policymakers on both sides of the Atlantic. The neighborhood's population and its packed and poorly constructed housing became an arena of dispute, just as happened in other large cities in the Americas.[12] Foreign governments worried that poor living conditions in Brazil would spread diseases to their citizens, who might then return home with their illnesses. Brazilian public health specialists agreed, although they worried that sick immigrants would spread disease to natives.

Concerns centered on working-class residential spaces as the number of cortiços exploded in the 1880s as central districts like Bom Retiro experienced population growth.[13] New municipal codes sought to control this kind of housing, and the informal commerce linked to it, but in 1920 more than 80 percent of São Paulo's residents were renting "houses that shelter or serve as a dormitory, even if temporarily, for several families or for many people from different families."[14] Even after World War II, half of Bom Retiro's population lived in cortiços, and in 1976 the many precarious residences led the city to tag it as "as one of the decaying areas of the central city."[15]

In 2000 almost 600,000 residents of the city of São Paulo lived in corticos, 6 percent of the total population, although the percentages skyrocketed to almost five times that amount in central neighborhoods like Bom Retiro.[16]

By the end of the nineteenth century, every street in Bom Retiro was lined with corticos. Close quarters combined with poor public services to create both discursive and real geographies of bad health in Bom Retiro. Corticos had high rental costs given the wages of the working classes, and families shared bathrooms, kitchens, and other service areas in internal spaces or in open courtyards. In most corticos, multigenerational families ate and slept in single rooms, with shared water usage and outdoor or corridor toilet and bathing facilities. Newlyweds often lived with, and worked in the same factories as, their parents. Many corticos had a central open area where residents met socially and where domestic work like washing clothes and preparing food took place. These common areas also were centers of commercial activity such as small-scale vegetable and nonhuman animal raising.[17] While cortico construction has changed, they continue to operate as they did in the past, with shared facilities and mixed residential and work spaces. Beginning in the interwar period, Bom Retiro had one of the highest numbers of buildings per square hectare in São Paulo and today has one of the highest percentages of residents living in corticos in center-city districts.[18]

Corticos filled with foreign workers attracted the attention of health officials. In 1892 the municipality established the Sub Secretary of Hygiene and Public Health to regulate "food, public safety, hospitals, retreats, slaughterhouses, markets or fairs, cleaning and cleanliness, laundries, fountains, water supply and sewage, gardens, immigration and accommodation, [and] cemeteries."[19] The 1894 Sanitary Code was the first of many that put public health functions in the hands of law enforcement.[20] As historian André Mota has shown, institutions and the policies they created othered immigrants and nonwhites socially and geographically. Corticos became "cramped, unsanitary, repulsive constructions" filled with diseased, often foreign, residents.[21] The language here is important. While conditions in corticos were poor, the Health Code suggested that the residents were the cause of bad health.

Officials criminalized health violations and treated them as moral transgressions. In the nineteenth century, the state increasingly used public health as an excuse to enter intimate and commercial spaces and enforce new forms of social control. "Health" helped to motivate changes to the built environment with the destruction of corticos.[22] Public health officials were so eager to rid the city of cortiços that in 1911 the São Paulo state Health Service eliminated the word from official parlance, replacing it first with *collective habitation* and later using words like *buildings with apartments* or *hotels*.[23]

Many cortiços were constructed in the large inner spaces of closed or abandoned factories. Others were within what had been single-family homes. These often became rental properties as the middle and upper classes separated themselves geographically from the working classes by moving to new neighborhoods. Cortiços and their residents became the targets of many city leaders, although Eva Alterman Blay has argued that this was a "fake problem."[24] The falsity may explain why decrees formalizing minimal building heights and the internal sizes of window and doors, and specifying that there should be at least one bathroom for every twenty residents, often went unenforced.[25] Cortiços were a "highly lucrative business," and property owners continued renting homes they moved out of or building new inexpensive housing, all with elevated rents.[26] Immigrants were charged a premium for the cramped and unventilated quarters close to their workplaces, and the generally absentee property owners included some of São Paulo's wealthiest residents and even some banks. The municipality also profited by taxing cortiços based on the number of internal residences rather than as a single property, with the cost always passed on to the renters.[27]

In the twentieth century, São Paulo's city geography included cortiço-filled neighborhoods that had been abandoned by the nonworking class and new neighborhoods considered wealthier, healthier, and whiter.[28] In 1893 Higienópolis, or Hygiene City, was built, which French diplomat Paul Walle described as the "meeting point for the richest and most distinguished in São Paulo where you can admire a large number of sumptuous houses, what the elite call mansions, and luxurious and comfortable villas."[29] Health outcomes in neighborhoods like Higienópolis were far better than those in Bom Retiro with its high population density, factories, and precarious housing.[30]

Public health leaders frequently accused the working classes, rather than industrialization, poor services, or inequitable access to care, for bad health.[31] Since cortiços and other nonelite housing did not fit the image of a proper home, policies and actions naturalized Bom Retiro and the people living there as dangerous, dirty, and diseased.[32] The shifting of blame can be seen during a smallpox outbreak at the Bom Retiro immigrant hostel in June 1887. A report citing São Paulo's provincial inspector of hygiene claimed, "After a thorough examination and inquiries, he found that the news was false, with no case of that terrible disease in that establishment or in its surroundings, although there were some cases of measles." After the inspection, smallpox was confirmed, and the patient was immediately removed to the isolation hospital although nothing was done about conditions at the hostel.[33]

While officials and residents agreed that packed, unventilated cortiços were conducive to health problems and other social ills, there was little agreement on solutions. Residents of Bom Retiro vacillated in their relations with the state, sometimes fearing public health officials and at other times relying on them. In 1884 a group of Bom Retiro's residents complained to local newspapers that they were "without gas, without police," and were living with "a lack of individual safety." They claimed that following the establishment of the immigrant hostel, bad health had increased in the neighborhood. There was the rape of a young German immigrant by two "foreigners" whom no one could identify, daytime robberies whose scared victims "reasonably seek to avoid dangerous conflicts," and even the "mysterious suicide" of an elderly man.[34]

I cannot emphasize enough that for the historical and contemporary residents of Bom Retiro, health, crime, and violence were part of a single equation. In this sense, having public health institutions within the Justice Department had some support across class lines, even if it also led to excesses, especially in the criminalization of disease. The 1898 arrest of Spanish immigrant Juan Moqueira is an example of how health, violence, crime, and population density all came together in everyday life. Moqueira lived in a cortiço at Rua do Areal, 42, just a block from the Central Disinfectory and next to what today is the Bom Retiro Public Health Clinic. According to police inspector José Pisa, Moqueira was running a counterfeiting operation out of his residence, but victims of the scams were unwilling to denounce the immigrant, perhaps out of fear of the criminals but possibly because of their distrust toward law enforcement. This changed in September 1898, when police convinced Moqueira's neighbor to let an officer hide in an oven and observe the fraudulent transactions. The *Correio Paulistano* fed the public image of Bom Retiro's residences as filled with danger with its provocative front-page headline: "More Fake Notes—Police in the Oven—Caught Red-Handed."[35]

Across the globe many officials and residents believed that neighborhoods with dense populations were prone to biological diseases, immorality, crime, and violence.[36] In 1893, following a yellow fever outbreak, the São Paulo city government commissioned a report on cortiços in the Santa Ifigênia district, which until 1910 included the Bom Retiro neighborhood. Health officials expressed disbelief at how immigrants and others in the laboring classes lived and demanded, "We need to do something about . . . the housing . . . where the working class accumulates, the inns where the working class swarms . . . in these unhealthy constructions, some repulsive, . . . [living] in the promiscuity that the economy imposes on them but that sanitation officials reject."[37] The commission proposed that the municipality construct new kinds of cortiços for rent. Called *casinhas*—little houses—the name and the structure were meant to be hygienic and modern. While this public proposal never was realized, urban planner Nabil Georges Bonduki points out that private enterprise often constructed workers' homes using this model.[38]

The 1893 report, while shocking to legislators, had little impact. In 1905 city councilperson and union lawyer Afonso Celso Garcia berated his fellow deputies about the lack of state intervention in working-class neighborhoods: "Gentlemen . . . let us at least be aware that we, having seen the city completely unprotected against the invasion and propagation of diseases and epidemics, know how to fulfill our duty." He proposed that the commission be reinstituted but only with physicians and public health engineers.[39]

Descriptions of Bom Retiro as diseased continued throughout the century, as did floods, overcrowded housing, and poorly functioning transportation, water delivery, and sewer systems.[40] "Colloque sentimental," a poem in Mário de Andrade's 1922 collection *Pauliceia Desvairada* (the title might be translated as "Frantic São Paulo," or in more contemporary language "São Paulo Unhinged"), tells of a "Count" from São Paulo who has only "heard of Paris" when asked, "Have you heard of Brás, of Bom Retiro?" A walk through the working-class neighborhood emphasizes the reactions of the wealthy to real conditions:

> Let me put my handkerchief over my nose
> I have all the Parisian perfumes,
> But look, under the doors, spilling out . . .
> Into the sewers! Into the sewers
> . . . spilling out
> A thread of tears without a name[41]

Disgust toward cortiços was also found among immigrants.[42] A 1906 report in the Italo-Brazilian newspaper *Fanfulla* complained about "the insufficiency of air and light . . . the many people in very small, poorly ventilated, damp, and low environments . . . in agglomerations of ten or twelve people in one or two rooms. . . . In poor neighborhoods . . . the tenements have become human anthills, where people live in promiscuity and sex."[43]

Speakers at a 1913 labor protest at the corner of the Rua dos Italianos and Rua Tenente Pena, directly in front of the Central Disinfectory, complained that the "major São Paulo newspapers involved themselves in everything except the cause of the exploited." As a result, workers "live their lives dying from factory work, on farms, and in workshops, where their paltry salary is barely enough for their meager daily bread."[44] Alfredo Cusano, an Italian journalist, spent five years in Brazil at the beginning of the twentieth century. He described São Paulo's cortiços as "huge warehouses, where residents live in a promiscuity that nurtures and feeds the most unpleasant vices and facilitates contagious diseases."[45]

It would be a mistake to imagine cortiços as only residential. The living spaces were (and are) often workplaces, and thus labor-related accidents frequently happened at home. The investigators who prepared the 1893 municipal study on cortiços expressed surprise at how what they thought of as two different built environments intersected: "Cubicles made of plywood and painted with tar, all raised from the floor by 0.70 m. The area is not tiled, it has a tap, and the kitchen does not have access to the outside [the shared kitchens in cortiços usually opened onto an open-air space for both ventilation and easy disposal of food waste]. The bathrooms are really for the workshop, not for the residents."[46] City councilperson Celso Garcia sat on the Commission on Hygiene and Public Health and the Commission on Justice and Police.[47] From these dual perches, he generated multiple policy proposals that linked housing to improving moral and biomedical health outcomes. In 1905 he worried to his politician colleagues:

> I have noticed that in certain neighborhoods of our capital, mainly in Bom Retiro and Braz, there are already innumerable collective dwellings. In these neighborhoods, families are made up of many people living in a single house, even in a single room, sometimes along a damp and infected corridor. In these rooms the air must be unhealthy. In each room there is an accumulation of people, furniture, objects, kitchen utensils, an unwashable floor; in these dens live the old person, the young person, and the child; there women give birth, then close their dead eyes; in more than one case, when families live in one room, the immodest sleeps beside the maiden, the drunkard beside the old man and the child.[48]

Celso Garcia was unusual in desiring to improve the quality of life in cortiços. Other politicians sought to demolish worker housing, and throughout the twentieth century, families were expelled from their residences in Bom Retiro.[49] Most legislators, however, seemed content to leave cortiços in place. The high rents were income generators for their often-wealthy benefactors or themselves. In spite of the tax revenue they generated, working-class districts were slow to receive municipal improvements like sewers and affordable transportation.[50] Jorge Americano remembers electric trams as for "high-class people and politicians," who sent their domestic workers to tram stops, demanding they run to advise the "patrão" (employer) that the vehicle was coming.[51] Jacob Penteado called the wealthy people who rode trams "caraduras" (cheapskates), since many who could afford the fares instead jumped on wagons transporting materials.

Tram prices began to drop in 1909 when a "worker's fare" was established at half the price of a regular ticket. Even so, the anarchist newspaper *A Lanterna* complained of the "insatiable interests" of the São Paulo Tramway, Light and Power Company (known colloquially as the "Light"), the "powerful Canadian company" that ran electric services in São Paulo. The Bom Retiro tram line, opened in 1911, was "not an improvement but a Trojan horse" because its stop was far from where the working class lived.[52] Those distant stops meant that horses, and thus stables and mosquitoes, remained a part of the working-class landscape longer than in more upscale locations. Indeed, it was only in the mid-1920s that São Paulo Tramway traffic maps showed intense daily movement to and from Bom Retiro.[53]

Cortiços were also linked to education. Almost half of the forty "Italian" schools that opened between 1887 and 1905 were in Bom Retiro, which Jacob Penteado called "a typically Italian stronghold, thanks to immigrants, who, fleeing difficulty and poorly paid rural work [on Brazilian plantations], came to try their luck in the capital."[54] While some of these schools received subsidies from the Italian government, all were obligated to follow the São Paulo state-legislated curricular model, including a focus on hygiene, as was the case in most of the Americas.[55] The Sempre Avanti Savoia! school opened in 1887, and fundraising events included performances of Italian opera at the German-immigrant operated "Turnerschaft" (gymnasium).[56] The Corsican anarchist and labor activist Angelo Bandoni (1868–1947) settled in Bom Retiro after arriving in Brazil in May 1900 aboard the *Città di Genova*.[57] In 1902 he founded Escola Libertária Germinal (The Libertarian School) at Rua Solon, 138, near the Central Disinfectory, although the school would only last for three years before running out of funds.

While schools were teaching hygiene to youth as a moral/scientific topic, other forms of health management emerged as well. The *Correio Paulistano* opened a Bom Retiro office in 1911 and offered new subscribers free medical care and reduced-price medicine as a carrot:

> In an attempt to capture the sympathy of the residents of Bom Retiro, we will open a free medical post in the newspaper building.
>
> There, every weekday, from 11 a.m. to noon, the distinguished clinician Dr. Simões Corrêa will assist all people who seek him.
>
> Our physician's prescriptions will be filled with a 20 percent discount at the "Romana" and "Italo-Brasileira" pharmacies, located on the Rua dos Imigrantes.
>
> The "Correio Paulistano," to help the admittedly poor classes, will also provide them with medicines free of charge.
>
> To obtain all of this for free, people in need of medical assistance must bring a copy of the Correio Paulistano to the doctor's office.
>
> Just yesterday Dr. Simões Corrêa treated a patient who came to clinic in the newspaper building with a copy of the "Correio Paulistano."
>
> We also have established an alms box for the poor of Bom Retiro. The "Correio Paulistano" branch in this neighborhood will receive any and all donations intended for the poor of Bom Retiro.[58]

Health dominated discourses about Bom Retiro and other central neighborhoods in part because they contained housing types that had worse conditions than cortiços. For poorer-than-average immigrants, pensões (singular: pensão) had only single rooms, often lining a dark hallway behind a small street entryway, with an open sewer and a single communal toilet. Pensões were (and are) often managed by widows, who sometimes provided meals. While traditionally for single people and often segregated by gender, many of Bom Retiro's pensões crowded entire families into single rooms.[59] Hotel-cortiços (hotel tenements) were (and are) another housing type found in Bom Retiro. Until the end of World War I, hotel-cortiços often functioned as inexpensive restaurants during the day and then transformed the refectory space into a dormitory where workers would rent a bed on a per night basis.[60] Even rooftops in Bom Retiro became residences, as rooms were built there using cheap materials.

One form of housing typical of central São Paulo, but much less so in Bom Retiro because of its flooding, was underground basement apartments (porões). These dark and musty residences received light only from tiny windows at ceiling level or ground level. Porões often housed Afro-Brazilians in the decades following abolition in 1888, but as rental prices rose in central districts, they were often forced to migrate to outlying areas of the city.[61] Liberdade, for example, is a neighborhood in walking distance from Bom Retiro. It is associated with Japanese immigrants, who occupied porões in the 1920s as Afro-Brazilians migrated to other parts of the city.[62] Today those same porões again house many Afro-Brazilians as well as recent arrivals from Africa and Southeast Asia.

Not all workers' housing in Bom Retiro was precarious. Some nineteenth- and early twentieth-century factory owners built "vilas operárias" (worker's housing) next to or near their factories to attract and retain skilled workers.[63] These single-family row houses were grouped together to create mini-neighborhoods for those making above-average wages. Michele Anastasi, born in Sicily in 1887, migrated as a fourteen-year-old to the "Italian city!!" of São Paulo.[64] In 1906, at age twenty, he opened a "prizewinning distillery" of syrups and alcoholic drinks at Rua dos Italianos, 1 (today number 21), purchased a home next door, and then opened a dry goods store nearby (Rua Silva Pinto, 23), all of which he owned until his death in 1937.[65] Over the years he became so well known that even his health problems were reported in the Italian-language press.[66] Anastasi built a small neighborhood of brightly painted villas for his skilled employees. Today the Vila Michele Anastasi emerges out of a dark tunnel at Rua da Graça, 381.[67] It is home mostly to Bolivian immigrants and their Brazilian-born children, and the workshops/residences work semicollectively, for example, in the receipt of textiles and delivery of finished products.[68]

By the middle of the twentieth century, Bom Retiro experienced low-altitude verticalization as small apartment buildings of five stories or less began to replace many former wooden single-family homes and abandoned factories.[69] These changes to the built environment eliminated neither cortiços nor their residents. Some contemporary cortiços in Bom Retiro are built on precarious wooden platforms inside parking garages where luxury cars sit as owners go shopping for clothes. There are "upscale" cortiços that resemble tiny studio apartments and include internet access. During my fieldwork I noticed that residents of Bom Retiro usually described themselves as living in pensões rather than using the word cortiço. Health care workers, however, frequently used the term cortiço, with some applying it only to immigrant residences. Despite the 1911 law eliminating the word cortiço from official parlance, today the municipality uses the term to describe all multifamily residences in working-class parts of the city.[70]

Many people in São Paulo believed bad health emerged from Bom Retiro's environment. The neighborhood's seemingly ever-changing immigrant and immigrant-descended populations also seemed sick and dangerous. In the late nineteenth century, health officials focused on Portuguese immigrants for alcohol use and their relations with Afro-Brazilians. Italian immigrants were negatively stereotyped as being overtly sexual, having inappropriate reproductive practices, and spreading trachoma. In the first half of the twentieth century, the lens shifted to eastern European Jews, who were linked to prostitution, uncleanliness, trachoma, and unmodern social mores, ranging from clothing to food. In the late twentieth and early twenty-first centuries, stereotypes of Bom Retiro as unhealthy are often linked to Bolivians (for tuberculosis and uncleanliness), Brazilians (for drug addiction and uncleanliness), Chinese (for COVID-19, sexual health issues, and uncleanliness), ultra-Orthodox Jews (for vaccine refusal and uncleanliness), and Koreans (for supposed consumption of dogs and uncleanliness).[71]

Public health officials through the Americas linked immigrants to bad health and therefore built health surveillance institutions. Offshore sites evaluated immigrants, quarantined those with contagious diseases, and deported those who posed political problems.[72] In Rio de Janeiro, processing often happened on the Ilha das Flores (Flower Island) while in the United States it was usually on Ellis Island on the East Coast and Angel Island on the West Coast.[73] Another immigrant control approach used processing centers at coastal ports of entry, such as in Halifax, Canada, and Buenos Aires, Argentina.[74]

While the processes of immigrant control in the state of São Paulo were typical of the Americas, the operations and their location were not. The on-the-ground approaches highlighted the tensions between the desires for labor, for "white" immigrants, and for public health. For example, immigrants entering at the port of Santos were immediately sent to inland hospedarias (immigrant hostels) for health control and to sign labor contracts. One of the first was the tiny Hospedaria de Sant'Ana, erected in 1877 in a repurposed building on an agricultural colony outside of São Paulo city.[75] Growing numbers of entries soon made this edifice obsolete. In 1881 a special commission of the state Legislative Assembly named Nicolau de Souza Queiroz, a scion of a family of large landowners whose laborers increasingly came from abroad, as head of a new immigration service.[76] Queiroz believed that a "modern" hostel was necessary to rationalize the entry, health, and initial housing of newcomers before sending them to São Paulo's coffee plantations. Unsurprisingly, this building was placed in Bom Retiro, which, like New York City's Lower East Side in the late nineteenth century, had become the geographic stand-in for controlling the ills entering the nation with immigrants.[77]

In 1882 the Bom Retiro Hospedaria dos Imigrantes (Immigrant's Hostel and Reception Center) was opened near the junction of São Paulo's two primary rail systems, the Central do Brasil Railway and the São Paulo Railway. The hospedaria was only one and a half kilometers from the Luz Railway Station, which had been expanded in 1870 and again in 1895 as immigrant arrivals increased. The hostel's physical location, public health officials believed, would allow them to easily quarantine ill immigrants even as they signed contracts and prepared for work on plantations. New arrivals walked to the hostel, often with their luggage. For immigrants disembarking at the Northern Railway Station in the nearby Brás neighborhood, the hospedaria was waiting with horse-drawn carriages for baggage. A donkey-pulled tram was provided for women and children, who then still had to walk a kilometer to the hostel since tram lines did not cover much of Bom Retiro.[78] According to reports, men had to be convinced by health officials to separate themselves from their families and walk over four kilometers from the station to the hostel (see figure 3.1 for the hostel's location).[79]

Managing health for those arriving from abroad morphed quickly into making Bom Retiro's bad health the first among equals within São Paulo's neighborhoods. The new hospedaria was on a plot of land owned by Manfred Meyer and Elvira Isabel de Souza Queiroz Meyer, who were also awarded the contract to supply the food.[80] As the value of their land skyrocketed, the couple then sold the land to the state for what would become the Central Disinfectory, the center of health control, in the city of São Paulo.[81] From then on, the connection of immigration and health on a single plot of land over time helped to cement Bom Retiro as a place where bad health was related to foreignness. Residues of the plot's past uses are thus found in contemporary immigrant-related health institutions at that location, which continues to be the property of the São Paulo Secretary of Health.

It is ironic that while public health officials and others complained about the bad health emerging from densely populated cortiços, the state itself placed newcomers in overcrowded structures where diseases frequently spread. The Bom Retiro hospedaria officially held five hundred people at any given time, but it had only two hundred and thirty beds. Furthermore, when large ships arrived, often more than five hundred immigrants were

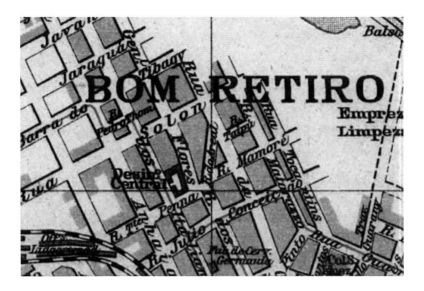

Figure 3.1 The main streets of Bom Retiro in 1913. The Desinfectório Central (Central Disinfectory) was constructed on the plot that previously housed the Hospedaria dos Imigrantes. Source: Alexandre Mariano Cococi and L. Fructuoso Costa, *Planta guia da cidade de São Paulo* (São Paulo: Companhia Lithographica Hartmann Reichenbach, 1913), https://www.loc.gov/item/2001620477/.

being processed, mostly Italians but with significant numbers also arriving from Portugal and Spain.[82] As a result, newcomers were frequently forced to sleep on the floor of the hospedaria's refectory, and when that space was filled, they were sent to a nearby ceramics factory.[83] While government officials emphasized that the main building had "good sanitary conditions, with no deaths," the reality was different. As the number of immigrants passing through the institution rose quickly, from a little under two thousand in 1882 to over six thousand in 1885, another building was built to house the dining hall, kitchen, pantry, and luggage.[84]

Almost immediately after the hospedaria opened, bad health there began to receive regular attention from the press. Outbreaks of croup, scarlet fever, and smallpox led to mutual recriminations between policymakers and health officials about the precarious physical conditions in the building.[85] There were reports that sex workers operated with impunity around the building.[86] Immigrants began to file grievances with Brazilian and Italian consular authorities.[87] Brazilian medical professionals working at the hospedaria were just as dissatisfied with the immigrants, and their reports often implied that foreign cultures were unhealthy.[88]

Disputes about the hospedaria were not just between immigrants and officials. The building and its inhabitants became a site of conflicts between an emerging political/economic class that favored immigration for social change and plantation owners, who sought to replace slaves with cheap labor. The former was represented by the Central Immigration Society (Sociedade Central de Imigração, SCI), founded in 1883.[89] Members of the SCI believed that abolition, which had taken place only in 1888, would create a labor crisis and that smallholdings would inevitably replace plantations. The supporters of the SCI believed that Brazil's bad health was related to its population of African and mixed descent and that expanding the white labor force would improve both public health and labor productivity. They were certain that Brazil's future lay with European immigrant colonies, which would in turn modernize Brazil.

The SCI positioned itself as the enemy of the landed oligarchy. Even so, both sides agreed that good health, which would emerge from public policy, was critical to ending European prohibitions on emigration and that immigrants would whiten Brazil racially. One of the most vocal SCI members was a central European immigrant who became a journalist and federal deputy from Rio Grande do Sul, Karl von Koseritz. He despised the large landowners, and his memoir described the SCI as "declaring war on the plantations" to create smallholdings.[90] By the end of 1883, SCI members included immigrant merchants from Portugal and England, a Swiss writer, a geologist from the United States, and a German teacher. Among the Brazilian supporters were the abolitionist André Rebouças and the modernizing technocrat Senator Alfredo d'Escragnolle Taunay. The SCI published its own newspaper, *A Immigração* , and its four hundred members critiqued some of the traditional ways that Brazilian society operated.[91]

One of the major disputes between members of the SCI and the landed elite was over the welfare of new arrivals at the Bom Retiro hostel. In March 1885 Ennes de Souza, one of the SCI's directors, inspected the hostel following complaints by immigrants that health conditions were so bad that they wanted to return to Europe. São Paulo's *Germania: Deutsche Zeitung für Brasilien* first published de Souza's highly critical report; it was reprinted in Rio de Janeiro's *Gazeta de Notícias* but not in the *Correio Paulistano*, which represented the landed elite.[92] De Souza complained that the location of the hospedaria, hailed by politicians for its proximity to the Luz Railway Station, was terrible because of flooding and its distance from the train stations and tram stops. Immigrants were packed in like "tinned sardines," and the building was "completely inappropriate for its purposes" and "does not even have the most basic hygienic conditions."[93] De Souza also saw bad health in the lack of private space for families, the thin walls separating unmarried women and men, and the lack of distance between beds. De Souza's concerns led the SCI to propose that a large new hospedaria be built in the port city of Santos so that immigrant health and labor processing would take place before the thirteen-hour train journey to São Paulo.

João de Sá e Albuquerque, the inspector general of immigration in São Paulo, responded to de Souza's attacks in the *Gazeta de Notícias*. Sá e Albuquerque claimed the report was "overly critical on some points and completely false on others."[94] He positioned the immigrant hostel as critical to good health, claiming that it was on the highest location in Bom Retiro and had excellent ventilation, making it uniquely hygienic. He also hailed the city of São Paulo's modern health system, rejecting de Souza's suggestion that a new hostel should be built at the port of Santos.

De Souza was quick to respond in the press. He claimed that while bad health might have been acceptable for slaves, it was not for free newcomers: "Poor immigrants! Their reception in São Paulo has been, until recently, more like the reception for blacks from the Coast of Africa than for Europeans, full of aspirations or tired of the old world, who seek a free America to exchange for their intelligent work, the advantages of liberty and property, and the guarantees of future prosperity for their families." How could Brazil attract such immigrants, raged the SCI director, with a hospedaria whose wooden refectory tables were impossible to clean and where "the flies are as black and grease filled as the floor."[95]

In 1884, as criticisms of the Bom Retiro hostel expanded, the São Paulo state government ordered another, larger hostel to be built in Brás, a district adjacent to Bom Retiro where the Northern Railway Station was located.[96] Construction began in 1885, and two years later, the new, much larger hospedaria opened. The Bom Retiro building and its adjacent land were put up for sale, but there were no takers due to its reputation for bad health, reinforced by constant outbreaks of diphtheria and smallpox at the hostel. Stuck with the building until 1889, public health officials doubled down, creating a quarantine site for sick newcomers and a location for immigrants wanting repatriation, leading to formal complaints by immigrants to the Italian consul.[97]

The Brás hospedaria operated until 1978; after World War II, it mainly housed and processed internal migrants from Brazil's northeastern states to São Paulo.[98] As was the case with the Bom Retiro hostel, the new one focused on health and labor, and the architectural style made the power of the state clear to newcomers. The hospedaria building today houses a museum and an archive, and the disinfection rooms and isolation quarters remain visible.[99] When the esteemed historian Warren Dean visited the Brás hospedaria in 1963, he compared the different ways that immigrants were received in New York and São Paulo:

> The Hospedaria de Imigrantes is Brazil's Ellis Island [yet] unlike the grim old institution in New York Bay, the Hostel has not been closed down for lack of clients. Now it receives an even larger swarm of people, peasants from the Brazilian Northeast who come to São Paulo to find work on the cotton or sugar plantations or to harvest coffee or oranges.
>
> A high fence of iron pickets, broken by a wide gateway, then a broad courtyard, and one faces the Hostel itself. A stupendous façade, three stories high and two hundred yards wide, plastered and painted with São Paulo's ubiquitous cream-colored whitewash, and relieved only by rows of great windows. The Hostel is a surprise among the shabby working-class tenements that share its streets.
>
> One passes through an arched vestibule whose walls bear maps showing where São Paulo's immigrants have come from—Italy, Portugal, Spain, Japan and lately from [the Brazilian states of] Minas, Bahia, and the Northeast. Passing through the archway one finds a large square of buildings; along their unplastered brick walls runs spindly wooden porticoes. In the midst of the square are two more buildings—a small hospital and a newer looking commissary. About the courtyard, leaning against the porticoes, sitting on the porches, or simply standing or squatting on the cobbles, are hundreds of ragged people, men, women, and children. The whole scene, the aged brickwork, the peeling paint, even the sunshine, a cold winter morning sun, is an instantaneous revelation of utter despair.[100]

Saving a Sick Neighborhood

Bom Retiro's hospedaria, while short-lived, helped to cement the neighborhood's connections with sickness and otherness. Fears among politicians and health care bureaucrats that bad health would spread to other parts of the city grew as street extensions and new transportation lines brought more mobility to the lower and working classes.[101] While the state often responded with increased vigilance and repression, some immigrants battled the negative images. A paradigmatic example was Ignácio Emílio Achiles Betholdi. Born in Milan in 1810, he fled with his parents to Brazil in 1831 following his participation in the same Carbonari secret society insurrection that led Giuseppe "The Hero of the Two Worlds" Garibaldi to immigrate to South America. Betholdi moved frequently in search of better opportunities, from the southern state of Santa Catarina to Rio de Janeiro to Campinas, a city in São Paulo state. He settled in São Paulo city in 1864 as a successful middle-aged physician known for producing and selling constipation pills. Betholdi was also a philanthropist and the first president of the Società Italiana di Beneficenza in San Paolo (Italian Charitable Society in São Paulo), which aimed to build a hospital. He is credited as one of the founders in 1868 of the "América" Masonic Temple and was named to the São Paulo Academy of Medicine.[102]

Betholdi's residence and clinic were located at Rua do Bom Retiro, 3 (on today's Avenida Couto de Magalhães), an elevated area on the south side of the Luz Railway Station, on the "good side of the tracks."[103] In the 1860s and 1870s, the Rua do Bom Retiro boasted mansions, and Betholdi's home/office sat well above the floodplains, in contrast to the working-class residences across the rail lines. By the 1880s the spatial relationship between the healthy Rua do Bom Retiro and the sick neighborhood of Bom Retiro began to change. Many in the dominant classes believed a pedestrian underpass allowed diseases to spread from Bom Retiro to other parts of the city.[104] Within a decade, some of the former mansions, many owned by well-off immigrants like Betholdi, were subdivided into cortiços, and other precarious housing sprang up in open lots close to the train station.[105] The São Paulo Sewer and Water Distribution Company built its headquarters on the Rua do Bom Retiro. While Alfred Moreira Pinto hailed the company's infrastructure as "one of the glories of Brazilian engineering," it was one of the most accident-prone employers in the city.[106] Today the area south of the Luz Railway Station (Avenida Couto de Magalhães, Avenida Casper Libero, Rua Maua [formerly the Rua da Estação, or Railway Station Street) has the same feel as it did at the end of the nineteenth century, filled with short-term residences and cortiços.[107]

Perhaps the proximity of poor immigrants to his home/clinic, and the fear that their poor health would affect his reputation, led Betholdi to offer medical treatment to "the poor" at no charge. But it was not only highly educated immigrants like Betholdi who reacted to the increasing attacks on immigrants as diseased. In the New and Old Worlds, newcomers also battled prejudice, often through physical activities.[108] Charles Dimmit

Dulley's love of sports made his Bom Retiro chácara a hub for cricket, golf, and rugby in the latter decades of the nineteenth century.[109] Many of the athletes were immigrant railroad laborers, and the São Paulo Athletic Club, inaugurated on the Chácara Dulley in 1888, continues to host English sports like rugby.[110] Legend has it that Brazil's first formal soccer match took place on the grounds of the Chácara Dulley in the mid-1890s, and over the next decades, soccer games often took place on the grounds (an area that today includes the heavily trafficked Rua Três Rios).[111] Injuries were typical in these games, and could be treated at the chácara's own medical clinic, which also included a maternity ward. These health services, however, were not enough to save the life of Charles Dimmit Dulley. He died in 1878 while trying to rescue a railroad engineer and a gardener who had fallen into a pit filled with formicide-contaminated water.[112]

Athletic activities were an important part of immigrant Bom Retiro. In 1910 a group of English railroad workers founded the Sport Club Corinthians Paulista, named after the London-based Corinthians Football Club, on what was then the Rua dos Imigrantes. Soccer quickly became popular, and within a decade the police were often called to remove children who were interrupting traffic with their games.[113] The club would become the greatest soccer team in the galaxy, and contemporary residents of Bom Retiro root for Corinthians at a higher-than-average rate in the city.[114] Today a small monument at the intersection of the contemporary Rua José Paulino and Rua Cônego Martins forces all passersby to negotiate the team's continued physical presence.

Sports, and the Corinthians soccer club, emerged as an important trope during my very first home health visit with Team Green, led at the time by someone I'll call Dr. Jacob, in 2016. We had just visited a dank oficina staffed by Bolivian immigrants, including multiple pregnant women. The supervisor, a Korean immigrant, had been reticent about giving the women time away from sewing to attend legally required prenatal visits with Dr. Jacob. This made the visit a negotiation for future health care as the physician made clear that if the women did not appear at the Bom Retiro Public Health Clinic for their appointments, law enforcement might visit the oficina. The pregnant women were given the time off, and the unusual threat of using law enforcement shows the seriousness of the incident. As Dr. Jacob and I walked back to the clinic, he used a soccer metaphor to help me to understand Brazil's public health system, which both providers and patients complain is not as agile as it should be: "Imagine a game between

Corinthians and [their rivals] Palmeiras at Pacaembú Stadium [at the time the Corinthians' home turf]. Now, imagine if the fans of both teams entered through the same stadium gate—people would get hurt [because they would fight]. So [at the stadium] you need a different entryway for fans of each soccer club. It is the same for health care—when all aspects of health must go through one entrance [the Brazilian Unified Health System], things don't work well."[115]

Bom Retiro continues to be the home of athletic activities and structures linked to immigration. The Mie Nishi Municipal Baseball Stadium was inaugurated in 1958 with the presence of Japan's royal family and Tokyo's Waseda University baseball team. The stadium was originally used for baseball and sumo (both practiced in Brazil primarily by those of Japanese descent), but more recently the focus is gateball, a croquet-like game that followed the US military to Japan and then Korea.[116] Today the sport is practiced by many of Bom Retiro's older Korean immigrants (others play intense badminton in the Jardim da Luz). The Mie Nishi Municipal Baseball Stadium also houses a recently built (in 2019) X-Sport Park and the municipality's Friends of Refugees Club, which provides athletic activities to the growing numbers of refugees in Bom Retiro and the city more broadly.[117]

This chapter has discussed two types of buildings that connected health and immigration. Immigrant residences were often poorly made, and immigrants had little access to public services like sewers or trash collection. Many politicians and health officials blamed the inhabitants for the real illnesses, and imagined moral sickness, that they observed or believed were spreading, in Bom Retiro and similar neighborhoods. One response by policymakers was to construct health buildings from which public health policy was enforced. In São Paulo the Central Disinfectory was located in Bom Retiro on the same plot of land as the city's first immigrant hostel. Linking foreignness, urban space, and illness, some in the dominant classes targeted immigrants and their descendants; as a result many policies were tinged with racist stereotypes. Such attitudes did not go unnoticed by immigrants, who often challenged policies in individual and collective ways ranging from sending petitions to diplomats to expressing hostility toward health agents. The vicious cycle of policies and responses meant that Bom Retiro, like so many working-class spaces with high numbers of immigrants in the Americas, became part of long-term discourses about danger, violence, and sickness.

In 2016, to great fanfare, the higher-end Lombroso Fashion Shopping Mall, built with a Miami Vice *tropical aesthetic of mauve and teal, opened in Bom Retiro.*[118] *The sixty glitzy clothing shops were constructed by demolishing an entire block of cortiços and small factories. The mall is named after the Jewish Italian criminologist Cesare Lombroso (1835–1909), who believed that lawbreaking was an inherited trait that could be identified through physical examinations. Lombroso, despite his own heritage, was racist and anti-Semitic, and his theories found wide purchase among the educated classes in Brazil.*[119] *His ideas were critical to firming up scientific racism in Brazil, influencing policies in policing, health, and immigration.*

One entrance to the Lombroso Fashion Shopping Mall is on Rua Professor Cesare Lombroso. The street was renamed in 1958; formerly named Rua Itaboca, it had been associated with procuring and sex work since the 1920s.[120] *The residues of immigrant sex work in Bom Retiro, however, remained. Contemporary fiction, walking tours that memorialize and give agency to trafficked women and girls, and press reports about vice raids often naturalize Bom Retiro as a place of sex work.*[121]

That Bom Retiro would be a place of impurity, danger, and bad health related to commercial sexual activity should not come as surprise given stereotypes about immigrants as disease spreaders. Alexandre Marcondes Machado (1892–1933) was a student at the polytechnic school on the Rua Três Rios in Bom Retiro; his alter ego, Juó Bananére, was a satirical poet who wrote in the Italianized Portuguese (what he called "macaroni talk") so common in the city. His 1915 poem "Sodades de Zan Paolo" (Yearnings for São Paulo) featured a sexy refrain focused on the "beautiful daughters of Bom Retiro," no doubt related to stereotypes of Italian women in the neighborhood. By the 1920s Bom Retiro had become associated with eastern European, usually Jewish, sex workers. The fight against geographic and ethnic stigmas would become one of the dominant themes among Jewish Brazilians for the next three decades.[122]

The relationship of immigration and sex work in Bom Retiro returns us to the location of the Lombroso Fashion Shopping Mall. In 1940 Adhemar de Barros, the São Paulo state governor (appointed by then dictator Getúlio Vargas), created a sex-work zone, over the objections of residents. The decision was, ironically, part of a "Moralization Campaign," in which Barros pressed the municipal vice squad to target Bom Retiro. According to the historian Guido

Fonseca, Barros boasted to Vargas that the police were actively repressing "drug abusers and dealers, fortune telling, the terrible macumba and spiritism [. . .] the centers of social corruption, the illegal exercise of professions and, in particular, pimping and prostitution."[123] To clean up the city, Barros thus created a sex-work zone "on two discreet public thoroughfares. Numerous benefits have accrued from these measures, not only for facilitating policing, but also for allowing the study of society, while defending public order and morality."[124] Barros was not being hyperbolic, and research on the prostitution in Bom Retiro was even done by undergraduate social service majors at the time.[125]

The two streets that Barros mentions, but does not name, were Rua Itaboca (today's Rua Professor Cesare Lombroso) and Rua dos Aimorés, named after an Indigenous nation devastated by Portuguese violence and smallpox in the eighteenth and nineteenth centuries.[126] From 1940 to 1953, these streets housed an authorized red-light district, eventually containing 161 small brothels, 650 sex workers, and large numbers of often-drunk males. Both streets ended at a wall over which the train lines passed, allowing police easy control of entry and exit. According to one account, Barros said about the neighborhood, "It [prostitution] is your product, so it stays with you [in Bom Retiro]."[127] The final closure of the zone, on December 31, 1953, included armed police and a "rebellion" by hundreds of prostitutes that spilled out into the neighborhood, leading to vandalism and injury.[128]

4

Enforcing Health

Antonio Baruf woke up feeling ill. As he had many times before, he went to the Santa Casa de Misericórdia hospital for treatment. This time was different, as his early October 1914 visit was transformed from a medical consultation to a security incident. An immigrant from Italy, Baruf lived in a cortiço close to the railroad track on the Rua dos Aimorés, the same small Bom Retiro street that decades later became the center of legal prostitution in São Paulo. Baruf, like so many in the working classes, went for free medical treatment at the Santa Casa, founded by the Jesuits in 1562 and São Paulo's main public hospital for the impoverished.[1] In the waiting room, Baruf met eighteen-year-old Zegio Costa, a resident of Mooca, like Bom Retiro a working-class neighborhood that emerged from the subdivision of estates and industrial growth. Mooca's residents included many Italian immigrants in the early twentieth century and Syrian refugees in the early twenty-first century.[2]

Baruf and Costa were awaiting treatment when the police arrived. A nurse reported that the pair had committed a crime and demanded they be forcibly removed from the hospital. The misdeed was serious indeed, reading A Lanterna, a self-described anarchist "Anticlerical Combat Newspaper." In the aftermath of the incident, the editors proudly reported on the duo's expulsion: "This does not surprise us at all. It is natural that A Lanterna causes terror among the Vatican's minions."[3]

That two ill immigrants were expelled from a hospital for political reasons typified the ways bad health and policing were part of everyday lives in Brazil's cities. Health and law enforcement intersected in the home, in the workplace, and on the street. The convergence can be seen in disputes between citizens and noncitizens, between tenants and owners, between workers and bosses, between neighbors and between coworkers. Policing was just one form of state-driven institutional violence in Bom Retiro. Factories, where bad health was often caused by machines and industrial pollution, saw frequent law enforcement interventions, as did residences, where police-affiliated public health professionals often appeared without invitation. Since Bom Retiro played a central role in multiple revolts, the state also created bad health via military actions. In the name of controlling space to control behavior, enforce order, and eradicate disease, the state entered people's intimate lives, often violently. The state targeted immigrants as disease vectors, labor agitators, and political provocateurs from the moment they disembarked.

The Pains of Revolt

Public health officials in São Paulo focused their policies and interventions on disease prevention and eradication. Residents of Bom Retiro, however, had a different view of what we might call the public's health. For them, violent interactions leading to injury, death, and trauma were as much a form of bad health as were illnesses. Violence at home and in the workplace created many bad health outcomes. So did the regular conflicts between the armed state and immigrants fighting for labor rights. While cortiços dominated the discourses about Bom Retiro, the biggest and most imposing buildings were health institutions and military barracks. The designation of Bom Retiro as a security zone was not just historical: in 1992 police took my camera and confiscated the film because I had taken pictures inside the Luz Railway Station.

Bom Retiro has a long history of violence. The 1896 "Italian Protocols" are one example of how the neighborhood became a focus of bad health that was not connected to disease or illness. In that year the Brazilian government indemnified Italian immigrants whose businesses were ransacked or destroyed by members of the Brazilian Armed Forces during two military-led uprisings, the Revolução Federalista (the Federalist Revolt of 1893–95) and the Revolta da Armada (the Brazilian Naval Revolt of 1893–94). Non-Italians complained that they, too, had suffered, and on the evening of August 22, 1896, groups of armed "Brazilians," many of them students, took to the streets of central São Paulo to protest the protocols. According to news reports, Italian immigrants and their descendants responded by shouting "Viva Italy" and "Death to Brazil." Businesspeople closed their shops, and authorities shut down all entertainment and trams. Some of the worst bloodshed occurred in Bom Retiro, where the shootouts ended with the Brazilian cavalry violently restoring order.[4]

The organized violence that consumed Bom Retiro and other central neighborhoods in 1896 was repeated three decades later during the three-week São Paulo Revolt of July 1924, sometimes called the Forgotten Revolution. The violence emerged as a reaction to a national economic crisis and many soldiers' perception that President Artur da Silva Bernardes was antimilitary. Inspired by junior military officers known as "Tenentes," who demanded the secret ballot, free access to justice, and compulsory public education, many in São Paulo joined the rebellion against the federal government.[5] "Massive" numbers of immigrants participated because the revolutionaries promised to end high costs for basic goods and because of what Boris Fausto termed "eloquent evidence of dissatisfaction in the new country and open opposition to the oligarchy."[6] Class conflicts between immigrants were noticeable during the uprising as working-class newcomers and their descendants looted the food warehouses owned by the immigrant bourgeoisie.

Bom Retiro was bombed from planes and occupied by federal troops. In response, the neighborhood was filled with trenches where residents defended themselves with "machine guns, pistols, and grenades, aimed at random."[7] On July 17 a grenade exploded in front of a house at Rua dos Aimorés, 60 (where Antonio Baruf had lived and just a block away from the contemporary Lombroso Fashion Shopping Mall I discussed in the postscript to chapter 3), where an Italian immigrant was playing with his two children, both of whom were killed.[8] Another Italian immigrant from Bom Retiro was "Major" José Molinaro, the neighborhood political boss of the Partido Republicano Paulista (São Paulo State Republican Party), the dominant political party in the state. Molinaro supposedly controlled nine thousand votes in the district, a number that represented most of the electorate since women were not enfranchised until 1932. The author and cultural critic Oswald de Andrade once asked, "Who is more popular, Major Molinaro, Republican Party boss and direct representative of a huge number of people, or the magnates who squandered a fortune to buy seats in Congress?"[9]

In 1928, after Molinaro was assassinated on the steps of the State Congress by a political opponent from Bom Retiro, Deputy Carlos Cyrillo Júnior remembered the major this way: "[He was] a very popular figure. . . . [He was] a true soldier of the Republic. During the July revolution he fought for legality, with a brave spirit full of conviction and beauty. He had had a price on his head in the Dantean hours of the rebellion, and he had fought bravely in the most dangerous locations."[10] Molinaro's funeral was huge, and the *Correio Paulistano* needed a full page to list those in attendance.[11]

Violent state actions in Bom Retiro, like everywhere else, always led to bad health outcomes. Thus, memories of the São Paulo Revolt often focus on suffering, not political ideals. Marcos Faerman's feature-length literary "new journalism" articles on Bom Retiro in São Paulo's *Jornal da Tarde* were published over two days in 1981. Like contemporary creative nonfiction, Faerman combined his own memories of the "Good Old Days" with interviews with elderly Bom Retiro residents. In one of his unconventional reports, Faerman linked 1924's violence to the children's gangs I discussed in chapter 3:

> —Those were good times, when the boys from Bom Retiro fought in the streets, caught canaries on the floodplains (where the Tiête's banks are today), fished in the river, then clean and beautiful.
> —The old residents of Bom Retiro like to tell these stories, from the first decades of the [twentieth] century, when so many Italian immigrants settled in the neighborhood.
> —Bom Retiro: from the beginning of the century until the thirties.
> —It was the time of the trocinhas—gangs, gangs of boys. The boys made war in the street—real war; they used stones, which became the tactic [that residents] used in the Revolution of 1924. . . . How many children's lives have not been ruined in your wars, Bom Retiro?[12]

Vitor Nicolau Montanaro, like so many early twentieth-century residents of Bom Retiro, was the child of Italian immigrants. An amateur soccer player who played for the Palestra Itália team (what would become the Sociedade Esportiva Palmeiras), he was fourteen years old in 1924. Fifty years after the revolution, he remembered the bad health caused by violence: "My family was terrified. I saw that a lot of bombs were dropped on Bom Retiro. Many people died. My family did not go hungry because we took food with us [when we fled]. But there were people who sacked the markets."[13]

Luiz Sérgio Thomás also grew up in Bom Retiro, a descendant of the Thomasi family that had left Italy in 1878. One brother went to Australia, another to Argentina, and Pietro Pacífico, Luiz Sérgio's father, settled in Brazil. Pietro first rented a room from a brickmaker on the Rua do Areal but accumulated enough wealth to buy a large lot of land on Rua Solon. He built a brick and tile factory, small houses for workers, and the first two-story building in the neighborhood.[14] Today multiple streets in Bom Retiro have the family name.

In 1981 Luiz Sérgio Thomás, then a bedridden ninety-six-year-old, told his daughter Alcina about the violence of the Revolt of 1924 and another revolt in 1932.[15] He focused on neighborhood solidarity to express the trauma of being bombed and occupied.

> No neighborhood was more political than Bom Retiro. When the Revolution of 1924 came, the soldiers wanted to use our house to place their weapons. I didn't let them. So we fled at dawn, to Santo Amaro. I was at a party when the news of the Revolution of 1932 arrived [another uprising in the state of São Paulo, this time against the federal regime of the often anti-immigrant president Getúlio Vargas]. I joined immediately. And all Bom Retiro enlisted when they found out that I was in the fight, that I was the head of the Second Detachment of the Civil Guard. . . . They came rushing in. . . . It was Bom Retiro in the war! Our house was the branch of the headquarters of the Revolution of '32—there in Bom Retiro. Yeah, nothing like '24, when we went, in that old Ford, that angry boom.[16]

Policing Immigrant Health

The armed state was only one of the purveyors of violence and its associated bad health in Brazil. The incident reports of the Posto Médico da Assistência Policial (Police Assistance Medical Clinic), home to São Paulo city's Police Medical Assistance Unit (known colloquially as the Medical Police), are filled with quotidian aggression on the street, in the home, and in the workplace. The Medical Police first emerged as a state health-enforcement organ in mid-eighteenth-century Germany, and an early Brazilian version appeared in 1854 within the Imperial Secretariat of the Police.[17] The São Paulo Capital Medical Police Service was inaugurated in 1885 with two physicians. In 1894 a new imperial decree created the Sub Secretary of Police and Hygiene within the Central Police Division, tasked with policing health in the streets, in homes, and in prisons.[18] Three physicians, who were allowed to have foreign medical degrees, were hired. Depending on the situation, each acted as a coroner pronouncing death, a medical examiner trying to determine cause of death, a forensic investigator working with police, and an emergency care physician.[19] While these professional categories are distinct today, physicians throughout the Americas (and elsewhere) continue to be compelled to report various types of medical incidents to the police, including abuse, sexual crimes, and injuries resulting from violence (like gunshot wounds).[20]

In the five decades following the 1894 decree, the connection between health and policing would expand as the working-class, Black, and immigrant populations grew.[21] In 1906 the coroner's office was established, and five years later the Medical Police was created within the Secretary of Justice and Public Security.[22] Fábio Dantas Rocha, playing on the comment that the "the *social* question [i.e., the labor movement] is a matter for the police"— attributed by immigrant labor activists to Brazilian president Washington Luís Pereira de Sousa (1926–30)—notes that "health administration in the capital [São Paulo city] . . . also became a matter for the police."[23]

In 1911 the Medical Police, whose activities I examine below, was formalized as a municipal emergency health service with direct links to the police.[24] The physicians, nurses, and ambulance drivers, while not having law enforcement training or ranks, became part of a broader security and moralist regime and were present in the formal and informal experiences of working-class residents. Between 1911 and 1940, when their services were transferred to the Secretary of Health, the Medical Police recorded tens of thousands of individual cases including the entire range of bad health. The reports detailed workplace accidents, street violence, pregnancy-related complications, injuries from human interactions with the nonhuman animals that roamed the streets or buzzed in homes, food that left people ill, attempted and successful suicides, and people found dead in homes or on the street.[25] Most ended with the Medical Police sending patients home, but there were other outcomes. Those with serious health issues were sent to hospitals or mental health facilities. Patients deemed criminals were handed over to the police or sent directly to jail. Women and girls were frequently remanded to male guardians like fathers and husbands. São Paulo's Medical Police thus fit into broader global patterns where "the ideas and practices of investigation, regulation and prosecution, and inspection, information gathering and intervention, were central to medical police practice."[26]

The connection of health, immigrants, and policing was highly racialized. The Medical Police files show how "whitening," a widespread belief among those in the middle and upper classes that eliminating Brazil's African heritage was critical to establishing the country's place as a "modern" world power, was operationalized under the guise of science. Many nineteenth-century politicians and health specialists, in Brazil and elsewhere, were enamored with now-discredited academic methods that claimed to cure social ills by controlling genetics and heredity.[27] Using scientific language to justify their racism, politicians implemented formal and informal restrictions on immigration and immigrants, including on those from Africa, those of African descent, Chinese, South Asians, Portuguese, and European non-Christians, each deemed at times by different parts of the population as outside of the "white" category. For example, in 1935 Brazil's House of Deputies decided to subsidize Japanese but not Portuguese immigration; one deputy summed up his vote by noting that Japanese colonists were "even whiter than the Portuguese [ones]."[28] Racist ideas and pseudoscience were acceptable parts of discourse and policies, buttressed by academic production from esteemed institutions—typical was the psychiatrist Paulo de Azevedo Antunes, whose oft-cited book *Eugenia e imigração* (Eugenics and immigration) emerged from his 1926 doctoral thesis at São Paulo's Faculdade de Medicina e Cirurgia (University of Medicine and Surgery).[29]

Public health specialists often embraced the combination of racism and fake science to target immigrants, nonwhites, and women. As policing become part of state health interventions, new health institutions like the Central Disinfectory began to dominate the built environment.[30]

> The primary way [for elites] to focus on the city of São Paulo as an "issue" was the hygienic-sanitary approach, combining the medical point of view with the observation/transformation of the engineer. . . . [T]ogether with [the] interventionist policy of a planner/reformer State, [it] sought in all forms to neutralize space, to give it a universal and manipulable quality, through the "rationality and objectivity" of science. . . . [This had] a key role in [the] struggle against "archaic [ideas of] order and progress," [working] together with the already latent desire of "being modern," . . . a synonym for progress in opposition to the countryside. Together with the urban issue, the social issue [was] built [on] the emergence of poverty and the identification of the other—the poor, the immigrant.[31]

Prejudices against immigrants and the working classes led many public health specialists, the press, and the police to believe that Bom Retiro's residents were particularly violence prone as the district was tagged as uniquely violent. Crime statistics played into these prejudices. When Olga Maria Panhoca da Silva, Rodrigo Prando, and Luiz Panhoca examined 1,350 evidence reports from the São Paulo Legal Medical Institute between 1910 and 1950, they found that immigrants were more likely to appear as victims of assaults than Brazilians.[32] Press reports on violence in Bom Retiro tended to the sensationalist, especially when related to immigrants. Articles on children injured by gunfire abounded, one as early as 1892, when three-year-old Virginia Sahú, a resident of a cortiço on the Rua do Areal, was shot while playing on the street.[33] These incidents, be they assaults or murders, generally ended with medical examinations at police stations and, at times, with bodies being transported to the Santa Casa hospital for confirmation of death before burial.[34]

Disputes between tenants and landlords were an arena of daily popular violence that led to both police and medical interventions. One landlord, Sixto Spina, first was reported to have trouble with the law in 1901 after he assaulted tenant Bernadino de Angelo.[35] In that case he avoided prosecution although the documents do not explain why (I surmise a payoff). Two years later Spina was back in trouble, this time for refusing to fix stuck windows in the cortiço he owned at Rua dos Imigrantes, 11A, despite resident complaints that they were getting ill from living in enclosed spaces. This time health authorities acted, forcing the landlord to pry open the windows to let air circulate. Even so, Spina's aggressive interactions with his tenants continued.[36] In 1906 Spina, whom the *Correio Paulistano* called the "Ferocious Landlord," committed yet another assault, this time against Francisco Bianca Stella, because the Italian immigrant had thrown "wastewater" into the courtyard of the cortiço, which did not have sewer access. While Spina's attack was ostensibly motivated by the immigrant's poor hygienic practices, the result was Stella's bad health. Indeed, Stella's injuries were so extensive that it took him three days to go to the local police station, where the physician on call confirmed the seriousness of the attack, leading to Spina's arrest.[37]

Another 1906 incident vibrantly portrays a different relationship between landlords and immigrant tenants with regard to health outcomes. Antonino de Lucca, an Italian immigrant, began using his room in a Bom Retiro cortiço at Rua dos Italianos, 30, as a small machining factory. The noise and dust produced in the workshop led the building dwellers, mainly Italian immigrants, to complain to the owner, who ignored them. The residents then filed a grievance with the police, but law enforcement authorities argued that health issues were not in their purview. Police and hygiene officers also did not act, claiming that neither dust nor sound was a pressing health action category. In frustration, the residents hired lawyers and contacted the press, which eventually led to Antonino de Lucca being fined—a fine that went unenforced and unpaid.[38]

Medical Policing

The establishment of the Medical Police in 1911 was part of a broader reorganization of the state and municipal health and law enforcement services. Health service employees now had new leeway in prosecuting those who sold adulterated food products and the right to use force and fine those who impeded disinfection of residences and businesses. The Medical Police were a municipal priority, expanding from a unit with three physicians in 1911 to one with sixteen teams two decades later, each with a male physician, a male nurse, and a male assistant.[39] The organization had its own space, denominated the *medical post*, and began to maintain detailed records that the state would use to justify health policies directed at immigrants, the poor, and the working class. A new on-call system meant the medical post was staffed twenty-four hours a day, and duties included providing care instruction for guardians or the injured and working with the mentally ill, physically challenged, or dead, all at no financial cost to the public. Housed within the Central Police Division headquarters, the Medical Police had ambulances and access to advanced technology like telephone and telegram services. Their responsibilities included first aid for accident victims and often-uninvited home visits "to the sick in the poor population, bringing them to hospitals."[40]

Health-related social control (both enforced and unenforced) was ever present throughout the Americas and often marked by "patronage, prejudice, and ineptitude."[41] Policies were buttressed by false objectivity, as is evident in the hundreds of thousands of incident reports filed by the Medical Police over its almost three-decade existence. The reports show a wide range of health issues among the working-class population, ranging from serious illnesses and work-related accidents to apparently less serious events like cuts, burns, and fainting spells. Traffic accidents, assaults, suicides, and murders appeared regularly.

The Medical Police forms utilized fixed categories that offered little information for complex health issues, putting the working classes and their health into simplistic boxes that were easy to interpret negatively. The one-page Medical Incident Reports included information such as the patient's name, age, profession, residence, and nationality; the location where the patient was found; the location of the incident; and where they were sent following the examination. Incident reports also included a space for "color," one of the few documents from this period of Brazilian history that includes the category. Katherine Ann Cosby, in her research on the geographic spaces of Black women in São Paulo, notes that the Medical Police were organized during the "apex of scientific racial thought [when the] theory that whiteness superseded all other races in racial mixture became widely accepted" by those in Brazil's dominant classes.[42] Incident reports thus reinforced citizenship categories like immigrant or Brazilian, racial categories like Black or white, and class categories like poor and working class.[43]

On many of the incident reports, a word was stamped in large letters over the top. For example, when the Medical Police suspected lawbreaking was the reason for an incident, the word *crime* was printed. Other categories were childbirth, help in a public space, suicide or a suicide attempt, disaster, or workplace accident. While many patients were walk-ins, the reports show that the telegraph and telephones were regularly used to dispatch a Medical Police vehicle to the incident site. The reports do not mention who precisely contacted the Medical Police.

Medical Police physicians had the power to determine fault prior to investigation. In some cases, like that of Amelia Marini, discussed in chapter 1, possible homicides were dismissed as suicides. In other cases, the Medical Police judged incidents as related to criminal behavior and sent patients to the police or even jail. That is what happened to twenty-two-year-old João Antônio Jorge. In 1916 the unmarried Syrian immigrant factory worker borrowed money from thirty-seven-year-old Anna Danzila, a married Italian immigrant who lived in the same cortiço on the Rua dos Italianos, which had multiple entrances, he in number 166 and she in 161.[44] One early November evening, as Jorge was returning home from work, Danzila (listed as Tansilla by the Medical Police) confronted him and demanded repayment. When he refused, she allegedly punched him in the head, and in retaliation he threw a bottle at her.[45] Both were taken to the Medical Police to be treated for apparently minor injuries, jailed, and then released.[46] We will meet João Antonio Jorge again in chapter 6, after he returned to the living following his death from the flu.

The Medical Police were a hybrid. On the medical side, they monitored and reported on intersections of health, geography, and criminality. When called to treat an accident or wound, they would report infectious diseases to the Health Service, and together the two units "inspected" hundreds of residences and commercial establishments every day, according to reports published in the *Diário Official da Cidade de São Paulo*.[47] With neither the training nor the equipment to care for serious health issues, the Medical Police funneled working-class immigrants into public hospitals like the Santa Casa, where the ill Antonio Baruf, who began this chapter, was hassled for reading a workers' newspaper. For the wealthy, things worked differently since a 1912 decree stated that if a private physician was present at a medical scene, the Medical Police should not involve themselves in treatment.[48]

Transportation technology helped the Medical Police connect health to law enforcement. The municipality promoted their horse-drawn and motorized vehicles as evidence of modern approaches to public health, using them to reinforce state authority (see figure 4.1). The public, not surprisingly, sometimes saw the ambulances as oppressive. A 1921 "Letters from Bó Ritiro" section of "Baolista Life," the macaronic Portuguese title of a section of the humor magazine *Vida Paulista* (São Paulo life), profiled popular relations with public health officials and mocked both the organization and its technology. Readers certainly related to the author's shocked experience of having to ride "on top of a Medical Police ambulance" to get medication from a clinic inside the Central Police Station.[49]

Communications technology such as in-house access to telephone and telegraph facilities allowed the Medical Police to quickly respond to health incidents. Telegraphists from the Fire Department received emergency calls from the growing numbers of "police telegraphic boxes" (figure 4.2) that began to be distributed throughout the city starting in the early 1910s.[50] These boxes looked similar to fire alarm call boxes and were produced by the Gamewell Company of South Carolina in the United States, which by 1910 supplied 95 percent of the US market for fire and police call boxes, likely a figure replicated globally.[51] In São Paulo the boxes were affixed to posts, and the keys to each box were held by a local police official and a single businessperson with a nearby store. Once the boxes were unlocked, the mechanism had a simple dial that was turned to the desired option: accident, central telephone switchboard, ambulance, or cadaver wagon. The "caller" then pulled a lever that sent a code to the appropriate department.[52]

Medical Police intervention in daily life grew along with São Paulo's population. A comparison of the organization in 1912 and 1930, two years for which Team Lesser was able to examine a full set of incident reports, shows the changes. In 1912, when the city population was estimated to be

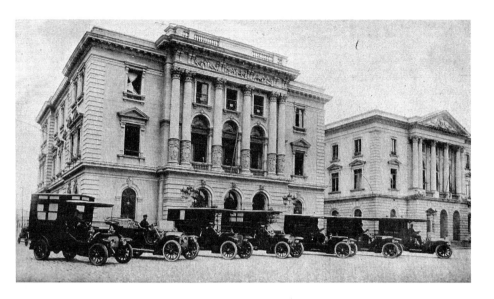

Figure 4.1 Ambulances and other vehicles in front of the Central Police Building in
1905. Source: Secretaria da Segurança Pública, Polícia Civil do Estado de São Paulo,
Fotos Históricas, accessed June 28, 2024, https://www.policiacivil.sp.gov.br/portal
/faces/pages_home/institucional/fotosHistoricas?_afrLoop=2609131526606252&
_afrWindowMode=0&_afrWindowId=tyzodfzb2_1#!%40%40%3F
_afrWindowId%3Dtyzodfzb2_1%26_afrLoop%3D2609131526606252%26
_afrWindowMode%3D0%26_adf.ctrl-state%3Dtyzodfzb2_25.

400,000, the organization had four physicians.[53] In 1930, when the population was about one million, the Medical Police had expanded to sixteen
physicians and an equal number of nurses and nurses' aides.[54] The increase
from 1 physician per 100,000 residents to 1 per 62,500 residents was reflected
in the overall numbers of incident reports. In 1912 incident reports filled
twelve volumes with a total of 6,146 reports. In 1930 they needed thirty-
eight volumes to hold 21,075 reports. The rate of increase was significantly
higher than that of population growth for two reasons. First, as politicians
and health bureaucrats watched the city expand and complexify in what
they believed were negative ways, they increased health surveillance. In
addition, the number of São Paulo residents who relied on the Medical
Police for basic health care grew over time. Each physician thus attended
about 1,500 cases in 1912 while that number dropped to about 1,300 in 1930,
as the increased staff allowed new triage systems to diminish the number
of citizens seen by physicians.

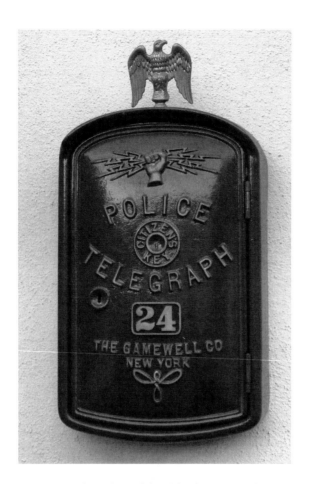

Figure 4.2 Police telegraph box like the ones used in São Paulo to call the Medical Police, undated. When the door of the box was opened with a key, the Medical Police official would find a listening device on a cord, a voice amplification device built into the box, and a dial that could be turned to call different emergency services. Source: Daniel Mayer, "Los Angeles—Historic LAPD Academy—Police Telegraph Box," July 2009, Wikimedia Commons, https://commons .wikimedia.org/wiki/File:Los_Angeles_-_Historic_LAPD _Academy_-_Police_telegraph_box.JPG.

The categories included in incident reports expanded markedly over the decades. While forms in the 1910s were succinct, with few details and large numbers of blank spaces, later ones were more elaborate. Citizenship was differentiated from birthplace to make clear who was a naturalized immigrant. Treatment was distinguished from diagnosis although sometimes this information was added later. As the numbers of public phones grew, incident reports for ambulance pickups included the names of the driver and attending nurse, the car number, and the times when the vehicle left and returned to the medical post.

The growing Medical Police staff, and the volume of cases, meant larger budgets and state attempts to lower expenses. Beginning in 1930, many Medical Police services had a charge attached although incidents in public spaces or for the "definitely poor" were exempt.[55] The prices for Medical Police assistance after 1930 were not cheap even though they remained a state organization and were not privatized. Simple injections cost between twenty and forty milreis; in comparison, in May 1930 you could purchase a nice jacket for sixty-five milreis and then go to the Maurice Chevalier film *The Love Parade* at the São Bento Cinema for three milreis for a matinee and four milreis for the evening showing.[56] Treating a fracture cost between one hundred and three hundred milreis, and an ambulance cost thirty milreis for the first hour and fifteen milreis for each additional thirty minutes.

While the legislation itself does not explain why the Medical Police began charging some people for treatment, we have several hypotheses, all of which may be accurate. One is that the Medical Police was becoming a kind of emergency room for a large segment of the population, including those with enough income to pay for private health care. Such use of public services intended for the poor is seen today, as those with private health insurance use the Brazilian national health system only for expensive medication and complex hospitalizations, something that also happens in the United Kingdom and Israel.[57] Another possibility is that the new charges for Medical Police services were meant to encourage employers to improve workplace safety in order to reduce the state's cost for worker health care. Finally, the new charges may have been an attempt to increase patient costs to the point that the state was effectively denying treatment for many ills.

The 1930 Medical Police expansion could not keep up with the demand for care. In 1933 the numbers of health professionals in the unit skyrocketed, to include thirty physicians, a head nurse, and thirty-six nurses.[58] Most services continued to have charges, with the same exceptions as before. One change in the regulations was that the word *poor* disappeared and was replaced by the word *indigent*, perhaps to force the working poor into payment. While there was no explanation of how a person could prove that they were indigent, the Medical Police clearly had the power to refuse treatment.

The Medical Police incident reports for 1911 to 1940 are held in 690 hardcover volumes in the São Paulo State Archives.[59] The 444,000 cases are organized by month and date, and each volume contains between a hundred and a thousand reports, with the number of incidents increasing every year. The reports allow different views of the relationship among health, immigration, and space as well as other topics like gender or class. To date, the three most in-depth studies of these documents show the links between class and "color," since this classification appears in Medical Police documents, but few other government-produced ones, in the first half of the twentieth century.

Each of the three studies used a different method to engage with the massive number of Medical Police incident reports. Ramatis Jacino chose twenty volumes (two per year for the years 1911–20) to study the relationship between occupation and color. Of the more than 55,000 incident reports he examined, about 43,300 included clear notations for both categories, while the others left one or both categories blank or listed them as "other." Jacino found that 87 percent of the incident reports referred to "white" people and 23 percent to "Black" or "Brown" people. Examining how color related to occupation, he concluded that "Black male and female workers were excluded from occupations with higher economic value and better social status."[60] His focus on the labor market also showed a "white invasion" in the health sector as Black providers were rapidly replaced in the first decades of the twentieth century by white ones (both Brazilians and immigrants) who had academic degrees, often from non-Brazilian institutions.[61]

Fábio Dantas Rocha used a different approach. He selected twenty volumes between 1911 and 1930 and then randomly chose 2,395 incident reports to make a quantitative argument based on his calculations of São Paulo city's population in those years.[62] He analyzed the incident reports by date (1911–15; 1916–20; 1921–25; 1926–30) and by nationality, including Brazilian, Italian, Portuguese, and Spanish. He lumped foreigners outside of the three southern European categories together as "others." Rocha concluded that the city's identity in the first decades of the twentieth century was constructed from "concepts of citizenship linked to an idea of whiteness that excluded the practices and lived experiences of Black people."[63] Katherine Ann Cosby took yet another methodological approach, examining almost three thousand incident reports of nonwhite women, most of whom were categorized as Black, from volumes in 1912, 1916, 1924, 1928, and 1930. For Cosby, the reports indicated that the Medical Police were more interested in incarceration than health, showing "the white imagination of cultural and economic backwardness and criminality. [Making the reports was] indispensable to whitening projects and narratives of progress and modernity in São Paulo."[64]

The Lesser Research Collective took multiple methodological paths in analyzing the Medical Police incident reports, arriving at different kinds of conclusions than Jacino, Rocha, and Cosby. Our first methodological choice was how to narrow down the large corpus of materials. We initially hoped to look for every Bom Retiro case in the 690 volumes, but after Delphine LaCroix, Juliana Casagrande, and I examined the fifty-one volumes from October 1911 to January 1916 (volumes 13954 to 14005), we realized we had neither the time nor the funding to follow through. Thus, we decided to examine every fifth volume from June 1916 to November 1940. We added these 126 volumes to our initial group of 51, meaning we found all incident reports from Bom Retiro (either as the patient place of residence or the accident location) in those 177 volumes (25 percent of the total 690 volumes).

One of our first examinations focused on the five streets around the Central Disinfectory to see how that building and the presence of health care professionals in everyday life might have affected residents (figure 4.3). The 256 health incidents between 1911 and 1940 overwhelmingly affected those who lived in Bom Retiro, showing that people often lived in or near their workplaces. In terms of age, most were between twenty and forty years old, with most tending to be thirty to forty years old. Of the 256 cases, the overwhelming majority (65 percent) were males. Most reports involved Brazilians (63 percent), with another 23 percent Italian immigrants. The rest were for Argentines, Portuguese, Yugoslavs, Russians, Lithuanians, Germans, Syrians, and Poles, with southern European cases higher before World War I and eastern European cases rising after Jewish immigrants began to settle in Bom Retiro in the interwar period. On the five streets examined, 94 percent of the incidents occurred among people denominated as "white" in the color category. This classification reflects how many Black residents of Bom Retiro had been pushed out by 1911. It also may reflect how the working-class population insisted on their own whiteness as part of negotiations for services with often-racist state representatives. Cosby, for example, tells of an incident report where a physician noted "White, I say Black," in the color category.[65]

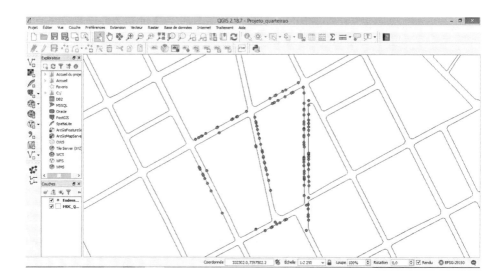

Figure 4.3 Medical Police incident reports plotted on the streets surrounding the Central Disinfectory, 1911–40 ($N = 256$). The street with the highest number of incident reports is the Rua do Areal. Source: Prepared by Delphine LaCroix and Juliana Casagrande, Lesser Research Collective, 2017.

The incident reports showed illnesses caused by poor sanitation, uncollected trash, dense living conditions, flooding, work-related accidents, and non-work-related injuries, usually from falling but from violence as well. Workplace injuries occurred in large and small factories, and some of the injuries treated at home may in fact have taken place at work. The number of street falling incidents show a lack of state care for the built environment. This inattention was the subject of constant complaints by residents to newspapers and to those municipal politicians who would listen; roads and sidewalks were poorly leveled, had holes, and often had impediments, just as they do today.

Forty percent of the 256 incident reports took place on the Rua do Areal, a street that has not changed in size and today borders the east side of the Bom Retiro Public Health Clinic. This one small street had high numbers because the Central Disinfectory building occupied large portions of the other four streets. Indeed, the only four cases listed as taking place in front of the structure were street incidents, not home based. Ironically, the streets around the Disinfectory posed environmental health risks for residents because of leaks of toxic materials and regular fumigation with what today are considered dangerous chemicals. Furthermore, given the often-negative views of public health actions among residents of Bom Retiro, we might surmise that being out of the sight line of the Central Disinfectory was seen as a residential upgrade.

Thinking about the Rua do Areal connects the built environment, health, and immigration. Before 1880 it was called the Areal de Sant'Ana à baixada do Tietê (Sant'Ana sandbank next to the lower Tietê River), and the sand (areia) was used for making ceramics and tiles. The Rua do Areal—Sandbank Street—already appears on 1894 maps from the São Paulo municipal water and sewer authority as an awkward extension of the Rua dos Imigrantes (today's Rua José Paulino).[66] The street is short, and its contemporary length is the same today as in 1894.

Living on the Rua do Areal may have been healthier than living directly next to the Central Disinfectory, but it was still a place of bad health. The street appears frequently in pre-1900 press reports for its litter piles, and the same are observable today. The street was a prime location for working-class protests because of the open space formed by the corners of the Areal, Tenente Pena, and Imigrantes streets. Today that corner is the location of the contemporary Bom Retiro Public Health Center. Lack of enforcement of teardown orders from the city Office of Police and Hygiene meant that the Rua do Areal's cortiços remained over long periods.[67] In the 1920s two- and three-story concrete apartment buildings emerged, many housing newly arrived immigrants from eastern Europe. Yet, as these families began to leave the neighborhood in the 1970s, the single-family apartments were often subdivided to create modern cortiços and oficina-residências.

A series of Medical Police reports about one resident of the Rua do Areal shows how health and race intersected. Fifteen-year-old Vinicius Bueno Prado worked as a shoemaker and lived in a cortiço at Rua do Areal, 30. He was seen by the Medical Police five times between 1935 and 1937, each time after passing out on the street because of his asthma. Bueno Prado was treated by a different physician for each incident. Three described him as "Brown," while the other two classified him as white.[68] We do not know precisely why Bueno Prado was listed in these different ways. Was the color suggested by the patient or his guardian? Might each physician have made a judgment based on where Bueno Prado had been found or what color the patient's father was judged to be? We will never know, but Bueno Prado's case brings to the fore that Brown and Black people (of the 256 cases, seven were listed as "Brown" and nine as "Black") were more likely be treated on the street than whites, who frequently were treated at the Medical Police post, just as in the present the Brazilian Unified Health System bureaucracy appears to treat Black Brazilians differently than others.[69]

When we examined the 256 cases by gender, we found that men were classified as suffering somewhat more work-related and violence-related injuries than women. Men were also categorized in a wide variety of professions: mostly as "factory workers" but also in jobs related to the textile industry, including tailor, hatmaker, shoemaker, and weaver.[70] Others had working-class occupations like bus driver, furniture maker, carpenter, mechanic, and bread maker, and there were even a few soccer players.[71] Many of the incident reports were for store owners, a reminder of the occupational variation in working-class neighborhoods.

Women on the five-street block were categorized overwhelmingly as "domésticas," a classification that does not have a fixed meaning when attached to labor. A woman called, or self-defining as, a "doméstica" might be employed in households other than their own or might be doing outsourced work like sewing or washing clothes in their own home.[72] The term might also describe someone working in their own home doing life-maintenance work such as preparing food and caring for their own children.[73] In Bom Retiro, where many women worked in factories, why was "doméstica" the single largest female category in the Medical Police records? One possibility is that women believed they would be treated better if they described themselves to Medical Police physicians in language that did not suggest labor activism, as the state formally registered eighty thousand female domestic workers by 1941.[74] Another possibility is that the Medical Police categorized women this way as part of their own interests in gender-based social control.

Luis Ferla has argued that "domestic workers operated in a gray zone on the borders of legality and illegality," and this may explain why women in these reports almost always brought along a male relative, always a father or husband.[75] Indeed, during the H1N1 flu epidemic of 1918, when the Medical Police kept particularly precise statistics of illness and death, the state did not assign any occupations to women, something that is discussed in more detail in chapter 6. After abolition the gray zone expanded to include foreigners, linking Black women and immigrants to the single category of "domésticas." This connection was expressed brutally in a popular saying, first mentioned in a text from 1711, that Antonio Candido analyzed in his famous essay on cortiços: "The Portuguese, the negro, and the donkey, all need three things: bread to eat, cloth to wear, and a stick [to make them] work."[76] The connection suggests that the racism that led to the whitening of the workforce simultaneously had an effect on immigrants.

Following our examination of the five streets around the Central Disinfectory, Team Lesser decided to reexamine our materials. Cintia Rodrigues de Almeida, Monaliza Caetano dos Santos, Luanna Gabrielly Mendes do Nascimento, Vitória Martins, and Bianca Almeida examined every volume (of the 690) that ended in zero, a total of sixty-nine volumes that encompassed every year except 1911 (recall that when the Medical Police were founded, one volume might represent a year's worth of incident reports, but by the 1930s each year's reports took up thirty volumes or more). The sixty-nine volumes contained a total of 49,956 incident reports, of which 1,619 took place in Bom Retiro.

In 2022 Fábio Dantas Rocha generously shared his materials with the Lesser Research Collective. This added more than four hundred Bom Retiro cases, increasing our database from 1,619 to 2,097 incident reports. We did multiple comparisons of the two datasets because some of our analysis took place with the set of 1,619 reports and some with the set of 2,097 reports. Fortunately, we found that the two sets matched tightly in terms of nationality, color, and gender, and thus we are confident of the analyses done with different totals. To use nationality as an example, we found the following for the set of 1,619 incident reports: Brazilian (57.0 percent; 923), Italian (14.5 percent; 234), Lithuanian (5.6 percent; 91), Polish (4.4 percent; 72), Russian (2.7 percent; 44), Portuguese (2.4 percent; 40), Spanish (1.6 percent; 27), and German (1.3 percent; 20). When we examined nationality using the set of 2,097 incident reports, there was little change except for an increase in Portuguese immigrants and a decrease in the percentage that did not list a nationality. The major groups continued to be Brazilian (60.6 percent; 1,271), Italian (17.5 percent; 366), Lithuanian (4.5 percent; 95), Polish (3.8 percent; 79), Russian (2.3 percent; 48), Portuguese (5.4 percent; 114), Spanish (1.6 percent; 34), and German (1.1 percent; 23).

We also compared the "color" and "sex" categories across the two datasets. For the former, the 1,619 incident reports categorized 90.2 percent of people (1,461) as white, 5.4 percent (88) as Black (preta/o), and 4.2 percent (68) as Brown (parda/o), with two reports leaving the category blank. When we reran the numbers for color based on the additional materials provided by Rocha, the numbers showed 87.9 percent listed as white (1,844), 6.8 percent as Black (142), and 5.1 percent as Brown (106), with five incident reports leaving the color category blank or unclear. For gender, the 1,619 incident reports listed 65.9 percent as male (1,067) and 32.6 percent as female (528), with twenty-four incident reports leaving that category blank. For the set of 2,097 reports, males represented 64.3 percent (1,348)

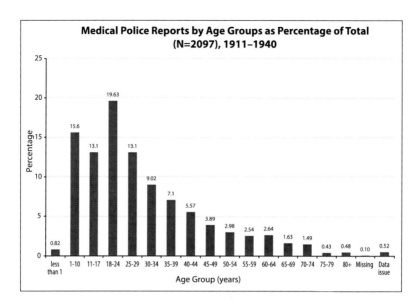

Figure 4.4 Source: Secretaria da Segurança Pública do Estado de São Paulo, Assistência Policial, Registro de ocorrências da Assistência Policial, 1911–40, Arquivo do Estado de São Paulo. Prepared by Cintia Rodrigues de Almeida, Monaliza Caetano dos Santos, Luanna Gabrielly Mendes do Nascimento, and Surbhi Shrivastava, Lesser Research Collective, 2023.

and females 35.0 percent (733), with sixteen incident reports leaving that category blank.

Using the larger dataset, Team Lesser member Surbhi Shrivastava began to break down the incident reports by nationality, by global region, and by age. Of the 2,097 incident reports, 820 (nearly 40 percent) were for immigrants. The largest groups were Italians (17.4 percent), Portuguese (5.4 percent), Lithuanians (4.5 percent), and Polish (3.7 percent). Other nationalities that appeared were Syrians, Argentines, Romanians, Austrians, Hungarians, Letonians, "Israelitas" (Jews), and Japanese. When we placed nationalities into broader regional categories, we generated the following results: southern Europe (62.6 percent), eastern Europe (29.7 percent), western Europe (3.7 percent), the Middle East (2.6 percent), and the Americas and Asia (less than 1 percent each). This period encompassed intense migratory change in São Paulo, and most eastern Europeans were Jews who emigrated after World War I, following restrictive quotas in the United States in 1921 and 1924 and the establishment of the new state of Poland.[77] In the 1920s Yiddish and Yiddishized Portuguese were as frequently heard in Bom Retiro as the Italian and "macaronic" Portuguese of the pre–World War I era. In terms of age, figure 4.4 shows that more than 78 percent of the neighborhood was younger than forty years old with almost half the population between eighteen and thirty-nine years old. Those under eighteen years old represented almost 30 percent of the cases.

Now that I have explained the numbers and the way we generated them, I explore some of our analyses. For example, we hypothesized that we might find spatial patterns; did violent crimes occur more frequently on some streets or blocks than others? This was not the case. We also hypothesized that we might find residence patterns based on nationality and/or color, but this was also not the case. We did find that bad health was distributed across age, gender, race, and citizenship status, with large numbers of incident reports ranging from asthma to nonhuman animal bites to infectious and noninfectious diseases.

Our data show that the Medical Police regularly entered homes, workplaces, and public spaces in addition to treating those who came to the medical post independently. More than 10 percent of incidents stemmed from human-on-human aggression, including fistfights, assaults (with everything from knives to rocks to tiles), and gunfights. Non-work-related accidents took place in the home and on the street. Many incidents in public spaces were transit related, and the press regularly reported on the serious injuries caused by automobiles running over those waiting for trams, with headlines like "Automobile Danger" or "It's Always Cars!"[78] Future research might examine how these accidents mirrored changes in the transport technology deployed by the city, from wagons to streetcars (both pulled by nonhuman animals and motorized) and finally to motorized vehicles like cars and trucks.

When we analyzed gender, our initial findings based on data from the five streets were confirmed. Women were almost always listed as "domésticas," a word loaded with a lack of clarity. It might indicate paid domestic work provided to a family or the nonremunerated activities carried out by women in their own homes. Given the high percentage of working-class women in São Paulo who worked outside the home, why this silence on female professional activity? Failing to specify female paid work indicates how the state saw women's health as related primarily to childbirth, not a surprise since the model of male "breadwinner" and female "housewife" was encouraged and hailed in early twentieth-century Brazil. Women understood these codes, and so did the men, who presented themselves as guardians. Those needing Medical Police aid likely described themselves in ways that they believed would lead to better care.

Women were more likely than men to be treated in the home or to tell the Medical Police that health incidents happened in the domestic sphere. Reports often mention specific rooms like the bedroom or the kitchen, suggesting that women's health was focused on private life and intimate space. When incidents did happen on the street, the Medical Police often categorized women as having a "hysterical crisis" or a "nervous crisis" rather than pointing to the cause. A significant majority of suicides or attempted suicides were by women, although, as we saw in the case of Amelia Marini, these labels may have hidden other issues.

Medical Police incident reports for men connected to factories and tell us something about state visions of male quotidian lives. Workplace accidents comprised 4.6 percent of the 2,097 cases between 1912 and 1940, and many other health incidents were labor related, taking place in residences or public locations. Work accidents took place in small workshops and workshop-residences, such as when José Bellotti lost a finger to a circular saw in a small woodworking shop that doubled as his home.[79] Numerous cases of what appear to be work accidents were not categorized as such by the Medical Police, although no explicit reason is given. Many were caused by foreign objects, which included everything from something small, like a grain of rice lodged in a child's throat to needles stuck in fingers. A typical example of how the "foreign object" category hid workplace accidents comes from February 1928, when Thereza Friate was treated in the late afternoon at the medical post. The fourteen-year-old Russian immigrant lived at Rua Silva Pinto, 55, and likely worked at the nearby textile factory at Rua José Paulino, 49. While she was at the factory, a needle entered the thumb of her left hand; after removing it, the Medical Police sent young Thereza home to be cared for by her parents. Defining the injury as a "foreign object" case rather than a "work accident" relieved the employer of fault.[80]

The Medical Police frequently attended to injuries linked to large factories and public works in Bom Retiro. The employees (many of them immigrants) of chocolate makers, coffee roasters and distributors, beverage makers, and utilities like the São Paulo Railway, the Light, and the Water and Sewer Authority all had frequent accidents. Workplace injuries were so frequent that the local Bom Retiro police unit (the 2nd Delegacia—Bom Retiro) kept, at least between 1934 and 1941, a separate file. Their form incident reports were very different from the Medical Police ones and included information like witness names, beneficiary information, salary, the name of the employer, whether the accident happened in a store or a factory, and a yes/no "Died?" question.[81] The questions lead me to believe that when the police became involved, they sought to relieve the state of care, try-ing to show either that the employers were responsible for treatment or that the employee was at fault, was not indigent, and thus could afford private health care.

One of the largest employers in Bom Retiro was the Germânia Beer Fac-tory, housed in a modern, block-encompassing six-thousand-square-meter "grandiose building" on the Rua dos Italianos (numbers 22 to 30).[82] Emilio Reichert, who arrived in Brazil from Württemberg, Germany, as a twenty-eight-year-old in 1889, just after Brazil's republic was established, founded the brewery. He and his brothers were typical of the immigrant bourgeoise discussed in chapter 1. While Manfred Meyer and Elvira Isabel de Souza Queiroz bought up plots of land and consolidated them to create the Bom Retiro neighborhood, the Reicherts bought up small beer factories. In 1907 the siblings consolidated their purchases and opened the Germânia Beer Factory, producing seven different types of beer, nonalcoholic drinks, soap, biscuits, and chocolates.[83]

In 1920 the Reichert brothers sold the business to Companhia Antarctica Paulista, today part of the Belgian multinational Anheuser-Busch InBev, owned partially by a group of Brazilian investors, including Jorge Paulo Lemann, one of Brazil's richest citizens and the son of a Swiss immigrant. The new owners changed the name of the company to Progresso Nacional (National Progress) and expanded the factory's footprint along the Rua dos Italianos. This new name was not loved by all because it seemed a rejection of the neighborhood in favor of the nation, as Luiz Sérgio Thomás remembered sixty years later: "[I liked] having a beer made in Bom Retiro, Germânia—that in one of those patriotic moments had to change its name . . . the beer began to be called . . . ah . . . 'Order and Progress!' Order and Progress Beer. . . . Jeez. . . . Things from Bom Retiro."[84]

As Antarctica's presence as part of Bom Retiro's built environment expanded through the 1920s, so did the number of accidents related to production and distribution.[85] Twenty-six-year-old Italian immigrant Luiz Maldi was transported by Medical Police ambulance in 1911 to the Samaritan Hospital after falling from his beer delivery wagon and frac-turing his right leg.[86] Another Italian immigrant, twenty-three-year-old Alexandre Domingues, also delivered Germânia-produced beers and lived just a couple of blocks away from the factory, at Rua Guarany, 34. In Novem-ber 1913 Domingues had his right leg pinned between a wall and the wheel of the beer delivery wagon he was driving. The Medical Police treated him at the factory and then sent him home, before sending the case to the police,

perhaps to force Germânia to pay the costs.[87] In mid-1916 workers from
the Germânia beer factory attacked Ferrucio Conte, a twenty-six-year-old
Italian who lived at Avenida Celso Garcia, 348. The motive for the attack,
which took place on the Rua dos Aimorés? Conte, who had been a wagon
driver for Germânia, now was a local distributor of Rio de Janeiro's Polonia
beer and represented the competition.[88]

The Germânia factory, like most in São Paulo, employed children, who
in the late nineteenth century may have made up as much as 25 percent of
the labor force. Only in 1919 was the legal minimum age for workers in the
city set at fourteen years.[89] One of those children was Guilherme Crivelarea,
whose job was to bottle beer. In 1916 the fourteen-year-old was badly injured
when one of the bottles exploded. Dr. Raul de Sá Pinto of the Medical Police
rushed to the factory, sending the boy to the Santa Casa hospital for treatment
since he was in danger of losing his vision. An initial report in the *A Gazeta*
newspaper stated that the factory was going to be fined for using child labor
and would also have to pay an indemnity to the minor. The following day the
newspaper retracted the second claim, noting that since all the medical costs
were being paid by the factory, "There is no claim for compensation."[90] In
another case, the Germânia factory appears not to have taken responsibility
in 1919 when one of its wagon drivers inexplicably threw a bottle at twelve-
year-old Atenor de Oliveira, sending him to the hospital.[91] In the 1920s the
company, which changed its name to Progresso Nacional (National Progress), remained a location of bad health. Adriano Francisco, a Portuguese
immigrant, had his arm sliced open by a bottle that broke during a delivery
on nearby Rua José Paulino.[92] Minors also continued to be regularly injured
on the job, leading to Medical Police intervention.[93]

The Medical Police judged more than 10 percent of the incidents in Bom
Retiro as crime related, sending patients to the police station for further investigation or directly to the *xadrez*, an officially used slang term that today
continues to describe a prison or jail. Alexandre Elias, a twenty-nine-year-
old Syrian immigrant, was transformed from peddler to criminal while being
treated by the Medical Police. In 1913 he fell and injured his head, arriving
by foot at the Medical Police clinic inside the central police station for treatment. According to the report, Elias was then jailed, perhaps for not having
an official work document.[94] Lola Zulbert, a married German immigrant,
had a different fate. When she fell ill in 1913, she was sent home even though
the Medical Police defined her profession as "prostitute."[95]

With some regularity the Medical Police were dispatched to deal with
death by natural causes, corpses found in unexpected locations, or the af-

termath of suicides and suicide attempts. The state considered this latter category a moral offense, and incident reports received a specific stamp for suicide or suicide attempt. While we do not know much information about the thirty-five cases in the Bom Retiro records, we can hypothesize that the stress of poverty, sexism, and xenophobia were partial triggers.[96] Some examples of suicide emphasize these points. Close to midnight on March 10, 1922, the Medical Police were contacted through a call box to go to a residence at Rua da Graça, 152, in Bom Retiro. There they found Rosa Pereira, an Italian immigrant, who had tried unsuccessfully to kill herself by drinking 100 proof alcohol.[97] Two weeks later, in the early morning of March 25, 1922, someone reported a gunshot near the Tamanduateí River. On the bank of the waterway, the Medical Police official found thirty-three-year-old Phelomena Charrates, a married Russian immigrant living on the Rua dos Aimorés, who had shot herself. The injured Charrates was brought to the clinic by ambulance, where she was treated and sent home to her husband rather than to a mental health facility.[98]

A decade later, in 1931, nineteen-year-old Brazilian seamstress Nicolina de Lima also attempted suicide, by ingesting ether at her home on Rua Matarazzo, a three-block street less than a ten-minute walk from the Central Disinfectory. As with Charrates, someone contacted the Medical Police, which sent a vehicle. Unlike in Charrates's case, de Lima's actions were considered criminal, and she was remanded to the police for further action after her stomach had been pumped.[99] We do not know what motivated the different Medical Police judgments, but some possibilities are worth mentioning: (1) different physicians treated suicides differently, (2) married women were treated differently than single ones, (3) how the male member of the family (father or husband) responded to the Medical Police modified the outcomes, and (4) between 1921 and 1931, state ideas about suicide changed, with increased focus on the act as criminal.

Suicide, of course, continues to be a challenge in Bom Retiro. In late 2019 Team Green, Dr. Emily Sweetnam Pingel (at the time doing fieldwork at the Bom Retiro Public Health Clinic), and I learned of a teenager who had leaped in front of a metro and lost both her legs. Over the following weeks, there were many conversations in the clinic about whether health professionals should, or were even trained to, see suicide warning signs. Another case, of a man who leaped to his death off a building at around the same time, also led to extensive discussion of how health professionals should think about suicide, again without resolution. As Pingel notes, the conflict over whether potential suicide represented a health problem or an individual moral/psychological failure led to conflict in a health promotion group about whether discussing violence would be allowed in meetings that focused on positive discourses among participants.[100]

This chapter has focused on the Police Medical Assistance Unit. It has tried to reconstruct how quotidian health challenges in Bom Retiro intersected with state institutions that merged public health and policing. Our database shows that disease, suicide, violent crime, and work-related accidents were common, making living and dying part of other structural issues like racism and sexism. I have also proposed that residents of Bom Retiro, like everywhere else in the city, created strategies to take advantage of the Medical Police and make it function like a single-payer health system. Yet catastrophes often broke systems, as they did during the late nineteenth-century bubonic plague outbreak and the H1N1 epidemic in 1918–19, the focus of chapter 6.

A POSTSCRIPT

Let's call him Tae-Hyung. He lives with his spouse in a building whose residents are Korean immigrants, Korean Brazilians, and Jewish Brazilians of European descent. In his youth Tae-Hyung loved mountain climbing but following a stroke he is confined to a wheelchair and receives regular visits from the health professionals at the Bom Retiro Public Health Clinic. Many of the full-time residents in Tae-Hyung's five-story apartment building, be they owners or renters, employ domestic workers, who are often of African descent and practice various forms of Christianity and spiritism. Next door is an eastern European Jewish restaurant opened by a Bulgarian couple who migrated to Israel and then to Brazil. Following their retirement, the space was purchased by investors who turned it into a hipster Jewish diaspora eatery that sits alongside other hipster Korean diaspora restaurants.

Tae-Hyung, like most immigrants, faces daily aggressions, both macro and micro. Some residents of Bom Retiro mockingly refer to the street where he lives, Rua Correia de Melo, as "Coreia [Korea] de Melo" because of the country of origin of many of its residents. Others believe that Korean immigrants have unnatural smells, are money hungry, and are unusually violent. One frequently heard stereotype is that Koreans in Bom Retiro regularly eat dogs. These claims gained force in 2009 when the press began to report on a couple who were arrested for slaughtering dogs, supposedly for sale to Korean restaurants in Bom Retiro.[101]

Reporters descended on the neighborhood's eateries, searching for menu items that included dog. Four Korean immigrants were arrested, and meat was taken to the city's public health laboratories for analysis.[102] I thought about the connection of nonhuman animal diseases and Korean immigrants while I was doing fieldwork in 2016; articles in the print and online media told of a mentally ill Korean immigrant who had murdered an elderly trash collector on the street with a crossbow. An article, from one of Brazil's most widely distributed news networks, described the killer as having "raiva," a word that means both rage and rabies.[103] Bom Retiro, as it was a century earlier, was in the public eye as a place of otherness and danger, where bad health could come from the food served in restaurants and from simply walking down the street.

Residual stereotypes emerged yet again during the COVID-19 pandemic when morbidity and mortality rates in neighborhoods with large numbers of immigrants skyrocketed.[104] Sidnei Pita is the director of a nongovernmental organization representing the tenement dwellers who make up a significant part of Bom Retiro's population. His frustrated 2020 comments criticizing public health attitudes about working-class immigrants and nonimmigrants could have been made a century earlier: "Many [in the working class] are fully aware of the pandemic, but they do not have [the money to buy] hand sanitizer, masks, soap, and cleaning products."[105] The lack of resources made the impact of disease on the residents of Bom Retiro intense. Yet the state's representatives rarely recognized bad health as the result of structural issues, and health policies rarely focused on the causes of disease or violence. Instead, many policies appeared punitive to immigrants, in effect blaming the victims—for example, suggesting that street litter and the diseases associated with it resulted from dirty or unmodern immigrant cultures rather than a lack of street cleaning or convenient locations for waste removal.

5

A Building Block of Health

There is a saying I have heard in Brazil: "Mosquitoes are democratic: they bite the rich and the poor alike." While insects generally do not have a highly developed sense of class consciousness, mosquito-borne diseases, from yellow fever to malaria to dengue, in fact differentially affect people of different classes. One result is that the application of state-sponsored health programs, and the communications surrounding them (see figure 5.1), can create conflictual interactions with the public, despite long-standing class-crossing agreement that mosquito-borne diseases are dangerous and that eradication, control, and cures are important. There was disagreement, however, about whether, when, and how control or eradication should take place.[1] While public health officials and those in the privileged classes believed the strategies were objective, science based, and fair to all, the working classes often saw those same policies as prejudicial. Public health actions often othered the built environment where immigrants lived as "over there" while regarding the more upper-class neighborhoods "over here" as healthy.

The *Aedes aegypti* mosquito, which one evolutionary biologist has called a "contender for most lethal animal," was likely introduced to the Americas when European enslavers sailed with their human cargo from West Africa.[2] *Aedes aegypti* found fertile ground in Brazil's expanding nineteenth-century cities, especially in high-density, often-flooded districts like Bom Retiro,

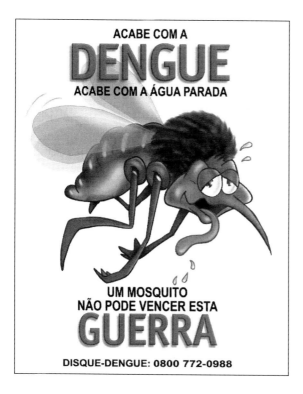

Figure 5.1 A caricatured image of a giant dengue-carrying *Aedes aegypti* mosquito, distributed by the city of São Paulo, Civil Committee against Dengue. The caption urges the population to eliminate standing water. This example comes from the Centro de Educação Infantil Vila Prado (Vila Prado Center for Child Education). The text reads "A mosquito cannot win this war: Finish off dengue, get rid of standing water." Source: CEI Vila Prado, "Um mosquito não pode vencer esta guerra," December 13, 2015, http://ceivilaprado.blogspot.com/2015/12/um-mosquito-nao-pode-vencer-esta-guerra.html.

where potential breeding sites included containers for drinking water, flowerpots, and street litter after rainfall.

The *Aedes aegypti* mosquito is just one of many factors that create health disparities where materially constructed spaces like residences and workplaces and socially constructed places like neighborhoods map onto each other. Built environments therefore connect to access to quality education, employment, affordable housing, and safe areas for children, all of which relate to health quality. Long-term inequalities emerged from geography, citizenship, ethnicity, gender, and race, and societal stressors ranged from state violence to unequal access to cultural, social, and labor opportunities. All buttressed long-term prejudices among public health workers and policymakers that residents of Bom Retiro were culturally and physically diseased. Thus, health policies and actions starting in the late nineteenth century were filled with ethnoracial and class-based assumptions as tools like nationalism and fear were used in education programs seeking to modify working- and lower-class people's health behavior.

Emílio Ribas began to work in the public health arena at the end of the nineteenth century, doing pioneering studies of yellow fever and becoming director of São Paulo's Sanitary Service in 1896. Much of his research assumed that health and national greatness were connected, as was clear in his 1901 flyer about the transmission of mosquito-borne diseases which used the phrase "The Public's Health Is the Best Guarantee of National Prosperity."[3] The arrival of immigrants who either were already sick or became ill in Brazil was thus one area of focus. For example, in 1902 Vicente Farcetta reported a strange death in the Bom Retiro cortiço where he lived, at Rua Marmoré, 21. Pedro Cassano, a twenty-year-old fish peddler who had recently arrived from Italy, was found dead at home without any apparent violence. Farcetta, a disinfector employed by the Central Disinfectory and likely an Italian immigrant, suspected yellow fever. Ribas, along with the Bacteriological Institute's Carlos Luiz Meyer, visited the cortiço multiple times but did not find *Aedes aegypti* mosquitoes. They concluded that the cortiço was safe and that Cassano had been bitten elsewhere. When Ribas later investigated the deaths of two Syrian immigrants, he again found that the cortiço where they lived did not have mosquitoes infected with yellow fever.[4]

In a series of early twentieth-century experiments authorized personally by the president of the state of São Paulo, Ribas examined *Aedes aegypti* (at the time known as *Stegomyia fasciata*) larvae from areas untouched by yellow fever that were brought to São Paulo to mature. In one set of tests, conducted in 1902 at the Isolation Hospital, today known as the Emílio Ribas Hospital, Ribas and other employees of the Sanitary Service, along with three recently arrived immigrants from Italy, volunteered to be bitten. Ribas did not contract the disease, but the immigrants did, fortunately surviving. A second 1903 experiment used three different Italian immigrants, who lived in "miserable conditions" and agreed to "volunteer" only after being remunerated.[5] These three slept in a closed room without mosquitoes but filled with bedding and clothes soiled with the blood and vomit of those with yellow fever.

The experiments led Ribas to multiple conclusions. First, yellow fever could not be spread via direct human contact.[6] Second, those who recovered from the infectious disease in childhood developed immunity. While both contentions have been borne out over time, the results tagged immigrants for their lack of immunity, merging health issues with xenophobia.[7] This led some public health officials to believe that the working classes were unable to understand their own health. Teaching immigrants how to be healthy led to new images in the Brazilian visual landscape. Posters with realistic-looking but giant rats became part of public health actions during bubonic plague outbreaks, and *Aedes aegypti*, while hard to distinguish from other mosquitoes, began to be presented as a terrifying demon, an approach that continues to the present (see figures 5.2 and 5.3).[8]

Control and eradication strategies for mosquito-borne diseases, in the past and present, have a correlation to policies about water. Disadvantaged districts in São Paulo, for example, have historically unpredictable water distribution. Before the widespread use of plastic, water-storage containers were often filled by rainwater or via hand-operated community pumps. Beginning in the eighteenth century, many Brazilian cities introduced public drinking fountains and taps as enslaved peoples transported water to wealthy residences while the broader public carried their own. In the mid-nineteenth century, municipalities began to inaugurate residential piped water supply systems and sewers, often constructed and managed by European-owned companies.[9] After World War II, individual wells were increasingly regulated by the state, forcing residents to use ever-larger containers to capture and store water.

Poor and working-class neighborhoods were the last to receive municipal delivery infrastructure; even then, water arrival was (and is) irregular. In the twenty-first century, affluent neighborhoods receive water regularly via large, building-owned tanks that are maintained by employees rather than by individual families. Less affluent neighborhoods, especially those far from central pumping stations, receive water only two or three times a week, on a random schedule. This means containers are filled when there is water and then drained as water is used. Historically, the arrival of water meant residents rushed to fill their wood or ceramic containers, which often had poorly fitting covers. More recently, drinking and bathing water is stored in plastic containers that range from about a meter

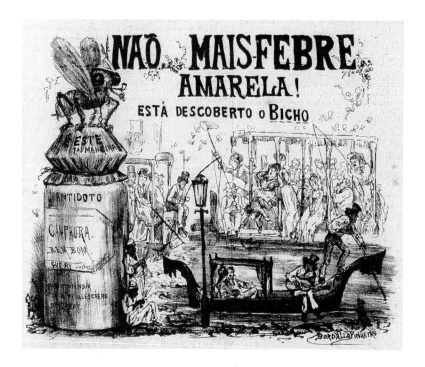

Figure 5.2 1876 poster alerting the population about yellow fever. The caption reads "No more yellow fever: The insect has been discovered." Source: Ricardo Westin, "No Brasil Império, chegada de vírus mortal provocou negacionismo e crítica a quarentenas," *Arquivo S* 68, Saúde, June 1, 2020, Agência Senado, https://www12 .senado.leg.br/noticias/especiais/arquivo-s/no-brasil-imperio-chegada-de-virus -mortal-provocou-negacionismo-e-critica-a-quarentenas.

in diameter for a single family to much larger ones for buildings. Today rooftop water tanks dominate the visual landscape in São Paulo, just as they do in all Latin American cities (figure 5.4).

When not properly capped or when broken, water tanks are highly productive sites for mosquito breeding, and uncleaned tanks can spread multiple diseases, as happened during the 2015 and 2016 Zika outbreak.[10] Zika is a kind of residual illness, a contemporary virus carried by infected *Aedes aegypti* and *Aedes albopictus* mosquitoes, just as are yellow fever and dengue. Zika brought global attention to how mosquito-borne bad health disproportionately affects those living in nonaffluent neighborhoods. People, especially pregnant ones without the privilege of moving away from mosquito-prone spaces or having the care of private doctors, were particularly affected by Zika. There were notable increases in both

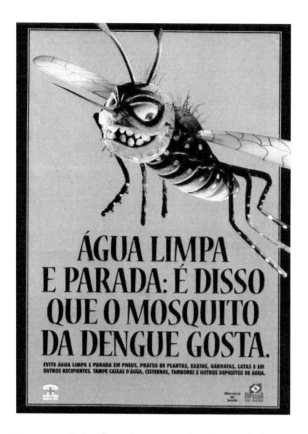

Figure 5.3 Poster from the 1990s urging the population to eliminate standing water. The caption reads: "Clean and standing water: this is what dengue mosquitoes like. Avoid clean and standing water in tires, plant holders, vases, bottles, cans, and other similar items. Tightly close water boxes, cisterns, drums, and other water containers." Source: Brazilian Ministry of Health poster used during the *Brasil em Ação* (Brazil in Action) program, 1996–99, Biblioteca Virtual em Saúde—Ministério da Saúde, Informação e Conhecimento para a Saúde. "Água limpa e parada: É disso que o mosquito da dengue gosta," accessed June 28, 2024, http://pesquisa.bvsalud.org/bvsms/resource/pt/mis-26796. Image courtesy of the Centro de Documentação, Museu de Saúde Pública Emílio Ribas, São Paulo.

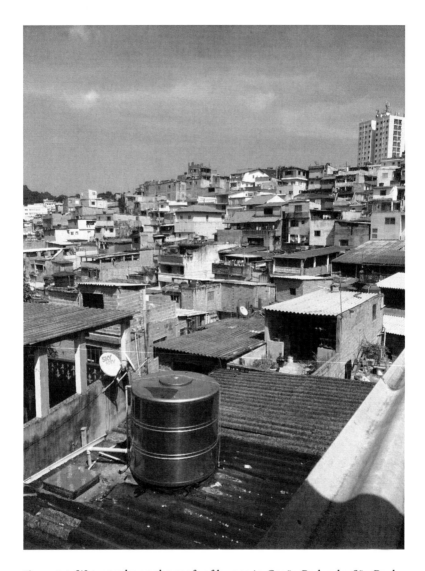

Figure 5.4 Water tanks on the roofs of homes in Capão Redondo, São Paulo, August 26, 2016. Source: Photograph by Jeffrey Lesser.

Guillain-Barré syndrome and microcephaly among newborns in north-eastern Brazil, an especially poor part of the country. Global attention to the Zika virus as a major public health threat followed the declaration of a public health emergency by the Brazilian Ministry of Health and the World Health Organization (WHO).[11]

Scientists, physicians, and politicians responded to the Zika virus with policies and actions, many of which aimed at eliminating standing water.

They focused on nonelite neighborhoods where public services had poor reach and where, many public health officials believed, homes were more likely to have conditions favorable to mosquito breeding. Yet these well-intentioned approaches sometimes appeared paternalistic to the poor and working classes since the actions often came without notice as public health officials arrived in neighborhoods and demanded entry to homes. Residents sometimes took the unrequested "help" as insulting since they believed they could care for their health in their own homes. At the most basic level, the fight against Zika often appeared to be part of broader systems of social control, residues of historical relationships in which the public views the state and its agents with suspicion.

The Brazilian Summer of 2015–2016

In 2015 I worked with Uriel Kitron, an epidemiologist and then chair of Emory University's Department of Environmental Sciences, to examine the relationship between mosquito-borne illnesses and international and domestic migration.[12] This research put us in contact with Dr. Eduardo de Masi, at the time a coordinator in the environmental health sector of the São Paulo municipal Secretary of Health.[13] De Masi focused on zoonosis control and generously invited Dr. Kitron and me to join municipal health surveillance teams as they were dispatched to check on complaints, called *denúncias*, of standing water that came in to a central office, usually via anonymous phone calls. Denúncias, we learned, rarely came from residents of middle- and upper-middle-class neighborhoods. Those residential spaces had single-family homes with full-time domestic workers who identified and eliminated standing water, along with sophisticated refrigerators without water catch basins that needed to be emptied.

Our observations were initially in geographically peripheral areas of the city where, like in Bom Retiro, precarious housing, lack of water and sanitary services, the urban heat island effect, prior exposure to mosquito-borne diseases, and other factors were observable problems. Disjunctions between state and public understandings of health actions were evident when we joined de Masi and the municipal health surveillance teams in Capão Redondo, whose 270,000 residents make it one of São Paulo's largest working-class districts.[14] Capão Redondo is almost twenty-five kilometers from Bom Retiro and the center of São Paulo. Yet like Bom Retiro, it has precarious housing, poor health outcomes, and higher-than-average indices of violence. The name of either neighborhood evokes both stigma and a sense of hipness: in contemporary Bom Retiro, the latter emerges from K-culture, and in Capão Redondo it is the artistic success of the hip-hop musicians Racionais MCs and the author Ferréz, both known for denouncing violence and racism.[15] While there are few recent immigrants in Capão Redondo, it is part of the Campo Limpo (Clean Field) district, settled in the early nineteenth century by a few German immigrant families and an important center of the Seventh Day Adventist religion. Following World War II, the district became more densely populated as rents rose in central São Paulo and Brazilians from the often drought-stricken northeastern regions increasingly migrated to São Paulo. In 2010 household incomes in Capão Redondo were below the median for São Paulo city, and more than 5 percent of residents had no income at all, a number that rises to 10 percent in Bom Retiro.[16]

During our observational research in Capão Redondo, the implications of population density were striking, just as in Bom Retiro. Most structures contained between six and eight households, each occupying two or three rooms. In other words, homes that in wealthy neighborhoods would have separate bedrooms, a family room, a dining room, and a kitchen were compressed here, like in Bom Retiro, into much smaller spaces serving multiple functions. Each family had its own plastic water tank filled on the unpredictable days when the pressure was high enough to move the water to the city outskirts. Living structures were constantly under construction, with the "roofs" filled with materials to be used for building new floors and thus rooms for more families.

The health surveillance teams worked with local politicians and clerics in Capão Redondo to inform residents about our presence. Standing water and *Aedes aegypti* breeding grounds were easy for the uniformed teams to find, and they tried to resolve the problem by eliminating standing water and educating residents on how to avoid recurrence. Typical problems were flowerpots with water pooled at the base, uncovered drinking-water containers, or old-style refrigerators with water-collection bins at the base. More challenging for the public health workers were streets filled with uncollected litter that would provide breeding sites following rain. Another problem was that the large and heavy materials on roofs were largely uncovered and, when filled with water, were attractive to *Aedes aegypti*.

Water tanks, as in the past, were the major source of trouble.[17] Many individual families had tanks made of durable, high-impact plastic, but some had older ceramic containers that would have been more typical before the 1970s. Whether plastic or ceramic, tanks with cracked or broken tops were another opportunity for mosquito breeding. While this was far from a scientific sample, during each day we spent in Capão Redondo, usually visiting about ten buildings, we found at least one tank with a broken top and *Aedes aegypti* larvae. Since mosquitoes generally remain within 150 feet of their birthplaces, a single breeding ground can put all the families in a structure at risk.[18]

Public health workers and the population at large recognized the importance of minimizing mosquito breeding grounds. Both knew that the state would rarely provide material solutions. For example, health surveillance officials advised residents to replace cracked tops or to seal holes and cracks with an epoxy-like solution, which was not provided by the municipality. Creative solutions included using old plastic bags to plug holes, yet when a top was badly cracked and needed replacement, families were in a bind. As I was told repeatedly, residents had neither the funds to purchase new tops nor the cars needed to transport the tops from a store to the home. When we found larvae in water tanks, health agents advised residents to clean the inside surface with a chemical solution that also had to be purchased. Yet the nonregular arrival of water made it hard to follow this prescription since emptying a tank for cleaning might mean going for days without water. When residents complained that the city no longer provided replacement tops, a kind of tarp that went over the tank and under a broken top, some of agents' responses could have come from nineteenth-century public health officers: that if the state provided help, individuals would become lazy and stop taking responsibility for their own health.

In the introduction I argued for the importance of interdisciplinarity. Yet convincing quantitatively oriented researchers that qualitative work was useful, and vice versa, was often a bumpy experience. Following our visits to Capão Redondo, Kitron wondered if our observations allowed us to make broader claims about health policy and actions or public responses. He challenged my comparative approach, noting that contemporary Capão Redondo was very different from historical Bom Retiro—spatially, residentially, demographically, ethnically, and in terms of transportation and water. My guess is that many residents of Capão Redondo and Bom Retiro would agree with Kitron. Even so, my research indicates that in some realms the two districts have similarities, even if it would be preposterous to suggest that they are the same.

Kitron's provocations are important ones for scholars in the humanities and led me to expand my data by working with municipal health surveillance teams in places other than Capão Redondo. Over the course of 2015–16,

I spent eighteen additional days doing observations in São Paulo's South Region, unaccompanied by de Masi. In one neighborhood where I participated in a health surveillance action, I was told that activities only take place with the blessing of drug traffickers.[19] In another neighborhood the housing was so precarious that I fell through a floor while looking for standing water. During this period the locations for actions emerged from phoned denúncias of standing water. Yet upon arrival, many of the calls seemed to reflect conflicts between neighbors, from dog control to property disputes. Residents had learned that making a denúncia about standing water and mosquitoes at their neighbor's house, at least in the Brazilian summer of 2015/16, would lead to a quicker response than calls to law enforcement about community conflict.

A Tale of Two Teams

In 2010 Bom Retiro had the highest incidence of dengue in São Paulo city, and in 2016 the illness returned in force, just as Zika was on the rise.[20] The dual outbreaks dominated the daily activities of the two health teams I was observing in Bom Retiro, one focused on health surveillance and the other on family health. My increased nonarchival time in Bom Retiro in 2016 gave me a better picture of the residues that contributed to contemporary bad health: flooding, poor litter collection, and poor water distribution.[21] The two different public health units that I observed worked physically close to each other, yet they had no contact and very different interactions with the public.

The health surveillance team to which I was connected was part of a large subprefectural unit that included Bom Retiro and other central city neighborhoods. Like those I had worked with outside the city center, team members were male; in the months I spent on this part of the research, I met only one female officer tasked with responding to denúncias. While there were no official gender restrictions, those I met responded to my questions about female participation by emphasizing danger in the field, including the possibility of harassment. I wondered if some male health care workers believe the often-punitive nature of health surveillance might be at odds with the "caring" health jobs often expected of women.

The health surveillance team wore uniforms and drove from place to place in official vehicles. Each member had passed a civil service exam that demanded completion of at least a middle-school education. All those I met were from working-class neighborhoods outside the city center, had little experience with immigrants, and did not have a direct relationship with those living and working in Bom Retiro or any of the neighborhoods in which they were investigating mosquito-related health issues. The team members portrayed themselves to me as having status because of their state employment. Agents often suggested that the public was not capable of taking responsibility for their own health, commenting on a lack of individual intelligence or will. They presented themselves to me and to residents as a kind of occupying force waging war against disease.

Some health surveillance team members made clear that my presence was a nuisance, something that had not happened with other teams when de Masi was present. De Masi's presence may also explain why those teams were education oriented when they found standing water. In one case, I observed de Masi intervene when he felt a team member was not giving a clear explanation to a resident. In Bom Retiro the lack of a "boss" covering for me meant that I was an irritant, especially because the official vehicle now was crowded with an extra person. Over time the team seemed to become comfortable with my presence and started to see me as a potential ally in expressing their work to higher-ups. They also saw me as providing free labor since I was familiar with Bom Retiro and able to provide help in everything from giving directions to indicating where the team could eat lunch.

There were numerous similarities in my experiences with health surveillance in Bom Retiro and other neighborhoods. For example, while teams were rarely denied entry into a residence, greetings were far from enthusiastic since the nonrequested interventions into private spaces meant the interruption of work and childcare. Residents understood that home visits from health agents would lead to demands to change or fix things that they could not afford. For example, many homes had older, highly inefficient refrigerators with water-collection bins at the bottom. While daily dumping of the water was possible, the suggestion of buying a new-model refrigerator without the collection bin always led to eye-rolling. I noted that residents seemed more comfortable asking me, rather than the uniformed agents, questions about health issues. I was frequently shown bugs and asked if they were mosquitoes, if Zika was the same as dengue, or if I could help get broken water-tank tops replaced. I think this was the result of various factors: I was not uniformed, I explained why I was with the team, and I was not a health surveillance agent. Perhaps most important, I did something the health surveillance teams almost never did: I always introduced myself by name and by citizenship status. Providing names is an important part of Brazilian social interactions, and the fact that members of the team did not introduce themselves emphasized their attitudes about the public and reinforced their status as part of the state "body" rather than individuals. To my surprise, my non-Brazilian citizenship status was rarely a point of conversation even though my twin sons insist that I have an accent in Portuguese.

My observation of the health surveillance unit in Bom Retiro coincided with my work as a member of Team Green at the Bom Retiro Public Health Clinic (BRPHC). Working simultaneously with two very different units in the municipal public health sector meant constant comparisons. One area of significant difference was related to social control. The health surveillance team portrayed their job as one of enforcement, while members of Team Green and other health professionals that I observed at other health clinics in São Paulo used a discourse of partnership, even if their actions were sometimes less than collegial.[22] The differences between the teams were even expressed in clothing. Health surveillance agents wore uniforms, while health professionals from the BRPHC used blue vests or white coats over everyday clothing. Contact with the public was also radically different. Following a denúncia, surveillance workers arrived at a building or home unannounced, in official vehicles, usually without any information other than an address to be entered. Professionals from the BRPHC used a different approach since many team members, especially community health agents, live in the neighborhoods where they work. When Team Green went on a home/workplace visit, they had appointments, arrived on foot, and began the interactions with personal introductions if they did not already know the patients.

Health States

The differences in how these two arms of the health state engaged with the public were highlighted following a denúncia at a Bom Retiro address that I knew well. Occupying almost an entire block of Rua Tenente Pena, the seven-story building is on the same street as the BRPHC and the former Central Disinfectory. The lot had held cortiços and small factories through much of the nineteenth and twentieth centuries, but after World War II, developers built more formal residential structures. The current building has five entrances and street-level businesses, and it originally had twenty-four multiroom apartments intended for middle-class families. When I began to spend time in the building in 2016, most of the apartments had been transformed into oficina-residências where textile workers lived and worked in the same space. Walls had been torn down to create large open areas filled with sewing machines and piles of fabric, ringed by small plywood rooms where families lived. Most of the residents/workers in the building were Bolivian immigrants in extended family groupings who had entered Brazil legally and then overstayed their visas.

I began visiting the building as part of a Team Green project to "bring health" to immigrant textile workers by creating pop-up basic health clinics inside oficina-residências. During these about two-hour visits, a long table was set up with different stations—to check that each person was registered with the Brazilian Unified Health System and to register newcomers; take their weight, height, and blood pressure; and check that prescriptions were up to date. At the end of the table sat the physician, and each resident had an opportunity to discuss their health with him in an open setting that was not confidential. Prenatal and maternal health was a priority, and pregnant people, and those who had recently given birth, received special attention, including reminders about upcoming appointments.

Team Green visits ended with group repetitive stress exercises. One of my main functions, since I was usually the tallest person in the room, was to tape A4-sized sheets with exercise information in Spanish high on the walls. Taking regular short breaks from sewing for stretching, while a very good idea, did not strike me as realistic since workers were paid by the piece, and even five minutes of self-care represented a loss of income.

US-based readers may find the idea of a medical team bringing health to patients with uncertain visa status surprising and perhaps inspiring. But the pop-up health clinics were not without complications. For example, some health care workers believed the Portuguese and Spanish languages were close enough linguistically to be mutually intelligible. Yet female patients from the Andes frequently sought out Spanish-speaking women on Team Lesser to discuss health issues they believed Portuguese-speaking medical workers had misunderstood. Overall, the pop-up clinics appeared to be appreciated, and access to free health care was a frequent topic during oral histories with Bolivian, Paraguayan, and Korean immigrants in Bom Retiro.

Given my experiences with Team Green in the huge building on Rua Tenente Pena, I was curious when the health surveillance team was sent to that same address one morning in 2016. I assumed we would be welcomed with open arms, but I was, as usual, wrong. We pulled up in an official vehicle filled with uniformed male health surveillance agents. Even after the team leader had been ringing the building doorbell for ten minutes, a porteiro (a door attendant/gatekeeper/security guard typical of residential buildings in Brazil) did not appear. Members of the health surveillance team began banging on the door, and eventually someone leaned out of a window on the third floor. One member of the team shouted that they had come to the building because of a denúncia, provided his identification number, and asked the resident to call the city health office to confirm its legitimacy. This approach was ineffective. A combination of distrust of authorities, a distrust of unknown people, perhaps language barriers (since the resident spoke Spanish), and the price of a phone call meant that no one was willing or able to confirm the identity of the team.

A stalemate ensued. The team leader became increasingly frustrated, insisting on his legal right of entry because of the Zika health emergency. Other surveillance workers explained to me that a failed investigation had to be noted and would make the team look bad. Eventually the police were called, which may have reinforced fears that the team was really from law enforcement since Bom Retiro has the third-highest level of reported police aggression in the city of São Paulo.[23] The police officers who arrived at the building were assigned to Bom Retiro and thus familiar with the space and the place, even if they were not beloved by all residents. To my surprise, the officers in effect sided with the residents, explaining to the team that entry might be dangerous to both the health professionals and the police. Thus, the law enforcement officials refused to accompany the team into the building, and the visit did not take place. In my multiple visits to the same building with Team Green—including one where Emory administrators stood out by wearing ties and jackets—there was never difficulty in entering, and I never sensed danger or hostility.

My observations highlighted the different ways that representatives of the health state see the immigrant public and create meaning out of space to make judgments, often based on distrust, about place. Historically, as in the present, the public did not passively accept attitudes that linked health policies to residential disruption and expulsion.[24] One of the most vibrant examples was found in Rio de Janeiro's 1904 Vaccine Revolt, versions of which occurred in other places and at other times.[25] The story began in 1900 when epidemiologist Oswaldo Cruz founded the Oswaldo Cruz Institute as a national public health organization. The institute's goal was to address health challenges at a time when many Brazilians believed that the poor, immigrants, and those of African descent were "naturally" sicker than others.[26] Using at-the-time widely accepted "scientific" methods like phrenology and eugenics, scholars, physicians, and others concluded that many in Brazil's population were "degenerate," a word that is found consistently in medical and health studies prior to 1945 and continues to be used in popular language about the poor, including by the poor and working classes themselves.[27]

In 1904 Brazil's House of Deputies approved Oswaldo Cruz's proposal for wide-ranging sanitary improvements, including a mandatory vaccination law. As in many countries, including wealthy and highly industrialized ones, health workers were given the legal right to enter homes to vaccinate people for smallpox, by force if necessary. Cruz also created "Mosquito-Killing Brigades," modeled after the rat-killing brigades discussed in chapter 6. The military designation—a brigade is a combat subdivision of an army—was part of a broader state approach that forced the public to build up health defenses to protect itself from being bombarded by diseases.[28]

The public reaction to the new health policies was mixed, although many Brazilians were eager for state-driven eradication and control measures. Indeed, in the second half of the twentieth century, vaccination rates in Brazil were very high. Members of the dominant classes generally welcomed health projects they believed would improve national "problems" of race, culture, labor, and poverty among immigrants and the African-descended citizenry. Disadvantaged populations often saw things differently, especially when health workers entered their homes with armed police escorts. Their frustration, and lack of confidence that the state could be trusted to develop a safe vaccine, led to the weeklong 1904 Vaccine Revolt, a Rio de Janeiro–centered civil uprising that left thirty people dead and hundreds more wounded or imprisoned.[29]

Residues of the kinds of conflicts that led to the Vaccine Revolt were clear in the health vigilance team's 2016 failure to enter that large building in Bom Retiro. Another example of tense state-public health relations came that same year when the Brazilian military, whose slogan is "strong arm: friendly hand," was tasked in February 2016 with conducting Zika mosquito eradication campaigns. This meant that uniformed military physicians were sometimes sent to public health clinics in the same neighborhoods where civilian deaths had occurred during "pacification" actions against drug trafficking (figure 5.5). The use of armed forces to fight disease appears to have been largely accepted by the targeted population, and there were no reports of violence against the doctors. Reports that the high command did not authorize entry into neighborhoods that they believed were controlled by criminal organizations, one of the clearest ways in which geographic areas are stigmatized in Brazil, may also have minimized violence against health care workers.[30]

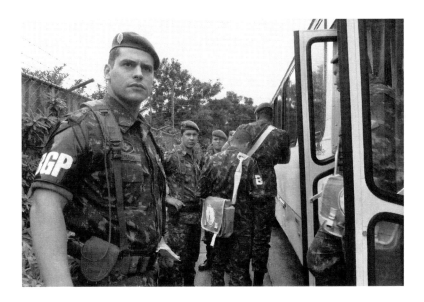

Figure 5.5 Soldiers from the Brazilian Armed Forces preparing to enter a neighborhood in search of the *Aedes aegypti* mosquito during the Zika outbreak of 2016. Source: Official Brazilian Ministry of Defense photograph by Tereza Sobreira, *Brazilian Army in Combat against the Aedes Mosquito*, Brasília—DF, January 15, 2016, Wikimedia Commons, https://commons.wikimedia.org/wiki/File:Ex%C3%A9rcito _Brasileiro_no_combate_ao_mosquito_Aedes_%2824653041645%29.jpg.

Sacred Spaces of Health

The actions discussed thus far began in health buildings ranging from the relatively small BRPHC to larger municipal health district offices. Health structures emerged in the nineteenth century as the state remade the built environment to give legitimacy to public health decisions. New neighborhoods had names like Saúde (Health), Higienópolis (Hygiene City), and the aforementioned Campo Limpo.[31] Such imprinting was not limited to the first decades of the Brazilian republic. In 2022 the Saúde Metro Station was rebranded Saúde-Ultrafarma, a nod to the profits generated by one of Brazil's largest drugstore chains.[32] New health buildings allowed laboratory testing and drug development. Hospitals and university training programs overlapped and dialoged with, and then slowly replaced, religious health institutions and colonial medical schools, just as happened throughout Latin America.[33] Architect Donatella Calabi's arguments about how urbanism emerged in early nineteenth-century Europe along with sanitary engineers

and medical hygienists is fully applicable to Brazil, where modern professions created novel health structures.[34]

Bernardino José de Campos Júnior, twice governor of the state of São
Paulo (August 1892–April 1896, July 1902–May 1904), was at the forefront
of modifying the built environment to achieve public health goals. A fawn-
ing tribute in a magazine focused on science and literature that was read
by many state leaders, laid out his approaches: "He organized the police
force, took over the reservoir and sewer services, developed the hygiene
and sanitation services . . . created the service for isolation and disinfection of ill people, founded bacteriological, pharmaceutical, and chemical
laboratories . . . and ordered the construction of isolation hospitals, created
the Vaccine Institute, and began building the Central Disinfectory."[35] The
latter was located in Bom Retiro, where immigrants were feared as disease
vectors and the geographic epicenter of bad health in São Paulo. The block
where the Central Disinfectory, the city's central health institution, was located was among the first to receive a sewer system, in 1893, although Bom
Retiro more broadly did not.[36] A decade later, the School of Pharmacy,
Dentistry, and Obstetrics was opened in Bom Retiro, further emphasizing
the neighborhood's connection to health.

Rafael Martins de Oliveira Laguardia has used cartographic analysis to de-
fine São Paulo's "sacred geographies," beginning in 1850 with a spatial analysis
focused on the elevation of Christian churches. As he shows, churches were
privileged spaces, and thus geography showed that they were of a higher
order, both religiously and financially. This connection of elevation to elite
status was also found among the small group of wealthy citizens who in the
late nineteenth and early twentieth centuries had enough capital to build
single-family homes. As Laguardia shows, the rich often built their homes in
a sacred geography of "higher elevations, over 750 meters [and] distant from
flooding."[37] In doing this, wealthy residents used geography and elevation to
reinforce the social gradient in which those with socioeconomic advantages
have better health and longer lives.[38] Thus, it may seem odd that I argue that
São Paulo's "sacred space of health" is in Bom Retiro, with its largely poor
and working-class population, low elevation, and constant flooding. Yet the
same wealth that created sacred residential areas of good health also created
spaces of bad health that they tried to control with an almost religious fervor.

To understand why one block in Bom Retiro has remained a center
of health activity for the entire city over time, I borrow from scholars of
European religion to view residues of Brazilian health institutions as part
of "sacred spaces of health." In Iberia, synagogues, churches, and mosques

were often built over each other rather than in new geographic locations. In São Paulo, religious sacred space also includes the placement of ostensibly Catholic churches on African memorial sites. The Igreja Santa Cruz das Almas dos Enforcados (Church of the Holy Cross of the Souls of the Hanged) is on the location of the whipping post in the Liberdade neighborhood.[39] The Templo de Salomão (Temple of Solomon) of the Universal Church of the Kingdom of God was constructed on a block filled with churches from competing Protestant and Catholic sects in the Brás neighborhood. A residue of the religious nature of health institutions from Brazil's colonial period is found in modern secular hospitals and clinics, where patients put their faith in biomedical solutions.

Bom Retiro's sacred space of health is bordered spatially by Rua Tenente Pena (where the health actions that began this chapter took place), Rua General Flores, Rua Solon, and the Rua dos Italianos. The residues of the faith imbued by politicians and public health officials in this health geography are found in the contemporary Museum of Public Health and Municipal Health Service warehouse, denominated an official heritage site in 1985. Both are in the former Central Disinfectory building, itself built on the grounds of what had been the Hospedaria dos Imigrantes and later was São Paulo's military hospital.[40] The contemporary BRPHC, opened in 1990 as part of a new national health plan that emerged after the overthrow of a military dictatorship, is also a residue of the original faith placed in that small space as a cure for the city's ills.[41] In the 1970s the municipality designated the site, which had previously housed a vaccination clinic and a treatment center for those with Hansen's disease, as the focal point of the much larger Santa Cecilia health district.[42]

By the turn of the twentieth century, no structure in São Paulo was more important to health policy and action than the Central Disinfectory. The institution's emphasis emerged from a still-prevalent seventeenth-century public health theory that diseases had their origin in miasmas, stinking odors that came from putrefying organic materials found on the ground in litter or in bedding and other residential materials that became contaminated and transmitted disease.[43] If the urban environment could be controlled, public health officials believed, the population would be cured via the elimination of material items that caused bad health. As Janes Jorge has shown, that goal was not achieved, and the connection of Bom Retiro with sickness persisted.[44]

The Central Disinfectory, like so many health buildings in this period across the Americas, was the physical manifestation of the fight against miasmas via public hygiene and its more contemporary residue, environmental medicine.[45] Disinfectories could be found throughout the Americas and Europe and were part of an operational public health arsenal since their leaders rarely made policy. G. W. McCaskey, an ear, nose, and throat specialist and professor at the Fort Wayne School of Medicine in Indiana, a state in the center of the United States, promoted the use of the word *disinfectory* in 1890 to make the nonpolicy work clear: "In view of its great importance and the desirability of having a single appropriate term to take the place of 'quarantine apparatus,' 'disinfection station,' 'disinfecting apparatus,' etc., I will venture to suggest the word *disinfectory* as applicable to the various institutions designed for practical disinfection."[46] McCaskey's article was republished in a number of medical journals in the United States, and disinfectories began springing up. Rio de Janeiro's first disinfection building was inaugurated in 1890, in the Praça XV de Novembro, next to the docks looking toward Niteroi, and another was opened in 1904.[47] San Remo, Italy, began constructing a "spacious public disinfectory" in 1892; following disease outbreaks, "whether occurring in hotels, lodging houses, or villas, the entire clothing outfit, linen, bedding, etc. . . . [would] be subjected to the action of super-heated steam, applied in the efficient manner of modern science."[48] In the United Kingdom, disinfection rooms began to be added to hospitals in the 1890s, and in 1912 Brazil's official representatives at the New York International Rubber Exposition promoted the need for disinfection rooms in Brazilian hospitals.[49]

São Paulo's Central Disinfectory changed the meaning of *disinfection* from a scientific process applied to material items to a social and cultural approach to controlling people. The floor plan included large sections for vehicles, used to expand the Disinfectory's reach far beyond the structure's walls, not just areas for receiving and disinfecting objects.[50] These vehicles were initially horse drawn, until the municipality paved the roads around the building so that motorized health enforcement vehicles could spread the sacred health power. Those vehicles did not just pick up materials to be disinfected (see figure 5.6) but took patients to isolation hospitals, transported cadavers to cemeteries (see figure 5.7), and brought disinfectors to the home of residents who had been denounced.[51]

The "vast" Central Disinfectory opened on November 1, 1893, as the first among equals in the state's Serviço Geral de Desinfecção (General Disinfection Service).[52] The director of the new institution, the physician Diogo Teixeira de Faria (1867–1927), was a typical public health official of his time. Born in Rio de Janeiro, Teixeira de Faria visited São Paulo as a medical student to participate in health actions to eliminate yellow fever in

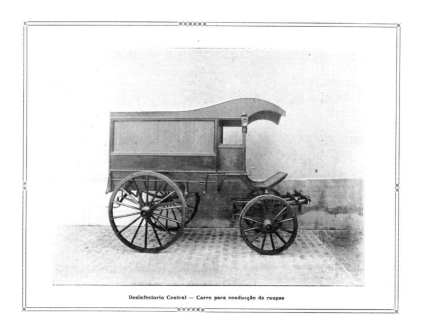

Desinfectorio Central — Carro para conducção de roupas

Figure 5.6 Vehicle used by the Central Disinfectory to remove infected clothing and bedding from homes. Source: *Álbum Serviço Sanitário do Estado de São Paulo: Algumas instalações do Serviço Sanitário de São Paulo* (São Paulo: Impresso gráfico, 1905), Fundo Serviço Sanitário de São Paulo, Acervo Instituto Butantan/ Museu de Saúde Pública Emílio Ribas.

the state's interior cities.[53] Upon graduation, he became the head of the Sanitary Commission in Campinas, a city less than a hundred kilometers from São Paulo that had been a slavocracy through the mid-nineteenth century. After abolition in 1888, Campinas continued to have a small landed class, a large population of African descent, and growing numbers of European immigrants. The city grew from about 17,000 in 1888 to almost twice that in 1896 and to over 115,000 in 1920, and with population density came infectious diseases.[54] In 1896 yellow fever killed more than seven hundred of the city's approximately thirty thousand residents, and in 1918–19 another four hundred died from the flu.[55]

With this background, Teixeira de Faria took leadership of the block encompassing the Central Disinfectory.[56] James Roberto Silva notes in his analysis of photographs of health institutions in São Paulo that "the Disinfectory was the embodiment of the sanitary police and photographs emphasize its military barracks-like construction, displaying the equipment, employees, vehicles

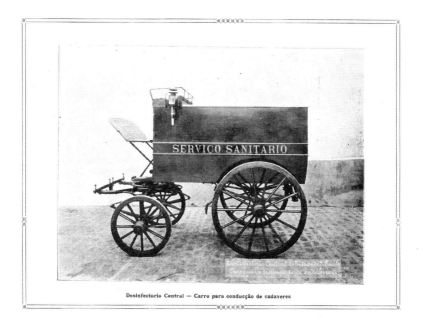

Desinfectorio Central — Carro para conducção de cadaveres

Figure 5.7 Vehicle used by the Central Disinfectory to remove cadavers from homes and public spaces. Source: *Álbum Serviço Sanitário do Estado de São Paulo: Algumas instalações do Serviço Sanitário de São Paulo* (São Paulo: Impresso gráfico, 1905), Fundo Serviço Sanitário de São Paulo, Acervo Instituto Butantan/Museu de Saúde Pública Emílio Ribas.

and animals, all in a position of readiness, with the gates open and the way clear."[57] Indeed, when I take colleagues and students on walking tours of Bom Retiro, they always think that the former Disinfectory building is related to the armed forces because it looks like a garrison(see figure 5.8).

The Disinfectory's operations were defined by a political decree. The twenty-one articles outlined everything from when to send sick patients to special hospitals, to how cadavers would be picked up, to how much potassium should be used to disinfect bloodstained clothing and sheets, to where official vehicles should park.[58] Agents had the right to enter private spaces and public buildings when they had even a suspicion of disease (figure 5.9).[59] The decree created two different types of health surveillance teams. One squad entered homes and removed sick people, items suspected of being infected, and dead bodies. A different crew was responsible for returning disinfected items like bedding, towels, and clothing to the population. The teams were available twenty-four hours a day, although the expectation was that actions

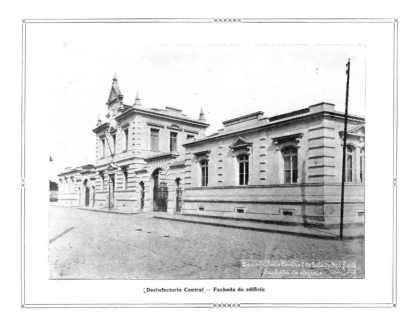

[Desinfectorio Central.— Fachada do edificio

Figure 5.8 The front of the Central Disinfectory, with its military-like facade, 1905. Source: *Álbum Serviço Sanitário do Estado de São Paulo: Algumas instalações do Serviço Sanitário de São Paulo* (São Paulo: Impresso gráfico, 1905), Fundo Serviço Sanitário de São Paulo, Acervo Instituto Butantan/Museu de Saúde Pública Emílio Ribas.

would take place during the workday. Later decrees expanded the reach of the Disinfectory; during the 1918 flu epidemic, health officials decreed that any residence with more than two deaths would be entered and disinfected.[60]

Disinfectory-related health actions frequently led to tense relations with the public. Jacob Penteado moved to Bom Retiro as a seven-year-old in 1907 and lived less than two blocks away from the building in a row of three connected cortiços owned by a Portuguese immigrant. He remembered how public health workers accompanied by police entered and disinfected residences with suspected cases of smallpox "and executed those tasks with such zeal and perfection."[61] Penteado wondered if an early twentieth-century slang word, *desinfete*, which meant that someone had suddenly disappeared, might have emerged from the forced removal of sick people from their homes.[62] Yet the removals of people were not mirrored by the removal of street waste, a primary cause of bad health in central São Paulo. A 1910 petition by immigrant residents of Bom Retiro (and the adjacent Luz district) complained that the Sanitary Service was not enforcing local laws regarding garbage collection,

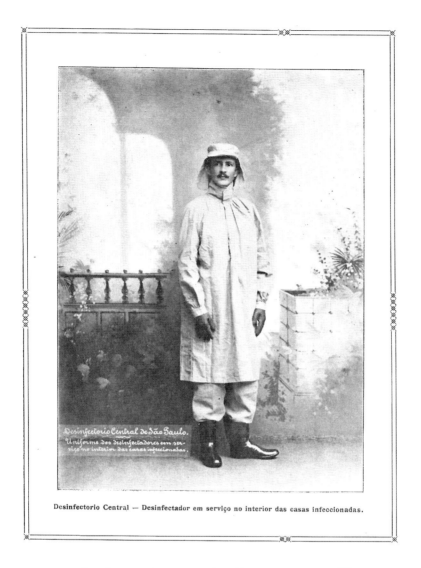

Desinfectorio Central — Desinfectador em serviço no interior das casas infeccionadas.

Figure 5.9 A disinfector working in an infected home, 1905. Source: *Álbum Serviço Sanitário do Estado de São Paulo: Algumas instalações do Serviço Sanitário de São Paulo* (São Paulo: Impresso gráfico, 1905), Fundo Serviço Sanitário de São Paulo, Acervo Instituto Butantan/Museu de Saúde Pública Emílio Ribas.

meaning that residents were "threatened by grave diseases and possible epidemics."[63]

Monthly publications and reports in newspapers highlighted the quantities of home disinfections and cadavers removed in horse-drawn carriages that resembled police paddy wagons, with entry from the rear and benches along the interior.[64] The vehicles emphasized social control as health officials took sheets, mattresses, curtains, rugs, and other textiles for disinfection by heat in large ovens. Leather, rubber, paper, and wood items were chemically disinfected, while bloody clothing was soaked in a mixture of water and potassium permanganate "to prevent permanent stains."[65]

For the working classes, the Disinfectory's actions were intrusive and militaristic. The upper classes saw things differently and believed the building and its employees reinforced their interests. Invited visitors were impressed by the modern technology in huge rooms, the large spaces for horse-drawn and motorized vehicles, and an attention to cleanliness that they believed separated the upper classes from the riffraff. As Daniel Reichman argues in a discussion of the artist Benedito Calixto's early twentieth-century painting *The Beach of São Vicente*, "modern" technologies were held in an almost religious reverence by the Brazilian upper classes, and even a sewer pipe could become "a thing of beauty."[66] Journalist Alfredo Moreira Pinto expressed a similar awe after visiting the Disinfectory in 1900, waxing poetic as he watched the "huge iron gates" open and close to let cadaver wagons and patient transports enter and exit.[67]

The wealthy's enthusiasm for the Disinfectory was more than visual or discursive. Health actions that emanated from building were different for the lower and upper classes. "Doentes de classe" (sick elites) were transported to the Isolation Hospital in a Berlinda, a spacious carriage with individual seats and a suspension system that made it particularly comfortable (figure 5.10). Everyone else used a cramped and uncomfortable wagon (figure 5.11).[68] The Isolation Hospital itself had a separate elegant pavilion where wealthy families could be accommodated, and a central atrium allowed sunbathing without leaving the building.[69] The Disinfectory thus mirrored and reinforced broader residential and transportation inequities. While the dominant classes lived in single-family homes that they owned, the working class resided in cortiços and informal housing. Elites used monogramed privately owned carriages driven by frock-wearing, top-hat-using, gloved employees. Carriages that worked the streets, on the other hand, were often helmed by cigar-smoking Italian immigrants in coconut-leaf hats.[70] Most people, of course, could only afford to walk.

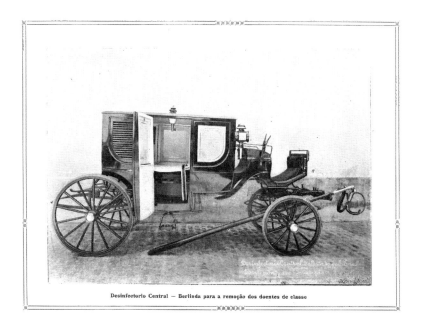

Desinfectorio Central — Berlinda para a remoção dos doentes de classe

Figure 5.10 Vehicle used by the Central Disinfectory to transport elites to health care facilities. Source: *Álbum Serviço Sanitário do Estado de São Paulo: Algumas instalações do Serviço Sanitário de São Paulo* (São Paulo: Impresso gráfico, 1905), Fundo Serviço Sanitário de São Paulo, Acervo Instituto Butantan/Museu de Saúde Pública Emílio Ribas.

The Central Disinfectory's use of space to control public health was not limited to the block on which it sat. The building's sacred geography meant that the sight lines from the tall building created a "Health Landscape," to paraphrase Thomas Rogers, whose groundbreaking coefficient you will learn about in chapter 6.[71] The Disinfectory also had an intensely reciprocal relationship with the Luz Railway Station, the large train station a little over a kilometer away.[72] Originally just a platform, the station expanded in 1888, just as the Disinfectory was being constructed. By 1893 the station and the Disinfectory, buildings with some of the largest footprints in São Paulo, worked together to control the health of the tens of thousands of immigrants from Europe, the Middle East, and Asia (in 1895 numbering about 140,000) who arrived at Luz Railway Station on their way to plantations or work in the urban economy.[73]

The interdependent dynamic among the built environment, health, and immigration emerged because officials considered newcomers the human vectors of disease, and their clothing and baggage the material vectors. Bom

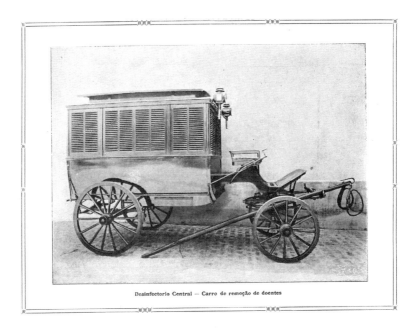

Desinfectorio Central — Carro de remoção de doentes

Figure 5.11 Vehicle used by the Central Disinfectory to transport nonelites to hospitals. Source: *Álbum Serviço Sanitário do Estado de São Paulo: Algumas instalações do Serviço Sanitário de São Paulo* (São Paulo: Impresso gráfico, 1905), Fundo Serviço Sanitário de São Paulo, Acervo Instituto Butantan/Museu de Saúde Pública Emílio Ribas.

Retiro, whether as a temporary place to pass through or as a more permanent residence, was a dangerous place, according to public health specialists, as non-Brazilians brought new and old diseases to the city. Policies and machines from the Disinfectory were linked to the Luz Railway Station in a 1896 decree that mandated that immigrant luggage be removed from arriving trains and "cleaned" in mobile disinfection units waiting at the station (figure 5.12).[74] Mobile public health vehicles had emerged in France in 1887 to control outbreaks of yellow fever and other diseases and to transport ill people from their homes to segregated locations without contact with the general population.[75] The Central Disinfectory's round disinfection chambers were first mounted on horse-drawn carriages, but in 1911 motorized vehicles, which remain on display today, diminished the time needed to move between the Disinfectory and the railway station (see figure 5.13).

Public health leaders in São Paulo were proud of the Central Disinfectory complex and what it represented. A 1905 Sanitary Service publication had more photos of the structure than any other health institution

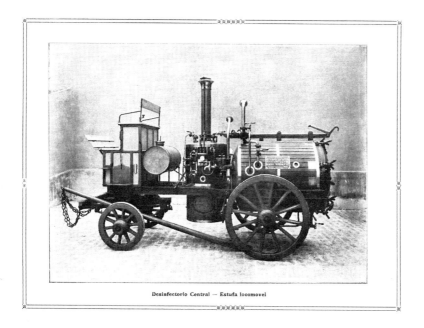

Desinfectorio Central — Estufa locomovel

Figure 5.12 A mobile disinfection vehicle, 1905. Behind the driver's seat is a tank with chemicals that are heated by a boiler, forcing the resulting gas into a wooden tank at the back. The boiler has controls for pressure, which in turn regulates the intensity of the chemical discharge. The wooden tank has pipes emerging from it that spray chemicals along the street as the vehicle passes. Source: *Álbum Serviço Sanitário do Estado de São Paulo: Algumas instalações do Serviço Sanitário de São Paulo* (São Paulo: Impresso gráfico, 1905), Fundo Serviço Sanitário de São Paulo, Acervo Instituto Butantan/Museu de Saúde Pública Emílio Ribas.

in the city.[76] Many images emphasized the authorities' readiness to disinfect and remove living and unliving people from their homes. Everything in the building, including ovens, laboratories, vehicles, scientists, and policymakers, was modern and reflected education and technology unavailable to most of the population. Many of the motorized vehicles were purchased from the Alma Manufacturing Company in Michigan, United States, the largest global manufacturer of trucks in the early twentieth century.[77] Mechanics in São Paulo converted the Hercules Trucks (later known as Republic Trucks), originally used for agricultural work, into mobile disinfection units.[78]

Vehicles acted as tentacles of health power as they traversed the streets between and around the Central Disinfectory and the Luz Railway Station and then reached into all parts of São Paulo. The presence of these vehicles,

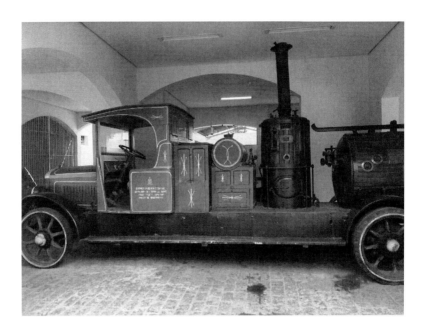

Figure 5.13 A mobile disinfection vehicle on display at the Emílio Ribas Public Health Museum, located in the building that was the Central Disinfectory. Source: Photograph by Jeffrey Lesser, May 2016.

especially during epidemics, made them part of the built environment, even if mobile. This was made clear in official photos from the late nineteenth to mid-twentieth century showing vehicles in front of the building, ready to move into action (see figures 5.14–5.16). The Disinfectory thus reterritorialized the city and its residents into "sick" and "well" spaces, ranging from the neighborhood to the home.[79] As health vehicles moved through urban spaces, they reminded the public that state control of the national body was intrusive and would become more so as transportation and communication technologies changed. Residents of Bom Retiro were particularly aware of the state's presence because their neighborhood was a primary target for health actions. The parade of vehicles going to and from the Disinfectory was a reminder that the built environment could be occupied at any time.

The public often resisted aggressive actions emanating from the Disinfectory. Refusing entry, as we saw at the beginning of the chapter, was typical in Bom Retiro and other working-class neighborhoods. Health agents who tried to enter homes were sometimes attacked, and residents also used the political apparatus, calling the police and petitioning

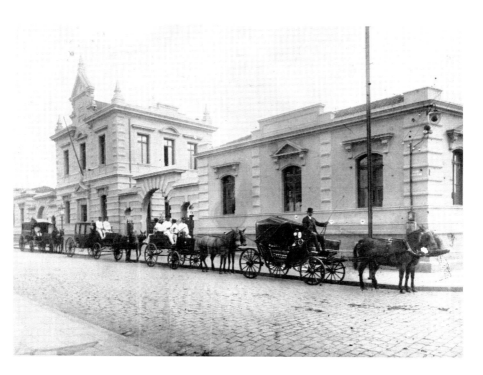

Figure 5.14 Facade of the Central Disinfectory with horse-drawn health service vehicles at the ready, ca. 1893. The vehicles have drivers whose white disinfection suits stand out visually. The vehicles are lined up in the following order: an elite passenger carriage, a transport vehicle filled with disinfectors, a people's passenger carriage, and a cadaver wagon. Source: Emílio Ribas Public Health Museum: Fachada do prédio do Desinfectório Central, R. Tenente Pena, Ampliação fotográfica, pb. [ca. 1893], Fundo Serviço Sanitário de São Paulo, Grupo: Desinfectório Central, Acervo Instituto Butantan/Museu de Saúde Pública Emílio Ribas.

municipal deputies. For example, residents refused to accept a state action in 1919, when Disinfectory officials proposed new stables for horse-drawn carriages at an intersection across the street from the Disinfectory, in front of the contemporary BRPHC. Since motorized disinfection units and cadaver wagons frequently needed repair, health officials argued that having backup vehicles would ensure continuity in removing the sick and dead from public spaces and private residences. Residents of Bom Retiro fought against stables since they were "breeding grounds for mosquito-borne diseases."[80] Why not, they argued, build a play area for children since many Brazilians agreed that youth hanging out on the streets was a problem?[81]

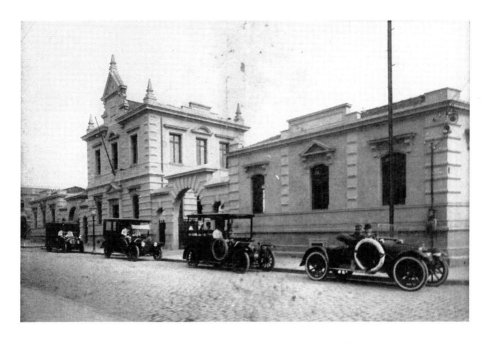

Figure 5.15 Facade of the Central Disinfectory with motorized heath service vehicles at the ready, 1900–1920. Source: Emílio Ribas Public Health Museum: Fachada do prédio do Desinfectório Central, R. Tenente Pena, Ampliação fotográfica, pb. [ca. 1900–1920], Fundo Serviço Sanitário de São Paulo, Grupo: Desinfectório Central, Acervo Instituto Butantan/Museu de Saúde Pública Emílio Ribas.

Residents petitioned municipal deputy Armando Prado, a member of the Justice and Police Commission and a long-term advocate of eliminating cortiços as a threat to the public's health. He argued to his colleagues that the erection of these stables would lead to fatal illnesses in "that populous neighborhood," which at the time had almost twenty-seven thousand residents and an average of nine people living in each home.[82] In 1919 Bom Retiro was one of the six neighborhoods along the Tietê River where officials shut down 345 stables and ordered the renovation of 149 more (out of a total of 1,418) to control mosquito breeding sites and the corresponding diseases.[83] While municipal health officials hailed the elimination of "insect clouds" near the rivers in 1919, residents of the neighborhood knew this claim was false and must have wondered why the Disinfectory wanted to build another large stable.

In the end, the residents won, and the stables were not built. Even so, the geographic location of the proposed construction remained part of São Paulo's sacred health geography. In 1925 a model health clinic (one of only

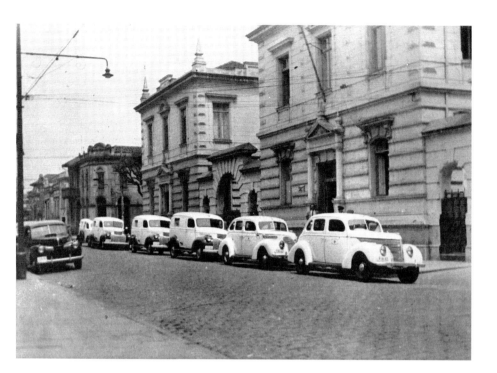

Figure 5.16 Facade of the Central Disinfectory with motorized ambulances and Sanitary Service vehicles at the ready, likely from the 1950s. The four larger vehicles have a door at the back for carrying materials or cadavers. Source: Emílio Ribas Public Health Museum: Fachada do Desinfectório Central com ambulâncias e carros de vigilância, data ca. 1938–75, Ampliação fotográfica, pb, Fundo Serviço Sanitário de São Paulo, Acervo Instituto Butantan/Museu de Saúde Pública Emílio Ribas.

two in the city at the time) was established in the space to much fanfare because of its free vaccinations.[84] Starting in 1940, legal sex workers went to a building on the lot for weekly venereal disease checkups, and in the 1950s it became a Hansen's disease treatment center.[85]

This chapter has argued that buildings and vehicles were as critical as people in creating and expanding the health state in its multiple guises. Imposing health buildings were surrounded by armed guards and dominated the built environment (as is still true). Yet, as I have shown, health workers were as intimidated by immigrant-occupied tenements and unregistered microfactories as residents of Bom Retiro were by health buildings and vehicles. The chapter has wandered between the past and the present, focusing on tensions between the state and the population over disease control and mosquito eradication to show how the residues of public health workers' attitudes about immigrants continue into the present.

The residues of the Disinfectory are easy to find in Bom Retiro. The building today houses the Emílio Ribas Public Health Museum, opened in 1979, the same year that four major municipal public health units were placed in the structure.[86] *The building remains a location for the spread of health power throughout the city as the transportation center of the Secretary of Health. One side of the building has a courtyard where early twentieth-century mobile disinfection units are displayed.*[87]

In 1979 Bom Retiro became the central location for the new Santa Cecilia health district, becoming the "Dr. Octavio Augusto Rodovalho" health district in 1983 in honor of a physician and faculty member at the University of São Paulo's School of Public Health.[88] *Health services today are delivered by the* BRPHC, *located on the plot of land that led to the 1919 stable dispute. While contemporary Bom Retiro's residents do not have the same contentious relationship with the* BRPHC *that others had with the Disinfectory, it is hard not to notice that the guarded building has a floor plan that could easily be mistaken for that of a nineteenth-century military hospital.*[89] *The western wall of the* BRPHC *is on the Rua do Areal, which today has three-story buildings that previously were home to eastern European, primarily Jewish, immigrants in the years around World War II. Today most of those buildings contain oficina-residências. One exception is a small precarious dwelling built out of cardboard that uses one side of the* BRPHC *as a fixed wall. That tiny shelter houses one man who sometimes uses the clinic lavatory facilities but whose health care takes place in a Unified Health System–operated ambulatory clinic since public health clinics are officially for residents with formal addresses.*

The contemporary BRPHC *is filled with immigrant patients. While health professionals today, as in the past, are overwhelmingly monolingual in Portuguese, the languages of their patients have changed, from Italian, Greek, and Yiddish to Chinese, Guarani, Hindi, Korean, and Spanish. Occupation of space by health workers also continues, although the aggressive modernity of vehicles transporting disinfection workers accompanied by armed police has been replaced by health teams that move through the neighborhood on foot, wearing blue vests over street clothing. Whether in 1890 or 2020, the health state is ever present.*

6

Unliving Rats and Undead Immigrants

The Two Deaths of Quincas Berro Dágua

To this day, there remains confusion surrounding the death of Quincas Berro Dágua. Unexplained doubts, absurd details, contradictions in the testimony of witnesses, various gaps. There is no clarity about time, place, and last words.

Missing PM Is Found Dead, Naked, and Tied Up inside a Pushcart in Downtown SP

A military policeman who had been missing since Friday [November 16, 2020] was found dead, naked, and tied up inside a cart in the Cracolândia region, downtown São Paulo, this Saturday (17).

The case was registered as qualified homicide in the 2nd Police District (DP), Bom Retiro. Daniel Lima worked in the 1st Company of the 18th Battalion of the Military Police, in Presidente Prudente, in the interior of the state, the city where he was born.

After identifying the body, the Civil Police sought to understand what Daniel was doing in the Cracolândia region . . . known for drug trafficking and consumption. The preliminary information is that he went there with the intention of evangelizing addicts and other residents.

According to the incident report, military police officers were patrolling the region on Saturday and decided to approach the four men pushing the cart. . . . Initially, the suspects said they were carrying rubble. When the MPs found a cadaver in the wagon, the men claimed they didn't know there was a dead body inside. Some parts of the corpse were crushed, according to police. The body was hidden under blankets inside the wagon.

Physical and discursive violence rise during global health crises.[1] When infectious diseases are named for the supposed geographic locations where they originated, individuals linked to those places, like immigrants or ethnic groups, are often stigmatized and targeted. In the twentieth century alone, the Spanish flu, the West Nile virus, and the Middle East respiratory syndrome have become household names. Increases in anti-Asian violence in Brazil and the United States directly emerged from comments linking COVID-19 to China, for example, calling it the Wuhan virus, by the racist (and sexist and homophobic and . . .) one-term presidents of the two countries, Jair Bolsonaro and Donald Trump.[2]

This chapter analyzes why public health officials targeted Bom Retiro and its residents during the turn-of-the-century bubonic plague and 1918 influenza outbreaks. I show how the two epidemics led to similar discourses from health officials, often targeting immigrants.[3] The immigrant working classes responded to the two events in similar ways as well, ranging from using popular medicinal practices for care and cure, to rising from the dead to wander to and from Bom Retiro.[4]

We met the Syrian resident of Bom Retiro João Antônio Jorge in chapter 4 after his 1916 altercation with an Italian immigrant over a loan. Two years later Jorge still lived in Bom Retiro, in a tiny room called "a flea pit" by *A Capital*, at the back of a cortiço at Rua Barra do Tibagi, 70, about a ten-minute walk from the Central Disinfectory, close to the Tietê River.[5] His experiences in 1918, as a victim of the H1N1 virus, popularly known with names like the Dakar sickness or the Spanish flu, illustrate the discursive and physical racism that emerge during pandemics.[6]

Jorge was often referred to in the press as João Turco (João the Turk), just one of many João Turcos in São Paulo, where calling Brazilians by national names like German, Japanese, Italian, or Portuguese is part of the racialized quotidian discourse.[7] In 1913 the police profiled one João Turco, along with another Syrian immigrant, in a violent and sensational strangulation case, although they were eventually exonerated.[8] "Lord João Turco" appeared as lead "folião" (merrymaker) of a São Paulo carnival club during the 1919 carnival.[9] In 1921 another João Turco, a known counterfeiter, was involved in a shootout at the Ideal Club, where he ran an illegal gambling operation.[10] In 1927 *O Estado de S. Paulo* denominated a gang of Spanish immigrants running a horse-racing gambling operation "the São Paulo João-Turcos."[11] All of these João Turcos had something in common: they were marked as money hungry, untrustworthy, and violent, all accusations leveled against the "Syrian dentist" in the Amelia Marini case discussed in chapter 1.

Bom Retiro's João Turco contracted the flu in late October 1918. He was interned by relatives at an improvised hospital in Bom Retiro's Diocesan School, at the time located on the Avenida Tiradentes, just a few minutes' walk from the Tiradentes Prison. According to the anarchist newspaper *O Combate*, João Antônio Jorge stayed at the hospital for only a few days because he "could not stand the food." This explanation is unlikely. Probably Jorge, like many in São Paulo's working class, feared hospitals since infections spread through the cramped spaces and rumors of unnatural deaths were rampant. Anxiety about being in hospitals was so widespread during the flu that many beds went unoccupied despite the large numbers of sick people.[12]

A few days after leaving the hospital, Jorge had a relapse on November 9, 1918. His family returned him to the improvised hospital, where he was diagnosed with pneumonia as well as the flu. Newspaper reports then differ. According to *A Capital*, Jorge's condition was so bad that the physician on duty, who did "not believe in miracles" and was sure he would die, sent him to the room where bodies were viewed prior to burial.[13] *O Combate* told the story differently, linking Jorge's case directly to public health leadership actions. In this version the Bom Retiro resident was examined by the former director of São Paulo's Sanitary Service and the most famous physician in the state, Emílio Ribas, and his son, who had the same name and profession. Together, the two pronounced Jorge dead. While awaiting transport to the cemetery, however, the corpse came back to life, speaking and asking for water.[14]

Jorge's return from the dead reflected and reinforced a working-class belief that the public health services were at best incompetent and at worst malevolent. His story can be interpreted in multiple ways. On the one hand, the ostensibly incorrect and deadly diagnosis suggests that Jorge's life was unimportant, that he was the victim of medical ethnic and class profiling. A different interpretation might be that he returned to life because of "Arab" spiritual power. The two doctors Ribas saw things differently, telling *O Combate* that because of his pneumonia, Jorge had been sent to an isolation room, where he became confused after waking up in a space meant to prevent disease transmission.[15]

It is no accident that Jorge's return from the dead took place in Bom Retiro. His story, and earlier ones emerging from the 1899 bubonic plague, concretized the bad health imaginaries that had begun with the widespread illnesses suffered by those in the Hospedaria dos Imigrantes. As Ricardo Augusto dos Santos notes in his comparative study of popular symbols and disease in Brazil, "Whether the plague, flu, or cholera, the association between disease and divine punishment is present. Individuals with 'suspicious' behavior were and are identified as propagators of evil, whether poor, Jewish, Irish, or Black. But there is one element that is always constant: fear."[16] Health care workers, policymakers, and portions of the public showed their prejudices during health emergencies, often questioning the national identity shifts that emerged as the citizenry became more diverse. Immigrants expressed their concerns with state policies by rejecting and manipulating science, seeking alternative cures, and returning to life after dying. João Antônio Jorge's story, and others that connect immigrants with the epidemics that I explore in this chapter, emerged from racism, poor working and living conditions, and their associated stressors. All show how global and local issues—workers' strikes, climate changes affecting agricultural production, and wars and uprisings—reinforced xenophobia.

Rats!

As the twentieth century approached, the bubonic plague seemed to have disappeared in Europe and the Americas, with the last reported outbreak in Marseille, France, in 1720. Scientists celebrated the 1894 finding that *Pasteurella pestis* (today known as *Yersinia pestis*) was transmitted to humans by fleas living on rats, and in 1898 human trials of vaccines began. Perhaps, then, the small August 13, 1899, note in Rio de Janeiro's *Jornal do Commercio* that the Argentine consulate was investigating reports of the plague in the Portuguese city of Porto went unnoticed by Brazil's public health leaders.[17] That lack of awareness lasted less than twenty-four hours. As soon as Nuno Ferreira de Andrade, a physician and Brazil's inspector general of port health, received the information, he ordered that ships arriving in Rio de Janeiro from Portuguese and Spanish ports enter a twenty-day quarantine and receive deep cleaning.[18] Andrade knew what he was doing. He had been part of a team that contained an 1866 cholera outbreak by constructing a quarantine center on the Ilha das Flores, where Rio de Janeiro's Hospedaria dos Imigrantes was located.[19] Yet in mid-August 1899 the scientifically sound decision became controversial, and many Rio de Janeiro merchants questioned the quarantine policy even as the epidemic spread rapidly to other parts of Brazil.[20]

The plague's appearance in Santos, the São Paulo state port at which most immigrants to Brazil arrived, is often attributed to the ship *O Rei de Portugal*, which arrived from Porto in October 1899. Almost immediately after the ship docked, public health officials recorded an explosion in rat deaths. Yet attempts to declare a medical emergency were stymied, as had happened in Rio de Janeiro, by businesspeople who called fears of the plague "propaganda."[21] It did not take long, however, for illness to spread. Fernando Prestes de Albuquerque, president of São Paulo province, expanded the number of health personnel at the port, ordering them to use "every sanitary policing approach based in science."[22]

The preventative measures taken by São Paulo state's leaders were far too late since the plague was already in Santos. Four months before *O Rei de Portugal* had docked, large and unexplained increases in rat deaths in warehouses along the docks were observed following the June arrival of ships from Burma and Mozambique.[23] In September 1899 rat deaths again surged, this time in residences near the docks, and large buboes were discovered during the autopsy of a quarantined yellow fever patient.[24] The plague quickly spread from Santos to other places. One destination was New York City on the British steamship *J. W. Taylor*, which on arrival was quarantined, containing the disease.[25] Another destination was São Paulo as the disease traveled along the railroad tracks connecting the port to the city.

In early November 1899 São Paulo city officially registered the first case of the bubonic plague although the disease had already been spreading. Two of São Paulo's top public health officials, Emílio Ribas and Adolpho Lutz, began intensive research and control programs in Santos, and in 1902 São Paulo's Butantan Institute developed a vaccine.[26] While Ribas and Lutz focused on rats and fleas, other public health officials targeted the human vectors, including by quarantining immigrants. Landowners and factory owners rejected the preventative policies, believing that immigrant entry was necessary for the production of agricultural and manufactured goods. These competing positions put Bom Retiro in the crosshairs, just as happened in other immigrant neighborhoods in the Americas. Chinese immigrants were targeted in Sinaloa, Mexico, and Lima, Peru, during an outbreak of the bubonic plague, leading to a series of new immigration restrictions, including, in the Peruvian case, demands for a health passport for Asian arrivals.[27] A rumor that a Chinese immigrant had died of bubonic plague in San Francisco in the United States led public health officials to quarantine that city's Chinatown neighborhood in 1900, as some San Franciscans demanded the district be burned to the ground. The city's board of health even gave physicians permission to forcibly inoculate Asians with a vaccine, at the time still being tested for efficacy.[28]

The violent approaches in the United States took different forms in São Paulo, where the Central Disinfectory became the headquarters for plague eradication. Using the language of war, public health officials in 1899 increased surveillance of immigrants in public spaces. Agents expanded forced entry into intimate spaces as they searched for rats, extending the Disinfectory's physical and symbolic space beyond its material confines. Municipal administrators reshaped the subsoil geography via the sewer system, focusing on Bom Retiro because of its foreignness, poor sanitation infrastructure, high population density, and informal housing.[29]

The focus on disease transmission led the Sanitary Service to use a tactic mirrored in other global cities: pay the public to find dead rats and bring them to public health officials for study and incineration.[30] To promote the program, they filled newspapers with "We Need Rats" advertisements. The service published a multilingual health publication, one of the very few in a language other than Portuguese produced until the twenty-first century. It was titled *PESTE* (The plague), with "Kill the Rats" splashed across the cover in red, and the text was in Portuguese, Italian, German, French, and English.[31] *PESTE* and other public communications used militaristic language to motivate the public: "Mobilize in a war to kill rats and fleas." Yet the bellicose approach also connected to the many foreigners who lived in working-class neighborhoods, making immigrants as much of a target as rats.

While we do not know whether *PESTE* had a significant readership, we do know that the population was as aware of the connections among rats, fleas, and the plague. Jokes circulated about eating a "bubonic pastry," a play on "bubonic plague" based on the similarity of the words *pastéis* and *pestes*.[32] João do Rio (the pen name of the journalist and chronicler of everyday life João Paulo Emílio Cristóvão dos Santos Coelho Barreto, 1881–1921) wrote of a popular turn-of-the-century ditty:

> Os ratos fazem qui, qui, qui,
> Qui, qui, qui, qui, qui
> As pulgas pulam daqui
> Pra ali, dali praqui, daqui prali
> Os gatos fazem miau
> Miau, miau, miau
> Quem inventou a peste bubônica
> Merece muito pau.[33]

(The rats make the sound, qui, qui, qui
Qui, qui, qui, qui, qui
The fleas jump from them
From there to there to there
The cats say meow
Meow, meow, meow
Whoever invented the bubonic plague
Deserves a beating.)

Wars needed weapons, and the Central Disinfectory became an armory. Health agents distributed strong-smelling disinfectants to treat trash, sanitizers for textiles, and a paste-like venom that could be placed in pieces of bread or meat and spread throughout the home. Public health officials devised three approaches to communicate with the public about how to use these products. First, they used pamphlets like PESTE although I found little evidence of any significant distribution. Second, they had the press publish everything from formulas to make rat poison with grated cheese to global mortality information.[34] Information in newspapers demanded access, time, and reading knowledge of Portuguese, and it is hard to judge the impact of this material on the working-class public, especially immigrants. Third, the most direct "education" took place as health agents forced their way into homes, where language confusion created tension and limited impact, just as it does today when Portuguese-speaking public health workers work with immigrant patients.

Like many public health programs, deratification often had unintended consequences, leading to bad health outcomes. While dead rats in homes were to be reported but not touched, agents were slow to remove them. For the public, getting venom was not as easy as it seemed to officials, who boasted that a center-city pharmacy, located at Rua Florencia de Abreu, 21, would distribute the paste free of charge each day from 1 to 3 p.m. Yet getting to the pharmacy, during the middle of the workday, was not easy. For residents of Bom Retiro, the pharmacy was about a thirty-minute walk away, and the process would likely mean missing a half day of work and income, or risking getting fired. A horse-drawn trolley might be quicker, but the costs were prohibitive (more expensive than public transportation in Berlin and Buenos Aires at the time).[35] Those who did get free venom quickly realized that it could also make humans sick, and some people used it to attempt suicide or poison spouses.[36] The chemicals caused unintentional poisoning too, especially among children.[37] Almost a century later, the connection of rats, chemicals, and children continued, even appearing connected to Bom Retiro in popular music.[38]

New industries sprang up to take advantage of the antirat campaign, often playing on a lack of public confidence in government pronouncements. A front-page article in *O Commercio de São Paulo* argued that rats should not be killed with chemical poison since this would lead to environmental pollution and harm residents.[39] Not surprisingly, "green" rat-killing solutions became the rage. Typical was the "Paraná Formicide," made from forest plants from the state of Paraná, which received a government patent in 1899. Within a year its inventor had opened stores in São Paulo.[40] Rat killing also spurred scams, especially the commercial sale of false venom. José Álvares de Souza Soares, founder of a homeopathic laboratory in Pelotas, Rio Grande do Sul, promoted his rat-killing venom as a "splendid triumph" in his free 1889 pamphlet *O Novo Médico ou a medicina simplificada ao alcance de toda a gente* (The New Doctor or simplified medicine available to all). He was, however, termed a charlatan by the government.[41]

Offering bounties for dead rats was one of the most important municipal public health initiatives. The rodents, recognized by authorities as the vectors of plague, were then incinerated at the Central Disinfectory. The program and the prices were widely publicized in the printed press, often with notices next to the lottery advertisements.[42] The public responded enthusiastically, even though collecting rats for bounties contradicted the public health instruction to never touch dead rodents. Gnawers-for-money transactions, often by children, exploded along with incinerations at the Central Disinfectory (see figures 6.1 and 6.2). Fourteen thousand rats were sold in November 1899, when each one was valued at four hundred reis, an amount remembered by one chronicler as "good money at that time."[43] Given the cost and time of travel, even within the center city, I wonder if there were rat brokers in other working-class neighborhoods in São Paulo who transported them to Bom Retiro.

Over seventeen thousand rats were incinerated in both December 1899 and January 1900.[44] Over the next few years, the numbers of rats purchased and then burnt were carefully recorded by officials, who published the information each day. The monetary value of rodents decreased over the course of the antirat war, from the original four hundred reis to three hundred reis in early 1903 and then to two hundred reis later that year.[45] This final figure put São Paulo prices in line with those in Rio de Janeiro. There, Oswaldo Cruz led an eradication campaign using the public and vaccinated professional ratcatchers as cases of plague dropped from 48.74 per 100,000 residents in 1903 to 1.73 per 100,000 in 1909.[46]

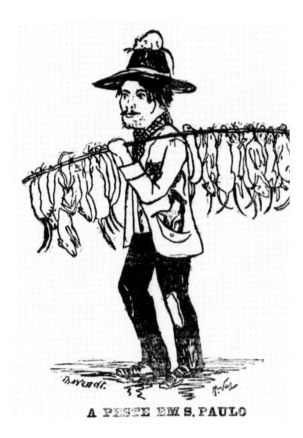

Figure 6.1 "The Plague in S. Paulo." Source: *O Commercio de São Paulo*, October 28, 1899, 1, http://memoria.bn.br/DocReader/DocReader.aspx?bib=227900&pesq=veneno%20ratos&pasta=ano%20190&hf=memoria.bn.br&pagfis=7943.

A PESTE EM S. PAULO

I wanted to get a better sense of the decreasing value of São Paulo's rats from the public's perspective. Thus, I used the Rogers Coefficient, which compares costs to the price of a bottle of beer from a case of forty-eight produced by the Companhia Antarctica Paulista.[47] Using this approach, I found the number of rats a person needed to buy a bottle of beer rose rapidly, from two to three rats per bottle in 1899 to five to six rats per bottle in 1903.

The differing ways that the public, and public health officials, understood health slowed the eradication of the bubonic plague. These multiple views became apparent with the 1903 end of deratification. Public health officials were disappointed that, as happened in other global cities, catching and selling rats had become an income generator for parts of the working-class public: "it is the daily bread for many people."[48] Another concern was that some enterprising Brazilians were breeding rats or catching them outside of São Paulo city and importing them. An audit of a huge payment for rats in

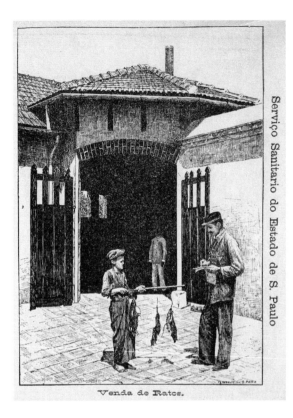

Serviço Sanitario do Estado de S. Paulo

Venda de Ratos.

Figure 6.2
Engraving depicting the sale of rats by children to the Central Disinfectory, 1900. Source: *Revista Médica de S. Paulo*. Ano III (São Paulo: Escola Typ. Salesiana, 1900).

Rio de Janeiro found that a "person of great business skills" was both breeding and buying rats for sale.[49] There were also accusations that the public was successfully selling false rats constructed from paper and wax.[50] These actions were not uniquely Brazilian. In Hanoi, Vietnam, some members of the public began raising rats, or freeing rats after cutting off their tails, to receive a bounty offered by the French colonial regime in 1902.[51]

Public health authorities complained that working-class populations were selling rats for the wrong reason—to make money—implying that immigrants were bringing the plague to Brazil for profit. The public was equally distrustful of authorities, and rumors abounded that those in working in the health arena were illegally profiting from rat killing and buying. Some pharmacists were accused of keeping the grated-cheese portion of the venom formula for themselves, creating a shortage of both in the city.[52] There were also allegations of an active rat-catching mafia, although there is no record of imprisonments. The *Lavoura e Commercio* newspaper claimed the deratification program was about enriching those with money, not promoting public health.[53] The newspaper posited that rat bounties had become a form of upward income redistribution to the wealthy and powerful. A 1900 front-page editorial dripped with sarcasm:

> In the news about public health that this newspaper receives each day, I read something really interesting—the rats incinerated each day are mostly brought from the countryside by a dedicated friend of our health—and the moneymakers at the Disinfectory.
>
> The little man wants to monopolize the rat hunt and is determined to cleanse the State of these rodents. Hygiene officials see rats as a danger, and this famous ratophobe, full of zeal for public health, also sees it as a danger. It is also a gold mine, and he tenaciously and calmly herds the harmful little animals and Sanitary Service funds.
>
> He brings a huge bunch every single day, with an English punctuality and a charming modesty, without complaint, just him and his mice. What an uplifting example of civility.
>
> Physicians working with the sanitary services, jealous perhaps of the selflessness of the ratcatcher—go on burning the animals, and quietly pay for each one, without remembering to tell the population what a great friend they have in that enemy of the rats.
>
> No. We need the hero's name to appear. Such examples of love for the public cause are rare, and therefore worthy of great tribute. How can mankind receive praise if we don't know how to direct the expressions of our gratitude?
>
> It is quite possible that he, always modest, would prefer to receive the Disinfectory's money instead of the homage, as he has done so far. But he is likely to prefer the gratitude of the public over the government's money, as he has humbly done to this day. But that is not a reason to leave him in the shadows where he insists on remaining.
>
> It is necessary, therefore, that the name of this devoted citizen be offered the grandness of our recognition. It is necessary to give him a place in our heart—and another with the police.[54]

The Disinfectory stopped paying for rats in 1903 as the bubonic plague was increasingly contained with vaccines. The rodents, however, lived on. In 1902 Casemiro Rocha, trumpeter for the Fireman's Band of Rio de Janeiro, composed the instrumental polka "Rato Rato" (Rat, rat), whose sound was intended to mimic the call to action of Oswaldo Cruz's rat-catching teams.[55]

Two years later São Paulo's Claudino Manuel da Costa composed lyrics to "Rato Rato," and the song became a hit at the 1904 carnival, leading the duo to release another health-related song, "Febre Amarela" (Yellow fever), three years later.[56] "Rato Rato" was an homage to antirat campaigns and even referenced rat-selling schemes. For our purposes, however, the critical lyric connected the bubonic plague to eastern European immigration:

> Who invented you?
> It was the devil, it wasn't anyone else, believe me.
> Who gave birth to you?
> It was a mother-in-law just before she died!
> Who created you?
> It was revenge, I think
> Rat, Rat, Rat
> Emissary of the Jew.[57]

Flu!

There is no consensus on the geographic origin of the 1918–19 global H1N1 epidemic, widely tagged as the Spanish flu. Yet countless public health officials, and many among the Brazilian public, connected diseases to newcomers and the countries from which they emigrated, a pattern that continued throughout the twentieth century (see figure 6.3). The linkage was more than discursive; physicians at São Paulo's Isolation Hospital inserted "Spanish Flu" after scratching-out the row previously reserved for the bubonic plague on mortality forms.[58]

The flu killed between twenty and a hundred million people worldwide and infected hundreds of millions in a few months.[59] The long-term global impact of the infectious disease stretched well beyond morbidity and mortality, yet the collective memory of the 1918 flu is surprisingly sparse, perhaps because the lack of control put it out of mind.[60] This does not seem the case in São Paulo. One of Brazil's most popular telenovelas, the 495-episode *Os Imigrantes*, (The immigrants) frequently referenced the flu, both for its impact on individuals and for the creation of negative public opinion about immigrants.[61] In the twenty-first century, an explosion of books and articles sought to link the H1N1 "Spanish flu" to the COVID-19 "Chinese flu," although the continuity of racialized geographic/ethnic terminology usually went unmentioned.

Centuries of widespread connections between outsiders and bad health in the Americas seemed to prophesize that immigrants would bring a

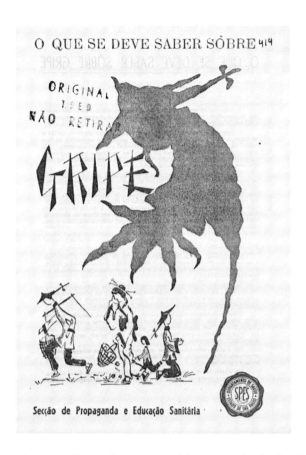

Figure 6.3 Cover of a 1958 pamphlet put out by the Section for Propaganda and Sanitary Education that uses stereotypes of Chinese and Japanese and the specter of a Chinese monster as educational tools about the so-called Asian flu. The text reads "What you should know about flu." Source: Folhetos de campanha de saúde, Gripe, Ministério da saúde, Seção de Propaganda e Educação Sanitária (do Estado de SP), Secretaria dos Negócios de Educação/Serviço de Saúde Escolar, Serviço Nacional de Educação Sanitária, Serviço de Educação Sanitária, Laboratório Sanitas, Acervo Museu de Saúde Pública Emílio Ribas/Instituto Butantan. Note: The archive shows the material as undated; the dating comes from Ademir Medici, "Asseio corporal. Combate à raiva. Noções sobre nutrição. Estamos em 1958 . . . ," *Diário do Grande ABC*, February 10, 2022, https://www.dgabc.com.br/Noticia/3829719/asseio-corporal-combate-a-raiva-nocoes-sobre-nutricao-estamos-em-1958; and Gilberto Hochman, "A gripe asiática vem aí! Crônica de uma pandemia antes de sua chegada (Brasil, 1957)," *Revista Ciencias de la Salud* 19 (July 2021): 1–22, https://doi.org/10.12804/revistas.urosario.edu.co/revsalud/a.10599.

Spanish flu–like malady.[62] In the United States, there was localized violence against newcomers since "when many Americans pondered health menaces from abroad, it was not *la grippe* that sprang to mind, but the millions of immigrants who had been flowing through the nation's ports and across its borders."[63] If immigrants *were* the flu, then the arrival of the "Spanish" in Brazil was terrifying as foreign entry surged in the aftermath of World War I. The disease made immigrants and their descendants in São Paulo, of whom Spaniards made up a significant portion, renewed targets of state policy and popular prejudice. The cartoon in figure 6.4 references Black-white relations, immigrant-native relations, and class relations with its play on the word *hespanhola*, used to refer both to an immigrant woman from Spain and to the flu.

In São Paulo the "Spanish Flu" epidemic officially lasted sixty-six days, from October 14 to December 19, 1918, although it likely began in March and stretched into 1920. While statistics, and the practices that underlay them, underestimate the demographic impact, they are still impressive: two-thirds of São Paulo's population of 528,295 became sick in 1918. One percent of the population (5,331 people) died.[64] During the peak, from November 1 to November 23, almost 4,200 people died in the city, in some cases entire families.[65] The year after the flu, there was a significant increase in infant mortality and stillbirths. Lessened literacy among women who stayed out of school because of the flu was apparent until 1940. The demographic shock had an economic impact as well, and "short-run agricultural productivity, as measured by the volume of coffee, rice and maize per capita, declined in 1920."[66]

One official story has the first Brazilian deaths from the flu among members of a medical mission leaving Dakar, Senegal, onboard the *La Plata* in September 1918. Even though the ship had eighty physicians aboard, 156 people died of what the mission chief called a "mysterious illness."[67] A report to authorities in Brazil was censored because of wartime rules but still reached the Academia Paulista de Medicina (São Paulo Academy of Medicine), which did not opine about the nature of the sickness.[68]

Another official story has the flu arriving in Brazil in September 1918 aboard the *Demerara*, owned by the British Royal Mail and named after a British Guiana colony often remembered for its 1823 revolt of enslaved peoples.[69] The liner steamed along the Liverpool–Buenos Aires route and carried mail, passengers, and goods such as sugar, returning to Europe primarily with meat and coffee. Digitalized records of immigrants, primarily from southern Europe, who registered at the São Paulo Hospedaria dos Imigrantes before being sent to plantations suggest that the *Demerara*'s first

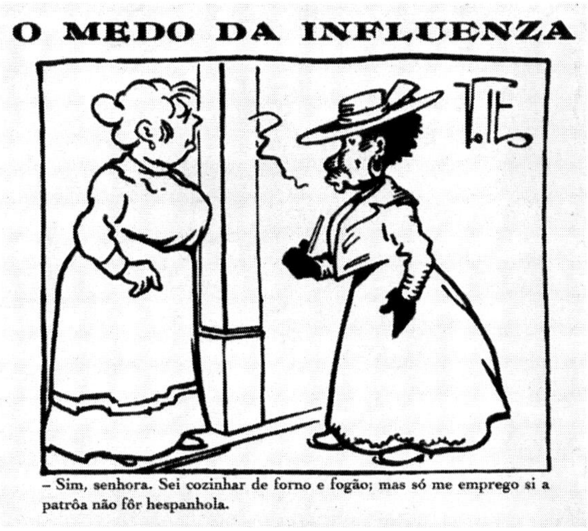

O MEDO DA INFLUENZA

– Sim, senhora. Sei cozinhar de forno e fogão; mas só me emprego si a patrôa não fôr hespanhola.

Figure 6.4 Cartoon entitled "The Fear of Influenza," linking the 1918 flu, popularly known as the Spanish flu, to race, ethnicity, and immigration. An Afro-Brazilian woman is drawn as a racist caricature with an exaggerated nose and lips, smoking a pipe. Playing on the popular name for the flu ("a Hespanhola" or "the Spanish"), she says to the potential employer, "Yes ma'am. I know how to cook with an oven and a stove, but I will only work for you if you are not a Spanish." Source: *A Gazeta*, October 19, 1918, 1, https://memoria .bn.br/DocReader/docreader.aspx?bib=763900&pasta =ano%20191&pesq=hespanhola&pagfis=10217.

voyage to Brazil was in 1912; it continued to ply that route through 1930.[70] While the trips before 1918 appear to have been uneventful, the 562 passengers and 170 crew that left Liverpool in August 1918 were not as lucky. Soon after departing Europe, the *Demerara* was attacked by German submarines and only saved by a Royal Air Force counterattack. The "death ship," as a 2020 BBC Brazil news report called it, continued its "cursed" voyage.[71]

The twenty-five-day journey from Liverpool to Buenos Aires included four Brazilian stops, first in Recife on September 9, then south to Salvador and Rio de Janeiro, and finally to Santos. Crowds waited at each port, hoping for news about the raging World War I. What many received as well was the flu. Arriving in Rio de Janeiro on September 15, the captain followed medical protocols by flying a yellow flag, indicating that there was illness on board. Even so, more than 350 passengers disembarked, and "Rio de

Janeiro [became] a giant hospital!," undoubtedly a reference to the physician Miguel Pereira's 1916 comment that illnesses rampant in rural Brazil made it "an immense hospital."[72] The illustrated magazine *Careta* (Grimace) made the linkage between the *Demerara*'s departure from Europe and its arrival in Brazil with a half-page caricature of a "bacillomarino" (a disease submarine) that merged advanced German weapons and H1N1.[73] Even recently elected president Francisco de Paula Rodrigues Alves became sick, dying before taking office. His passing reinforced both widespread fear of the flu and the false idea that the disease spread equitably throughout society, independent of class, living conditions, or access to health care.[74]

After the *Demerara*'s arrival in Santos, it took only a few days for the virus to spread to São Paulo city. Sanitary Service officials told yet another official story in their 1920 report, focusing on the flu's arrival in Rio de Janeiro and claiming that a soccer team and a student from that city brought the disease to São Paulo's center.[75] Regardless of who was patient zero, the flu quickly overwhelmed Brazil's precarious health care system as hospitals filled and mass graves were dug. The undercounted official national absolute mortality was 35,240 deaths (about 0.1 percent of the total population), with the percentages in Rio de Janeiro and São Paulo at 1.6 percent and 1.0 percent, respectively.[76] In São Paulo city, 4,790 of the 5,331 people who died lived in working-class districts with large numbers of immigrants or immigrant-descent residents. The records of the Medical Police show the stunning advance and decline of the flu (figure 6.5), which they labeled only as "sickness" for several possible reasons, ranging from timesaving in a crisis, to a lack of confidence in precisely what they were treating, to an attempt to hide the state's lack of control over the flu.

Incident reports for people reporting the flu to the Medical Police between October 23 and October 25 fill an entire volume in the archives, and another is required for just the next seven days. In October the Medical Police recorded more than 2,400 incident reports, about three times the usual monthly number. Many of the reports noted returning visits, and surnames were frequently registered simply as "so and so" (de Tal), an atypical formulation for these documents.[77] Entire families became ill, as did groups of residents varying in citizenship status, race, and age in single cortiços.[78] Since no treatment was available, many people reported their illness to the Medical Police but were not seen by physicians. In central São Paulo the numbers of deaths spiked quickly, from 301 (319 in the city overall) in October 1918 to 4,113 (4,580 overall) in November and then dropping to 376 (432 overall) in December.

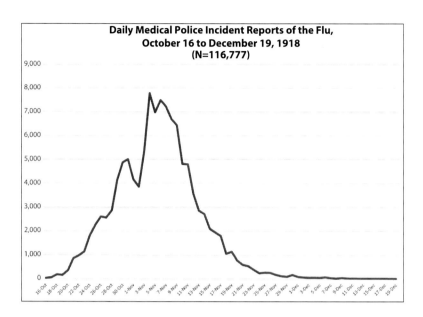

Figure 6.5 Source: Secretaria da Segurança Pública do Estado de São Paulo, Assistência Policial, Registro de ocorrências da Assistência Policial, 1911–40, Arquivo do Estado de São Paulo. Prepared by Monaliza Caetano dos Santos and Surbhi Shrivastava, Lesser Research Collective, 2023.

The director of São Paulo state's Sanitary Service, Artur Neiva, a microbiologist who himself would contract the disease, instituted measures to contain the flu on October 15, 1918. Many of his policies emerged from a new state health code implemented in early April 1918 and included shutting schools, theaters, cinemas, and other public gathering places.[79] Neiva's daily health bulletins and his "Advice to the Public" column were published in major newspapers and included information about handwashing, mask wearing, and social distancing. Traditional aspects of Brazilian social culture—for example, greeting people with kisses and hugs, walking hand in hand in public spaces, or even talking in public—became "almost acts of treason."[80]

Other physicians often contradicted Neiva, publicizing their own thoughts on preventing contagion and treating the flu in the press. The divergent information generated an atmosphere of confusion. The public often ignored regulations as myths about prevention and cure exploded, reinforcing ethnic and class issues. Contacts between immigrants and those in their countries of origin meant different sources of information, both scientific and less so. Like today, those with little or no literacy, non-Portuguese speakers, and those without access to media (whether in print in 1918 or via the internet a century later) heard about official information via word of mouth. As *O Combate* screamed in a front-page headline, "The Truth Is That We Don't Have a Sanitary Service."[81]

Distrust swelled as official attempts to downplay the crisis clashed with the "macabre spectacle of cadavers thrown on the streets because of a lack of coffins and burial spaces, creating indignation and fear."[82] Good advice, like social distancing, was often ignored, while bad advice, whether well intentioned or not, held equal weight. Contributing to the lack of trust was the disgust many residents of Bom Retiro and the rest of the city felt as they learned that São Paulo's governor, the mayor, and most of the political leadership had fled the city to their rural estates, often alleging that they had to take care of ill family members.[83] Major newspapers denounced "pharmacists, religious leaders, bakers, greengrocers, charcoal haulers, gravediggers and even police officers and doctors who evaded their commitments" and urged the public to boycott those making improper profits.[84]

Given the mediatic and viral nature of the epidemic, it is not surprising that Neiva, who in the 1930s would support various racist policies against immigrants and their descendants, expressed horrified memories in a 1920 report prepared by the Sanitary Service: "Future historians who try to describe the epidemics that have devastated Brazil will have great difficulty imagining the formidable calamity that was the epidemic flu. It is now known that the 'Spanish flu' was the largest known epidemic in history. It went around the planet [and] plagued the most populated centers to the . . . most remote regions."[85] Intellectuals were also shocked by the collective devastation. As Susanne Klengel notes, Mário de Andrade, a music critic for the *A Gazeta* newspaper in July 1918, "witnessed how the flu brought the international opera season to a standstill at the Municipal Theatre: singers, musicians and audience fell ill or stayed away out of fear, so that the theatre was finally closed."[86] Another participant in Brazil's modernist movement, Oswald de Andrade (no relation to Mário), wrote in his 1954 memoir, "The tragic episode of the flu shrouds the city. They call the disease 'the Spanish.' It took over the world. It also fell on São Paulo, putting everything in mourning. Six livid, interminable weeks. I feel that this plague is worse than war because it arrives quietly and disorients any defense. People don't know where the silent howitzer will come from. The city mobilized doctors, hospitals, nurses. Burial processions occupy the streets. Large hearses clutter the Center. Countless coffins parade through the neighborhoods."[87]

The first media reports of the flu in São Paulo appeared in newspapers like *O Combate*, whose working-class readers were concentrated in Bom Retiro and similar districts where labor continued even if the streets may have seemed empty in well-off neighborhoods.[88] Lola Mareira, a seventeen-year-old "Hespanhola" (Spanish) hatmaker, was run over by a cart as she returned home from her workplace in Bom Retiro on October 28, 1918, a day when about a quarter of the Medical Police incident reports were for injuries rather than the flu.[89] A few weeks later, *O Combate* noted that the "Hespanhola" was spreading under multiple names, including *grippe*, *puxa-puxa*, and *urucubaca*, the latter an Indigenous word associated with magic and bad luck. The flu was also known as "dengue," the name of a high-impact disease in Bom Retiro, perhaps a discursive residue of an outbreak of the mosquito-borne disease with flu-like symptoms that hit São Paulo in 1916.[90]

O Combate recognized that while the flu could potentially infect anyone, the disease did not spread equitably.[91] Unlike in upscale neighborhoods, corpses in Bom Retiro were often transported without coffins and buried in mass graves in cemeteries that "functioned day and night."[92] Factories and cortiços made the working classes particularly vulnerable even though the "Public Health Services—as everyone knows—do not have the means for the defense of the city against this invasion."[93] Indeed, public health leaders minimized the flu's impact by frequently categorizing morbidity in general terms, often simply noting that "the patient was sick." The Sanitary Service also manipulated mortality information by refusing to provide death certificates. Cláudio Bertolli Filho argues that the "flu's geography" shows a "democratic illusion" among officials, who treated it "as a disease that spreads independently of specific living conditions[;] it is understood as a kind of 'accident' linked more to individual luck or misfortune than to any other determinants."[94]

The flu had a higher-than-average impact in high-density working-class neighborhoods where there were also large numbers of immigrants. As with the bubonic plague, the Central Disinfectory took control of the crisis, and Bom Retiro became a central focus of health surveillance. Employees of the institution were told to lengthen their workdays by two hours to handle the influx of patients. Since the Disinfectory did not have enough vehicles for the volume of sick and dead, the São Paulo state vice president's and ministers' automobiles were reassigned. Taxis, which had begun to appear in the city around 1906, were also hired to support the efforts.[95]

The flu made space important in unexpected ways, often in connection with immigrants. Large numbers of deaths led the city to expand the Araçá public cemetery, founded in 1887. One reason was that foreigners were prohibited from being interred in the upper-crust Consolação Cemetery, leading one wag to quip, "When you go to the Araçá Cemetery, you might think you are in an Italian city."[96] There was also a growing need for beds in temporary infirmaries. One of the largest emergency hospitals was in the Hospedaria dos Imigrantes, where one thousand beds were available. So many people died at the hospedaria that the Mooca district registered the largest number of fatalities in the city by a large margin.[97]

The flu's impact was also visible in the death rate by profession, with the highest numbers among "factory workers." Yet the categories used by the Sanitary Service caused me to pause. For example, "unknown" was the largest specified professional category, suggesting that the public health officials were uninterested in getting a full picture of working-class lives during the epidemic. Unlike for males, female fatalities were lumped together regardless of age, showing the same paternalism discussed in previous chapters. Adult females were not categorized by profession even though they were a significant part of the waged workforce as factory workers and domestic employees.[98] The Sanitary Service separated boys under fifteen years of age out of the male category and listed them as having no profession although they were also active in the workforce. According to the undoubtedly sexist and ageist logic of the statistics, 1,601 of the 5,331 deaths (30 percent) were of adult males, and of these, 14 percent were "factory workers."[99]

About 29 percent of flu fatalities were not Brazilian, with the highest death rates among Italians (632), Portuguese (509), and Spanish (225). "Turco-Arabes" were lumped with "Asiatics" (52) into one category, and other Europeans comprised fifty-one deaths. High overall mortality rates in central districts suggest that many of the Brazilians who died were the children or grandchildren of immigrants. While a little over 52 percent of the total fatalities were male, this was not the case in Bom Retiro, where almost 58 percent of the 330 fatalities were female, a percentage found only in one of the other ten districts of the city (Bela Vista). This high death rate among women is almost certainly linked to the significant presence of women in the industrial workforce. The high number of cortiços, and thus the population density, in Bom Retiro was also a cause.

Over 90 percent of deaths recorded by the Medical Police were of those categorized as white, a surprise since Black and Brown Brazilians had significant presences in central districts and were overrepresented in state medical statistics before and after the flu. During the H1N1 epidemic, the Medical Police may have stepped back from using public health to criminalize the African-descended population in favor of a focus on flu-related activities. Or flu-stricken Black and Brown citizens may have been less likely to go to the Medical Police out of fear and because of their reliance on other types of prevention and cures.

The cultural connection of foreigners with the flu led many ethnic-immigrant institutions, including the Colônia Syria (the Syrian Colony, founded by Middle Eastern immigrants); the Cruz Vermelha Hespanhola (the Spanish Red Cross, founded by Spaniards); the Hospital Israelita (the Jewish Hospital, founded by European Jewish immigrants); and the Clube Germânia (the Germania Club, founded by Germans), to become provisional hospitals or become involved in care. In doing this, members of the immigrant elite sought to show that foreigners were helping to resolve a national crisis. The use of immigrant spaces as locations of curing also challenged the racist attitude that foreigners had caused the epidemic, an identity play that Carlos Dimas also found among nineteenth-century Italian immigrants responding to cholera in Tucúman, Argentina.[100]

Nonbiomedical interpretations of the flu abounded in districts like Bom Retiro with its lack of health care infrastructure; most residents there could not afford private medical services. When the Sanitary Service recommended citric acid as a possible remedy, limes suddenly became unavailable.[101] Officially sanctioned but ineffective medicines, like quinine, iodine water, and mentholated Vaseline, exploded in price and caused runs on pharmacies that "upped their prices in the same proportion as the numbers of sick."[102] In response, the Sanitary Service began issuing stamped and numbered prescriptions only accepted at state-approved pharmacies that were open twenty-four hours per day so that the poor and working classes would be assured of getting subsidized medicine like quinine pills.

Health authorities wondered if the smallpox vaccine might help to cure or prevent the flu.[103] When it did not, the use of already widespread non-biomedical cures skyrocketed, with immigrants and their descendants often combining pre- and postmigratory components.[104] Popular homemade remedies such as garlic, eucalyptus leaves, cinnamon, and limes, most of which could be mixed with pinga—sugarcane rum—were widespread. Many continue to be widely used in Brazil, including by me (along with bourbon, chicken soup, and Korean red ginseng extract). Ritual objects also became flu medications. One 1920 study of the plant-based cures sold by popular healers in the center of São Paulo, by a botanist at the Butantan Institute found that many people used amulets that were filled with pieces of wood and bark as cures, just as they would for simple colds.[105] False medicines also spread throughout the city, and some took hold among the upper classes. Sr. Antonio, whose parents immigrated to Brazil in 1900, was interviewed by Ecléa Bosi and remembered, "They treated the flu with benzoic acid, a medicine that a fashionable pharmacy invented, taking it out of the stomachs of animals."[106]

The Sanitary Service was ineffective in convincing the public not to use popular cures for illnesses, and to this day the media advertises them.[107] This lack of confidence in public health authorities resulted from several factors. Disputes among physicians created a sense that no one knew what they were talking about. Public health officials were often far removed from the lives of the working class, whose local health systems included people they knew and trusted. One self-reflexive article in *O Estado de S. Paulo* connected fake cures, immigrants, and fear as follows:

> The grippe that is invading the city has another name this year: it is no longer the "urucubaca" but the "hespañola." In other words, because of its new name, or perhaps because of its seriousness, the old and well-known influenza has caused real fear, as if it were an epidemic of a deadly disease.
>
> But it is not about the influenza epidemic that I write today: it is about the other epidemic, that of influenza-preventing medicines. In three or four days, how many "infallible medicines" do readers think have already appeared in newspaper advertisements?
>
> —Half a dozen?
>
> —Only half a dozen? . . . It's clear that you do not read the last pages of the newspapers. Well, in today's *O Estado de S. Paulo* alone I counted about thirty? And all of them are infallible.[108]

The general distrust of authorities and the devastation that the population observed each day led to various health-related rumors.[109] One was that Ermelino Matarazzo, director of the Italian-immigrant-founded Indústrias Reunidas Fábricas Matarazzo (Matarazzo Industrial Factories), was adding water to lard, making him "the only person who got rich" during the epidemic.[110] There was widespread speculation that health officials were using the flu for their own personal gain. The illustrated magazine *A Rolha* (The cork, as in a wine bottle stopper) denounced a Red Cross hospital for distributing prescriptions without health checks and claimed the physicians were having "debauched" relations with nurses and getting drunk at every meal.[111] Perhaps the accusations were true because the hospital fired multiple employees after the story appeared.

Medical institutions also became terrifying spaces, an inversion of the traditional idea that they were spaces of cures. There were widespread allegations of a bed shortage in the Santa Casa de Misericórdia hospital, where Bom Retiro's residents were usually treated. Each night, it was rumored, nurses would give a lethal "Cha da Meia-Noite" (Midnight Tea) to moribund patients to free up space. This belief was so widespread that in 1919 a samba school used a float in the shape of a teacup for carnival while singing about the treatment of poor patients in a song called "O Chá da Meia Noite."[112]

Another rumor, recounted by the well-known fiction writer and journalist Monteiro Lobato (1882–1948), was that getting sent to the infirmary at the Hospedaria dos Imigrantes was a death sentence. He had become concerned about Brazil's poor public health record and authored a multipart series on the topic for *O Estado de S. Paulo* in early 1918, before the flu outbreak. Two years later his collection of short stories appeared, with immigrants appearing in several. "Slice of Life" took place during an epidemic when it was rumored that the ill people taken to the provisional hospital at the Hospedaria dos Imigrantes were "the poorest of the poor and the treatment was what it should be, because the very poor are not really people." The result was that "nothing terrified the little people as much as being taken to 'the Immigration.'"[113]

Health rumors led to health humor. Jacob Penteado writes that his uncle, also named Jacob, frequently repeated a story about disease in the "Italian cities" of Naples and São Paulo:

> -Tomorrow morning, they can send patients of such and such bed numbers to the mass grave.
> —At daybreak, the nurses carried out the order. However, one of the dead protested:
> —Hey, where are you taking me? I'm alive!
> —Do you know more than a doctor, paisano? If he said you're dead, you're dead.[114]

Reports of deaths and serious illness caused what some called "Spanish flu delirium." Sometimes this took the form of visions. One child of Italian immigrants told Ecléa Bosi, "I remember as if it were today that during the Spanish flu I saw in the sky a carriage with white horses in front, pulling my coffin.

I really saw it, not that it was a miracle, but I saw it and I remember it like it was today."[115] Reports of what appeared to be deranged behavior circulated widely as front-page news in inexpensive newspapers that often were passed from person to person, in more traditional newspapers with wide circulations, and in publications outside of São Paulo. In Curitiba, in the southern state of Paraná, Manuel de Campos fell ill with the flu, leading to "a terrible bout of insanity" in which he killed four people and injured others.[116]

According to Liane Maria Bertucci, many residents of São Paulo were terrified that the flu would bring "shots, stab wounds, clubs, drownings, leaping to death. People with the flu attempted suicide or killed those closest to them." Many of the stories were about immigrants who leaped to their deaths from hospital or home windows or shot or drowned themselves.[117] João Gomari, a forty-eight-year-old from Argentina with four children, collected trash, but his wages were so low that he also received aid from a local church. According to *O Estado de S. Paulo*, he had tuberculosis, he had recently lost a child to the flu, and his other children were sick. Believing that he had contracted the flu, he committed suicide with a knife to the heart.[118] Some scholars examining the coverage of these "crazed" deaths mention media sensationalism and mass hysteria.[119] Other analytic approaches suggest that the responses to the flu ranged from increased social cohesion and well-being to suicide.[120]

Ordinary People

Intense pressures on those of immigrant descent (both foreign and native-born residents) by the majority of the population often lead to the growth of alternative belief systems among minority groups.[121] These beliefs are frequently health related and sometimes seem "crazy" to those in the dominant classes, even when widely held among less powerful sectors of the population. A mid-nineteenth-century Brazilian example emerges from the Muckers, a Christian-based religion practiced by some German immigrants and their descendants in Brazil's southernmost state, Rio Grande do Sul. The group lived separately from more conformist immigrants and believed that their leader, Jacobina Mentz, who cared for the ill with Bible readings and homemade medicines, was the reincarnation of Jesus Christ. Following accusations in 1874 that Mentz had ordered the assassination of those who had left the religion, a police battalion killed her and many of her followers in an attack on their rural compound.[122] Another alternative belief system responding to discrimination in Brazil emerged among the largest global population of Japanese descent outside of Japan. World War II–era repression of Japanese immigrants, including relocation and property confiscation, led about 100,000 Japanese immigrants to join a movement that proposed that Japan had won the war.[123]

To think about how the flu created identity challenges, I now examine some cases that might seem extraordinary but represent reactions to typical pressures that majority societies place on immigrants and their descendants. These "strange deaths" were an epidemic-related outcome created by stereotypes and their relation to national identity. On November 23, 1918, at the height of the flu, the often-sensationalist *O Combate* recounted the story of a "Japanese couple, victimized by the flu, dead without medical help."[124] According to the article, a Medical Police physician who was himself recovering from the illness received an urgent call to go to a home in Santana, a peri-urban district about five kilometers north of Bom Retiro. When he arrived at the location, a group of scared neighbors told the physician that they "suspected something abnormal" because the neighborly and friendly immigrant couple and their baby had been stricken by the flu and had not come out of their home for twenty-four hours.

The physician knocked on the front door but received no response. He and the crowd that had formed then broke down the front door and searched the home. Moving down a long corridor, they came to the couple's bedroom, where they found the "grim spectacle" of the immigrants "in complete death rigidity under the covers of a humble bed." More shocking was that the starving eight-month-old baby was lying on top of the mother's body, "sucking at her breasts and whimpering," and upon seeing the rescuers "sobbed movingly."[125]

The image of hardworking immigrants dying, with a living baby refusing to give up her life, was no doubt meant to invoke the fanatic inward-looking approach with which Japanese immigrants and their descendants in Brazil were and are frequently tagged.[126] The description of the physician winding his way through the dark corridor to a bedroom at the back of the home reminded readers of a hive-like cortiço. The story contained many of the tropes that would emerge less than two weeks later in another widely reported case. This time it involved an immigrant family from Württemberg, Germany, who had immigrated to Brazil in the first decades of the twentieth century.

Like the Japanese family, the Schonardt family lived in a rural district that was transitioning into an urban space. Father Ernst was a stonemason, and he and his wife, Elise, had two children, nineteen-year-old Ernesto, who worked at a hotel, and sixteen-year-old Rosa, a domestic worker living in the home of Rodolpho Weil about ten kilometers away. *O Estado de S. Paulo* reported the Schonardt past as one of individual success that improved Brazil: "He managed to save money with which he bought land. . . . He built a small two-story chalet with his own hands, in the middle of a plot of land that he carefully worked, planting and landscaping. . . . The Schonhardt family lived happily."[127]

In 1918 Ernst and Rosa contracted the flu. Rosa's employer interned them at the Clube Germânia's fifty-bed provisional hospital, an example of how immigrant-descent networks operate and how some ethnic minorities construct health institutions to promote their place within the nation.[128] According to newspaper reports (including the working-class *O Combate*; newspapers linked to industrialists, landowners, and the ascendant middle classes, like *A Gazeta* and *O Estado de S. Paulo*; and even newspapers and true crime magazines in Rio de Janeiro), the two recuperated from the flu. Soon thereafter, Ernst began exhibiting signs of mental instability that the media termed "insanity."[129] Symptoms included insisting that he was Catholic, although by all accounts he had professed Protestantism prior to his illness, and that his family had to "fight against the Devil by praying nonstop."

Ernst was correct about the devil's presence. After spending a day preaching on the streets, he returned home on the evening of November 30, 1918, possessed. Over the course of the night, Ernst sang, screamed, and destroyed everything in sight. He burned Elise with a kerosene lamp before holing up in the home's basement. Later in the evening, he came upstairs and again attacked his wife, leading Elise and Ernesto, according to *O Combate*'s account of the police report, to believe Ernst needed an immediate exorcism. To release the devil, they forced Ernst's mouth open by stuffing it with a whetstone, which suffocated him. Following his death from asphyxiation, Ernesto and Elise cut his neck. When the police arrived, the two confessed to the crime. Their claim that the flu had put "the Devil in his body" led the detective to remand them to the Juquery Psychiatric Hospital, which determined the crime was "the result of a lamentable act of insanity" and should not be prosecuted.[130]

There is much in common in the recounting of the two "Spanish" flu deaths, even though the two families, one Japanese and one German, seem different. In both cases, the media and police suggested that the disease unleashed a dormant premigratory fanaticism among what had seemed hardworking and neighborly immigrants. In both cases, much of the action took place in spaces hidden from sight and light, the bedroom deep in the house and the basement. All of this, I propose, suggested to readers that these were not momentarily sensational cases. Rather, insanity was a harbinger of what the Spanish flu was going to create in a city filled with foreigners. The two incidents played on the population's terror resulting from the societal upheavals caused by the flu, World War I, and widespread labor unrest in the city.

Bom Retiro was also the location of strange undeaths, often called *mortos-vivos*, where people declared deceased returned to life. The fascination with the unliving or zombies has a long history in Brazil, in the Americas, and globally. The seventeenth-century leader of the Quilombo dos Palmares, a runaway-slave community in the Brazilian state of Alagoas, was known as Zumbi (zombie), a word that some scholars link to western African words meaning a ghost or spirit who has risen from the dead.[131] In the twentieth century, zombies have become a global fascination, with zombie-themed books, comics, films, and television series produced in Asia and the Americas, including a not very good Brazilian one based on historical interactions between Blacks and immigrants.[132]

Widespread fear of being buried alive appeared as cholera epidemics spread globally in the nineteenth century.[133] Taphophobia led not only to stories of mortos-vivos but to the invention of "safety coffins" that allowed those accidentally buried alive to ring bells to alert the undead. In urban Brazil and elsewhere, mortos-vivos were also a form of entertainment. In 1912 the Bijou Theater presented the two-act comedy "O Morto Vivo," and a decade later "an extraordinary number of people" went to the almost two-thousand-seat Colombo Theater, in the building that had housed the Brás Municipal Market until 1908, to see Manuel Urbano, an artist known as "the buried alive," in a glass coffin.[134] There were also jokes, such as one published in *A Tribuna* (Santos) a few months before the 1918 flu consumed São Paulo: "The buried-alive industry is proliferating. It is everywhere. Soon, when a corpse arrives at the cemetery, the gravedigger will ask, 'Is he alive or dead?'"[135] Mortos-vivos are also part of the contemporary discourse about Bom Retiro's "Cracolândia," creating both fascination and repulsion. This geography of police-patrolled drug use in front of the Julio Prestes Railway Station emerged in the 1990s; the area was depopulated and then repopulated with addicts, sellers, and their families, widely referred to as *mortos-vivos*, a term that one scholar has called an example of "necropolitics."[136]

During the 1918 flu, tales of mortos-vivos were inspired by the real burials of victims in group graves with others who were not family members. Many funerals took place without family members present, rupturing the formal separation of the living and the dead that takes place at burial services.

Stories were "spread by thousands of mouths" in immigrant working-class neighborhoods. This was one result of the "disorganization of the Sanitary Services," which were unable to promptly remove corpses from the streets and often buried flu victims without informing family members. Popular wisdom was that the mortality numbers from the flu were "six times the official number. [Rumors abounded] of people buried alive, without coffins or official notice. Incredible things were said about the provisional hospitals."[137]

Bom Retiro's mortos-vivos reflected tales of immigrant survival and state incompetence and were remembered into the late twentieth century.[138] They were also stories of xenophobia, racism, and societal uncertainty. The story of João Antônio Jorge, whose return to the living opened this chapter, was one of them. There is no doubt that his rise from the dead was celebrated, especially since it prevented him from being buried alive. Another Bom Retiro resident, an immigrant stonemason from Italy, was not so lucky. *O Combate* began its coverage of the case cinematically on November 29, 1918, announcing "This Time It Is Not a Rumor." The teasing story recounted how a telephone call to the newspaper offices about a "morto vivo," something that apparently happened with some frequency, was so convincing that a reporter was sent to investigate.

The residential address that the newspaper received for the morto-vivo was wrong. The hardworking reporter, however, went door-to-door in the pouring rain trying to identify the perhaps-living person. Everyone he met had heard the story, convincing him it was true. When the reporter entered a store where customers were sheltering from the storm, the owner gave directions to a construction site where the morto-vivo was part of the crew (at Avenida Luiz Antonio, 187). The journalist's conversation with the morto-vivo was so amazing that *O Combate* could only reveal, "Tomorrow we will publish the statements made to our reporter by the man who . . . spent a few hours in a coffin, only escaping the horrible torture of being buried alive with . . . Providential help."[139]

Tomorrow arrived, along with the story. *O Combate* published it on the same day it began reporting on the João Antônio Jorge case, while *A Capital* focused on the morto-vivo. While some of the information differed in the two newspapers, the story was basically the same. Eugenio Benzana (or Bezzana) was a middle-aged (either fifty-two or fifty-five years old) stonemason from Italy who lived in the back of a cortiço at Rua Anhaia, 162, in Bom Retiro. Benzana was married to Luiza "So and So," his second wife, and had adopted two of her children and then had two more with her. Luiza "So and So" had died from the flu a little over two weeks before Benzana's resurrection; according to the reports, this led the immigrant to start drinking heavily.

On Saturday, November 23, 1918, Benzana and the other workers left the construction site at Avenida Luiz Antonio, 187, following hours of intense downpours. He went to a bar to have "a 'draught' to keep away the dampness and the 'Spanish.' He may have had a second drink" before heading down Rua Major Diogo in the direction of the centrally located Praça da República. That was the last thing that Benzana remembered since drinking led him to have epileptic attacks that left him "pale and cold like a corpse."[140]

Benzana woke up that evening inside a coffin in the Araçá Cemetery, "probably driven there in the Medical Police's cadaver wagon, called in by the patrolman in the vicinity." Forcing open the cover, Benzana found that he was next to a grave, surrounded by other cadavers waiting for interment. "Terrified," the stonemason leaped over the cemetery wall and ran down the Rua Rio de Janeiro for the five kilometers back to his home in Bom Retiro. The morto-vivo did not tell his family what happened. Indeed, when someone reported that they had seen Benzana's body being transported to the cemetery in a vehicle like the one in figure 6.6, his daughter-in-law did not believe it because he was already home.

O Combate did not let the story go. On December 2 it reported a failed attempt to find Benzana's file at the Gabinete Medico Legal (an early version of the coroner's office). The newspaper concluded that he had been brought to the cemetery at the request of a patrolman, without having been examined by a physician. The reporter then interviewed the gravediggers, who admitted they had moved forward with the burial without verifying that Benzana was dead.[141]

The story of Benzana's return to the living began to circulate in immigrant neighborhoods. On the one hand, it emphasized the neglect that so many in the working classes felt during the epidemic. On the other hand, it represented a sliver of hope amid death. A reporter from the illustrated magazine A Rolha claimed to have heard the story from Benzana's son while at the fish market in the 25 de Março neighborhood, which was associated with Arab immigrants. On the streets of Bom Retiro, "everyone was talking about Mr. Eugenio, the lucky worker who miraculously escaped from being forced six feet under." A worker attending a funeral at the Araçá Cemetery claimed to have heard the patrolman and the gravediggers discussing the case, saying they witnessed Benzana "running like a rabbit" out of the coffin.[142]

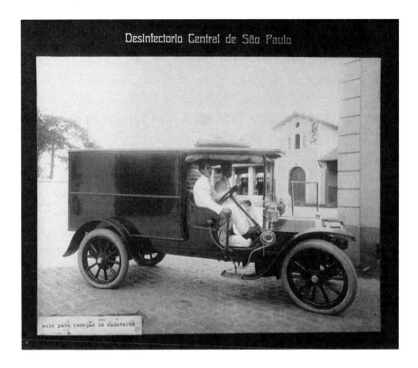

Figure 6.6 Central Disinfectory cadaver removal vehicle, likely from the first decade of the twentieth century. Source: *Álbum Desinfectório Central de São Paulo*, [1893–1913], Fundo Serviço Sanitário de São Paulo, Grupo: Desinfectório Central, Ampliação fotográfica sobre papel cartão, PB, Laboratório fotográfico Fotografia Alemã, Acervo Museu de Saúde Pública Emílio Ribas/Instituto Butantan.

Complaints about the collecting and burying of the dead without identifying corpses or informing family members were frequent and largely ignored by the municipality during the flu. The public outcry over Benzana's return from lifelessness, however, also led to a different response. Alarico Silveira had been appointed director of the city's Department of Public Cleaning in 1914, in part because of the need for a diplomatic connection between the city's health needs and the state Sanitary Service, led at the time by Emílio Ribas.[143] With the outbreak of the flu, Mayor Washington Luiz asked Silveira to supervise municipal services for the ill and burial services for the dead.[144] After being questioned by *O Combate*, just as the Schonardt story was making headlines, Silveira began an investigation.[145]

According to *O Combate*, Silveira personally visited the Araçá Cemetery and the Medical Police to hear their side of the story. He confirmed that there was no death certificate for Benzana. He found no written record of any bodies being picked up by the municipal cadaver wagon on the day of Benzana's first death. Silveira even went to Bom Retiro to speak with Benzana's family, but he did not discover who had reported that the immigrant had been transported with other bodies to the cemetery. Silveira, without intending to, confirmed widespread rumors and newspaper stories of unregistered deaths and mass burials, and the story ended there, except as a memory.[146]

This chapter has explored two global health crises, the turn-of-the-century bubonic plague and the 1918 influenza outbreak, from state and popular perspectives. I have shown that public health officials believed that immigrants brought diseases to Brazil and that the working-class neighborhoods where large numbers of foreigners lived encouraged the spread of disease. I have argued that residues of bubonic disease eradication policies in the nineteenth century could be seen both materially, in medical forms and in building usage, and discursively with the outbreak of the flu in 1918. Dissecting how life and death were negotiated by immigrants and state representatives shows the limits of biomedical approaches to cures and the residues of prejudice and xenophobia, critical factors for understanding public health policies and actions.

In both cases, public health officials made immigrants a focus. They used forced entry into homes as part of eradication programs that emerged from prejudices about immigrant filth, rather than resolving infrastructural factors like poor sewer systems, nonexistent litter collection, and flooding. Immigrants and others in the working classes responded in multiple ways to the increased incursions. Popular cures were one reaction to a distrust of official medical pronouncements. Some eradication programs, like catching and selling rats, became income generators rather than just public health actions. The state's inability to handle medical crises even led immigrants to return to life after being declared dead by state representatives.

A POSTSCRIPT

Eugenio Benzana's return to life did not end Bom Retiro's flu-related miracles. Antoninho da Rocha Marmo was born in the district on October 19, 1918, just a month before Benzana became undead. Antoninho's father was a police officer, and his mother worked at home. They were neither immigrants nor cortiço dwellers, living in a small house at Rua dos Bandeirantes, 24 (now number 188). Antoninho is reputed to have been born prematurely just as the flu became rampant. Living in a part of Bom Retiro where residents appear to have had money for private doctors led to a miracle because, as the story goes, "In the confusion caused by the health crisis, a doctor mistakenly knocked on the door of the Marmo family's residence, saving the life of the parturient and her child, as well as helping some neighbors who had been assaulted by the 'Spanish flu.'"

Doctors did not usually circulate in Bom Retiro because it was poor and flu ridden. That one unexpectedly appeared at the instant of Antoninho's birth is accepted among the faithful as the first miracle of a life that emerged from certain death. Like the cases of João Antônio Jorge and Eugenio Benzana, Antoninho's is a story of survival amid widespread death. As a child, Antoninho is said to have begun to build altars and play at Mass in his backyard. Many people believed he could predict the future and induce miracles. At age five he contracted tuberculosis and left Bom Retiro in search of treatment in other parts of São Paulo state. He is said to have predicted his own death, which took place in 1930, at the age of twelve.

Antoninho is buried in the Consolação Cemetery, São Paulo's oldest necropolis, opened as a municipal cemetery in 1858 following an outbreak of smallpox and a prohibition on burials on the grounds of religious institutions. Over the decades, Antoninho became a popular saint, especially for newborns and mothers with pregnancy challenges. Today his tomb is one of the most visited in the cemetery (Quadra 80/Terreno 6). His story was also used by some health professionals "because Antoninho served as a paradigm of the 'good patient,' knowing how to forgive medical shortcomings and, more than that, following with strict obedience the health teachings that prevented the spread of Koch's bacillus."[147]

Antoninho's life was investigated by TV Globo in 1982, as part of its "True Cases" series, which included reenactments of the story by well-known Brazilian actors. Marília Schneider's study of how Antoninho is remembered shows that place is critical to the story, from the Rocha Marmo home in Bom Retiro to the Santa Casa hospital, where so many of Bom Retiro's residents were treated.[148] Thus, while he was not an immigrant, his story follows a trajectory like that of others in this chapter as disease, citizenship, and space marked everyday living and dying in Bom Retiro.

A Conclusion

Light and Dark in a Saintly City

São Paulo is named after Saul of Tarsus, commonly known as Paul the Apostle, a saint often connected to the book and the sword. Those two different approaches to evangelism highlight the tensions in São Paulo city, where rich and poor, healthy and sick, and foreign and Brazilian often live and work in proximity. Bom Retiro is a microcosm of the larger city and of urban spaces around the globe, and an evening visit to the neighborhood highlights the distinctions. The positive names that policymakers and health officials attached to the built environment (Good Retreat, Luz [Light] Railway Station) slammed up against their recurring images of the neighborhood and its residents as unhealthy, dangerous, dark, and dirty.

Bom Retiro, after the sun sets, is anything but a light retreat—the streets are dark and largely empty since retail workers have returned to their own often-distant homes. Most residents stay behind closed doors in part because they are afraid, in part because they usually do not have the disposable income needed to enjoy the wonderful restaurants that have sprung up for those who can arrive and leave by car. The simultaneous light and dark descriptions and lived experiences are typical of immigrant working-class neighborhoods and remind us that while Bom Retiro may not be "the world," it does explain much of the world. Bom Retiro, as a geography of good and bad health, of race and racism, of ethnicity and prejudice, and of labor and oppression, teaches us about urban life in many places. While much of this book is about residues, I will be disappointed if readers think of the neighborhood and others like it around the world as unique or unchanging.

I have argued that thinking about people, actions, and space over time is more than an academic project that helps us understand the past. Engaging with the past makes the present better, for example, by helping present-day health care workers understand the long-term effects of poor housing conditions, flooded streets, and long workdays. By asking questions about continuities, about the residues that remain over time, I have proposed that the environment, both built and natural, is as much a force for social and cultural construction as are policies or long-term social structures like racism or migration. In Bom Retiro the residues are impressive. Many goods are still delivered by nonmotorized transport, often two-wheeled pushcarts. Sewing machines, while electric, would be instantly recognizable to those in the nineteenth century in ways that digital musical files would not be to someone who only knew record players. The presence of law enforcement and health care workers on the streets is constant, where they hear Portuguese, Spanish, Korean, Chinese, and Yiddish, among many other languages. Streets in Bom Retiro have names that are residues of peoples and structures of the past and present: Rua dos Italianos, Rua dos Imigrantes, Rua Aimorés, and Rua Prates-Coreia are just some of them.

As I wrote this book, the materials and my experiences in gathering them led me to increasingly consider my role in the story. This sense was highlighted in 2020 and 2021 when research travel was discouraged by Emory University (and many universities) even when the rate of COVID-19 spread in São Paulo was much lower than it was in Atlanta. When I finally returned to São Paulo in September 2021, during what seemed to be the end of the COVID-19 pandemic, I began to write the initial draft of *Living and Dying*. The eighteen months that I had spent away from one of my homes—I had been to São Paulo at least once every four months for the previous thirty-five years—made me see anew the relationships between past and present that this book highlights. One of the most important was the power and independence of Brazil's Unified Health System in distributing vaccines and encouraging mask use despite the right-wing president's claims that COVID-19 was no more than a cold.[1] My experiences of writing in the city of São Paulo, where many in the public appeared largely committed to both personal and communal health, contrasted starkly to my experience in Georgia, in the southern United States, where a widespread lack of concern for others meant large parts of the population refused vaccinations and masks. Indeed, in early October 2021, the state of São Paulo, with over forty-four million people, had almost 40 percent fewer total new cases of COVID than the state of Georgia, which has a quarter of its population.[2]

Returning to São Paulo after a year and a half also reminded me that having multiple homes is reflected in my research. While historians do not always focus on comparison, writing and revising in different places led me away from treating national, regional, city, and neighborhood specificities as unique. I searched for data that told stories of migrating and remaining, of state actors and the population re-forming the built environment and communities, and of enduring bad health and demands for well-being. I saw how global structures affected "health" spaces as small as a bedroom or a sidewalk. I met the world in the oficinas and oficina-residências where Team Green created pop-up health clinics for textile workers who might not be easily able to go to the Bom Retiro Public Health Clinic for regular checkups.

The pandemic frequently led me to reflect on my own past. One recurring memory was of a college seminar on Afro-Brazilian studies with the late great Professor Anani Dzidzienyo. Classes often took place in his apartment, and one week he opened a discussion of racism and resistance by asking the class, "What is a mikveh?" Only one student (yours truly) knew the answer, that a mikveh is a Jewish ritual bath. Even so, all the students struggled to understand the relationship of this small piece of the built environment to the African diaspora in Latin America. Professor Dzidzienyo's point was to suggest that many experiences of community making and migration, including surprising ones, were intertwined locally and globally, over time and space, as partners, competitors, oppressors, and resistors. Comparative analyses within broader national and transnational race, class, and gender relations, he argued, needed to be added to the often single-group, single-nation, single-city, point-to-point focus of immigration, ethnic, and diaspora studies. This book, then, is an homage to Anani Dzidzienyo and the messy complexities of time, space, and human identities.

A POSTSCRIPT

The mapping of ethnicity, labor, and class on Bom Retiro's geography takes place in all aspects of health and work. On a home visit, I met a grandchild of European immigrants—let's call him Moisés—who lives near streets with names like Lubavitch (Rua Corrêa dos Santos until 1991) and Talmud Thoráh (Rua Tocantins until 1993) that reflect a historical ethnic, and a more recent religious, Jewish presence.

Moisés, who has a mobility impairment, lives with his extended family in a small, simple apartment on the top floor of a two-story building without an elevator. This makes going to his small shop that extends to the sidewalk a daily challenge. The building is on a block whose residences range from cortiços to middle-class apartment buildings. It is steps away from a yeshiva and a religiously based nongovernmental organization that delivers food to the elderly. Just across the street is a geography of cultural difference whose divide is as wide as that in the biblical exodus across the Red Sea; there are self-denominated Korean supermarkets, Christian churches, and Brazilian snack shops. While Moisés is deeply faithful to only one religion, he could choose among many others if he wanted: Jehovah's Witnesses, Buddhists, Jewish Messianics and non-Messianics, Spiritists, and Christians across a spectrum of belief and practice.

Moisés and his father make part of their living repairing small mechanical items. They employ another multigenerational resident of Bom Retiro, who is of African descent. His job is to pick up broken items and then return them on a bicycle-powered cart, a long-used delivery method for goods and services ranging from sharpening knives to selling fruit and drinking water.

I met Moisés following reports from a Team Green community health agent that he had become increasingly depressed because of his physical impairments. My introduction to him showed how residues work on the ground. Even though Moisés is not an immigrant, he was treated like one by the health care professionals. Indeed, both Moisés and the health care workers believed, as would have been the case a century earlier, that among Jews religion was more relevant than nationality. The team also assumed that my ethnicity would help them relate to Moisés even though he and I engage with ritual and belief in different ways.

When we entered the apartment, I was introduced as a researcher from a university in the United States, and my "Jewishness," my foreignness, and my European ancestry were immediately communicated to the family by the health workers. These kinds of introductions are complex to analyze since home visits are meant to break down some of the distance between providers and patients. Thus, connections—whether via ethnicity, soccer team allegiance, or shared acquaintances—are often mobilized.

After the home visit with Moisés, which included prescription renewals, suggestions for a wheelchair upgrade, and encouragement to seek psychological counseling, the team walked back to the Bom Retiro Public Health Clinic, about fifteen minutes away. During the stroll different kinds of questions emerged that related to migrating knowledge: one had to do with Jewish ritual symbols in the home such as mezuzot or candelabras or books in odd writing, which was in fact Hebrew. Bom Retiro's health professionals see these symbols frequently but, according to them, never had anyone they could ask for explanations. A second group of questions might be called ethnosanitary and emerged from nineteenth-century European ideas about health and foreignness. I was asked about the cleanliness and odors in Moisés's home and if European Jews were like immigrants from Korea and Bolivia. Did Jews eat dogs like Koreans or refuse to bathe, like Bolivians? Another set of questions were class related, based on centuries-old stereotypes linking Jews to money that migrated from Europe to the Americas.[3] In some ways, the visit and its aftermath tell the story of this book, about how patient-provider relations influence and are influenced by what spaces we inhabit, who we think we are, and how others see us.

An Introduction

1   Malta et al., "Association between Firearms and Mortality."

2   Bastos, "A territorialidade portuguesa," 237.

3   Buechler, "Sweating It."

4   "Entregar voluntariamente arma de fogo, munição e acessórios," Justiça e Segurança, Governo Federal, https://www.gov.br/pt-br/servicos/entregar -voluntariamente-arma-de-fogo-municao-e-acessorios. Last updated May 1, 2023.

5   Willis, "Antagonistic Authorities."

6   Lovers of K-drama (like yours truly) will enjoy the scene of a police officer examining a fake gun in *Run On* (런 온), episode 1, original broadcast date December 16, 2020. I leave it to readers to decide which of the two main actors best represents my experience. Wikipedia, s.v. "*Run On* (TV Series)," last modified March 10, 2024, 3:50 (UTC), https://en.wikipedia .org/wiki/Run_On_(TV_series).

7   Isa Stacciarini, "Bandidos usam cada vez mais armas de brinquedo e de pressão em assaltos," *Correio Braziliense*, March 7, 2017.

8   E. Ribeiro, "Confiança política na America Latina"; Keefer, Scartascini, and Vlaicu, "Shortchanging the Future"; and M. Machado and Pimenta, "Authoritarian Zones within Democracy."

9   Vanderwood, *Disorder and Progress*; and French, *Drowning in Laws*.

10   Farias et al., "Tempo de espera e absenteísmo na atenção especializada"; and Moimaz et al., "Satisfação e percepção do usuário do SUS sobre o serviço público de saúde."

11   Graham and McFarlane, *Infrastructural Lives*, 2–3.

12   [Name illegible], Military Infirmary, to Inspector of Hygiene, São Paulo, January 11, 1892, Inspectoria de Hygiene da Provincia de São Paulo (Serviço Sanitário), Ofícios Recebidos, 1887 á 1898, vol. 138ª5, Arquivo Histórico Municipal Washington Luís (AHM), São Paulo; and Kleber Tomaz, "Suspeito de matar catador com flecha em SP esfaqueou homem em 2013," *Portal G1—Globo*, September 17, 2016.

13   Moszczyńska, *A memória da destruição na escrita judaico-brasileira depois de 1985*, 148.

14   Mateus, "Memórias de uma prisão"; and Freire, Almada, and Ponce, *Tiradentes, um presidio da ditadura*.

15   Ferrari et al., "Migration and Urban Development."

16   Reibscheid, "Plétzale," 51–58; Hamburger, *O ano em que meus pais saíram de férias*.

17   Our drive from the Praça da Sé to the Emílio Ribas Public Health Museum, mapped in Google Maps: https://maps.app.goo.gl/Z2CYRvPDgtEuS23VA. Accessed June 22, 2024.

18   Lei Estadual No. 1236, de 23 de dezembro de 1910, "Cria o distrito de paz do Bom Retiro, desmembrado do de Santa Ephigênia, no município da capital," Assembleia Legislativa do Estado de São Paulo (ALESP), https://www.al.sp.gov.br/norma/65400.

19   "No Bom Retiro e Santa Iphigenia," *Correio Paulistano*, May 10, 1911, 8.

20   Hayward, "Gamarra, Lima, Peru"; and Scranton, *Silk City*.

21   Taylor, "Performing the 'Thing,'" 58–59; M. Fontes, "Paisagens impermanentes"; and M. Santos, *Natureza do espaço*.

22   Bill Clinton, National Security Council, Speechwriting Office, and Antony Blinken, "Brazil—Speech to Business Leaders 10/15/97," Clinton Digital Library, https://clinton.presidentiallibraries.us/items/show/9732.

23   Britt, "'I'll Samba Someplace Else,'" 263.

24   "Time Out Names the Coolest Streets in the World Right Now," *Time Out*, June 9, 2021, https://www.timeout.com/about/latest-news/time-out-names -the-coolest-streets-in-the-world-right-now-060921. See also "From Lisbon to Tokyo via Lagos," *Time Out*, September 17, 2019, https://www .timeout.com/about/latest-news/from-lisbon-to-tokyo-via-lagos-arroios -shimokitazawa-and-onikan-top-time-outs-list-of-the-worlds-coolest -neighbourhoods-right-now-091719.

25 *Vida Paulista: Humorismo, Literatura, e Esporte* 2, no. 18 (June 16, 1921): 9.

26 Cidade de São Paulo, "Imigrantes na cidade de São Paulo"; and Baeninger and Fernandes, *Atlas temático*.

27 Baeninger, Demétrio, and Domeniconi, "Espaços das migrações transnacionais," table 2; and Bomtempo and Sena, "Migração internacional de africanos para o Brasil e suas territorialidades no estado do Ceará."

28 Shu and Tiashu, "Studies on Chinese Migration"; Mandelbaum and Buitoni, "Territorializations"; Shu, *Chinese Migration to Brazil*; and Piza, "Chinese Migration."

29 Jensen, *Color of Asylum*; Baeninger and Fernandes, *Atlas temático*; Daniela Bucci and Maiara Matricaldi, "Refugiados no Brasil, em São Paulo e região metropolitana: Desafios para o acolhimento," *Rede Brasil Atual*, September 26, 2021, https://www.redebrasilatual.com.br/blogs/blog-na-rede/refugiados-no-brasil-em-sao-paulo-e-regiao-metropolitana-desafios-para-o-acolhimento; and Caritas: Arquidiocesana de São Paulo and United Nations High Commission on Refugees, *Mapa de Georreferenciamento de Pessoas em Situação de Refúgio Atendidas pela Caritas Arquidiocesana de São Paulo*.

30 Césaro, "Uma etnografia da mobilidade internacional de senegaleses em Porto Alegre (RS, Brasil) e Atlanta (GA, Estados Unidos)."

31 Ball, *Navigating Life and Work*; and Sontag, *Illness as a Metaphor*.

32 Rezende and Heller, *O saneamento no Brasil*, 43.

33 Koselleck, *Sediments of Time*, 5–6; and C. Andrade, "Resíduo," 92.

34 Authors as diverse as anthropologist Claude Lévi-Strauss and music critic Greil Marcus have argued something similar, in very different realms. Lévi-Strauss, *World on the Wane*; and Marcus, *Lipstick Traces*.

35 Boudia et al., "Residues," 168.

36 Tsing, *Friction*, 74; and Gordillo, *Rubble*.

37 Jesus, *Quarto de despejo*; and Fernandez, *A poética de resíduos de Carolina Maria de Jesus*.

38 Anzaldúa, *Borderlands/La frontera*, 25–26.

39 Heathcott, "Infrastructure Designs," 1.

40 Cortinois and Birn, "What's Technology."

41 Young, "Postcolonial Remains," 19.

42 James, Jia, and Kedia, "Disparities in Cancer Risks."

43 Hochman and Birn, "Pandemias e epidemias." See also Birn and López, *Peripheral Nerve*; and Kropf and Hochman, "Science, Health, and Development."

44 Gandhi, "Catch Me," 48; and Americano, "O realejo e os macacos," 155.

45 Armus and Gómez, *Gray Zones of Medicine.*

46 Buechler, "Sweating It."

47 Vargas, "When a Favela Dared."

48 Cymbalista and Nakano, "São Paulo, Brazil."

49 Martes and Faleiros, "Acesso dos imigrantes bolivianos aos serviços públicos de saúde na cidade de São Paulo"; Park, "'Foxes' Outfoxed"; Kang et al., "Mental Health of Korean Immigrants"; and S. Silva, *Costurando sonhos.*

50 Link and Phelan, "Social Conditions."

51 Bosi, *Memória e sociedade,* 105.

52 Marcos Faerman, "O bairro de Szmul, de Isaac, de Jacob, do *beigale,* do arenque, das dez sinagogas: Ontem, na primeira parte da reportagem, mostramos o Bom Retiro dos italianos. Nesta página e na seguinte está outro Bom Retiro—o bairro dos judeus," *Jornal da Tarde,* November 24, 1981, 14–15.

53 Bernardo, *Memória em branco e negro,* 75, 119.

54 Pingel, "Immigrants, Migrants, and Paulistanos," 7.

55 Pingel, "Primary Care," 44.

56 "Círculo de Reflexão sobre Judaísmo Contemporâneo com Jeffrey Lesser," Casa de Povo, accessed August 29, 2023, https://casadopovo.org.br/en /circulo-de-reflexao-sobre-judaismo-contemporaneo-18/.

57 Portelli, "Uchronic Dreams."

58 Green, *Ready-to-Wear.*

59 Lisboa, "Insalubridade, doenças e imigração"; Colgrove, *Epidemic City*; Stepan, *"Hour of Eugenics"*; Markel and Stern, "Foreignness of Germs"; Barnett and Walker, "Role of Immigrants"; E. Jones, "'Co-operation in All Human Endeavour'"; Martin, Goldberg, and Silveira, "Imigração, refúgio e saúde"; and Vignie and Bouchaud, "Travel, Migration."

60 Farmer, *Pathologies of Power*; and Pegler-Gordon, *In Sight of America.*

61 מענטשן־פֿרעסער , *Mentshn-Fresser ("People Devourer"), 1916.* https:// opensiddur.org/prayers/collective-welfare/trouble/epidemics/mentshn -fresser-people-devourer-by-shlomo-shmulevitsh-1916/; and Shalom Goldman, "Yiddish Plague Songs," *Tablet,* April 29, 2020.

62 Vertesi, "Mind the Gap."

63 Monmonier, *How to Lie with Maps,* 1.

64 Doreen Massey, "Double Articulation."

65 Carlos Frederico Rath, "Planta da Cidade de São Paulo—1868." In "São Paulo antigo: Plantas da cidade," *Informativo Arquivo Histórico de São*

Paulo 4, no. 20 (September–October 2008). http://www.arquiamigos.org
.br/info/info20/img/1868-download.jpg.

66   Cosby, "Flowers Grew," 116–20.

67   Mapa Falk da Cidade de São Paulo (1951)—1, Acervo do Museu Paulista
da USP, https://pt.wikipedia.org/wiki/Ficheiro:Mapa_Falk_da_Cidade_de
_S%C3%A3o_Paulo_-_1,_Acervo_do_Museu_Paulista_da_USP.jpg; and
Joyner, "Planta da cidade de São Paulo levantada pela Companhia Canta-
reira e Esgotos, 1881." In "São Paulo antigo: Plantas da cidade." *Informativo
Arquivo Histórico de São Paulo* 4, no.20 (September–October 2008). http://
www.arquiamigos.org.br/info/info20/i-1881.htm; http://www.arquiamigos
.org.br/info/info20/img/1868-download.jpg.

68   Silveira et al., "O lugar dos trabalhadores de saúde nas pesquisas sobre
processos migratórios internacionais e saúde"; and Pardue, "I Only Know."

69   Plataforma Pauliceia 2.0, accessed June 22, 2024, https://pauliceia.unifesp
.br/portal/explore.

70   Research was conducted with the approval of the São Paulo Secretary of
Health Municipal Ethics Committee (April 5, 2016) based on prior ap-
proval by the Bom Retiro Public Health Clinic (April 1, 2016). The proj-
ect was also approved by the Emory University Institutional Review
Board as STUDY00002187 and by the Collaborative Institutional Training
Initiative—Human Subjects Protection (ID: 36799181).

71   Mele, *Selling the Lower East Side*; Shah, *Contagious Divides*; Truzzi, "Etnias em convívio"; Chalhoub, "Politics of Disease Control"; and Armus,
Disease.

72   *Unidade Básica*, created by Helena Petta, Newton Cannito, and Ana Petta
(Globoplay, 2016–18). See also *Sob Pressão*, created by Lucas Paraizo, Luiz
Noronha, Claudio Torres, Renato Fagundes, and Jorge Furtado (TV Globo
and Globoplay, 2017–22).

73   Gregg, *Virtually Virgins*; Monica Andrade et al., "Brazil's Family Health
Strategy"; and Pingel, "Primary Care," 38.

74   A. Cruz et al., "Estudo de análise," 2.

75   Pingel, "Primary Care," 36–37.

76   Lotta, *Burocracia e implementação de políticas de saúde.*

77   E. Santos and Kirschbaum, "A trajetória histórica da visita domiciliária no
Brasil."

78   História, Mapas e Computadores (HIMACO), accessed June 22, 2024,
www.unifesp.br/himaco; Plataforma Pauliceia 2.0, accessed June 22, 2024,
https://pauliceia.unifesp.br/portal/explore.

79   "Research Collective," Jeffrey Lesser, Department of History, Emory University, accessed June 22, 2024, https://jlesser.org/team/.

80 Toji, *Immensity of Being Singular.*

81 Low, "Empire and the Hajj."

82 Miéville, *City.*

Chapter 1. Naming a Death

1 In 1913 São Paulo city had a population of 480,000. There were 9,301 deaths in the city that year, for a rate of 18.9 deaths per 1,000 inhabitants. Bom Retiro, despite its reputation as a dangerous place, had a significantly lower death rate of about 13.5 deaths per 1,000 inhabitants. São Paulo, *Annuario demographico 1913*, 21–22.

2 Boletim de Ocorrência 13493, November 22, 1913, folder E13979 (MY 13979-1690), Registro de Ocorrência de Atendimentos Médicos realizados no Posto Médico da Assistência Policial, Arquivo Público do Estado de São Paulo (APESP), São Paulo.

3 Rocha, "Saindo das sombras."

4 "Suicídio ou crime," *Correio Paulistano*, November 23, 1913, 6.

5 In Brazil ethnic-national terms (such as Syrian) are as often applied to descendants as to immigrants themselves. Lesser, *Negotiating National Identity.*

6 Plínio Salgado's pseudorealist novel *O estrangeiro (Crónica da vida paulista)* (The foreigner [Chronicle of life in São Paulo]; 1926) was filled with references to neighborhoods like Bom Retiro where Syrians and other non-European, non-Christian immigrants preyed on women. Lesser, *Welcoming the Undesirables*, 61.

7 "Suicídio ou crime," *Correio Paulistano*, November 23, 1913, 6; and Bertolli Filho, *A gripe espanhola em São Paulo*, 45.

8 Boletim de Ocorrência 13493, November 22, 1913, folder E13979 (MY 13979-1690), Registro de Ocorrência de Atendimentos Médicos realizados no Posto Médico da Assistência Policial, Arquivo Público do Estado de São Paulo (APESP); and "Suicídio ou crime," *Correio Paulistano*, November 23, 1913, 6.

9 Penteado, *Belènzinho, 1910*, 35.

10 Miranda, "Ensaio de um método"; M. Araújo, "A escolarização de crianças negras paulistas"; and Peters, *Apartments for Workers*, 17.

11 Holloway, *Immigrants on the Land.*

12 "Saúde pública," *Correio Paulistano*, February 9, 1892, 1.

13 Romero, "Construção da nação e exclusão social."

14 Lei Estadual No. 12, de 28 de outubro de 1891, "Organiza o Serviço Sanitário do Estado," ALESP, https://www.al.sp.gov.br/repositorio/legislacao/lei/1891

/lei-12-28.10.1891.html; Blount, "Public Health Movement"; Márcia Silva, "História da assistência hospitalar em São Paulo"; Mascarenhas, "História da saúde pública no Estado de São Paulo"; and Kropf and Hochman, "From the Beginnings."

15   Nemi, "Charity and Philanthropy."

16   Blount, "Public Health Movement."

17   Mota, *Tropeços da medicina bandeirante*; and Márcia Silva, *O laboratório e a república*.

18   Caggiano, "Inmigrantes en la ciudad Buenos Aires"; Kidambi, "'Infection of Locality'"; Walcott, "Overlapping Ethnicities"; Shear, "When the Virus Came for the American Dream"; Dwork, "Health Conditions of Immigrant Jews"; Fee and Liping, "Origins of Public Health Nursing"; Yankelevich, "Migración, mestizaje y xenofobia"; and Monteyne, *Temporary Accommodation of Settlers*, 6–8.

19   Decreto Estadual No. 120, de 29 de outubro de 1892, published in *Diário Official do Estado de São Paulo*, November 4, 1892, https://www.al.sp.gov .br/norma/137615.

20   Alfredo Pinto, *A cidade de São Paulo em 1900*, 27; Bandeira, *Indústria no estado de São Paulo*; Galvão, *Parque industrial*; and Zequini, *O quintal da fábrica*, 185.

21   M. Ribeiro, "Engenheiro e o inquérito," 131. See also Decreto Estadual No. 233, de 2 de março de 1894, "Estabelece o Codigo Sanitario," ALESP, https://www.al.sp.gov.br/repositorio/legislacao/decreto/1894/decreto-233 -02.03.1894.html.

22   Rodriguez, "Inoculating against Barbarism?"; and Stepan, *Eradication*.

23   Mangili, *Bom Retiro*, 50.

24   Ferrero, *Nell'America meridionale*, 35. See also Constantino, *Italiano na cidade*, 38.

25   Dwork, "Health Conditions of Immigrant Jews"; Fee and Liping, "Origins of Public Health Nursing"; E. Jones, "'Co-operation in All Human Endeavour'"; and Stepan, *"Hour of Eugenics."*

26   [name illegible], Military Infirmary, to Inspector of Hygiene, São Paulo, January 11, 1892, Inspectoria de Hygiene da Provincia de São Paulo (Serviço Sanitário), Ofícios Recebidos, 1887 á 1898, vol. 138ª5, AMSPER; and Magnani, "Rua, símbolo e suporte da experiência urbana."

27   Penteado, *Belènzinho, 1910*, 259.

28   See the typical case of Italian immigrant Antonio Quamatri, who was run over by a horse-drawn cart. "Factos diversos—accidente," *Correio Paulistano*, July 2, 1906, 2; Sposati, "Mapa exclusão/inclusão social do município de São Paulo—III (2010)" In 2018, Team Green mapped socioenvironmental

challenges to health in Bom Retiro as part of a larger sus project in the city of São Paulo.

29 Antunes, "Eugenia e imigração"; Formiga, Melo, and Paula, "O pensamento eugênico e a imigração no Brasil"; and Penteado, *Belènzinho, 1910,* 42.

30 Guimarães and Hirata, *Care and Care Workers*; and Georges and Santos, "Olhares cruzados."

31 Martinez et al., "Equity in Health"; Ferreira, Veras, and Silva, "Participação da população no controle da dengue"; Figueiredo, "Dengue in Brazil"; and Ferraz and Gomes, "A construção discursiva."

32 Azevedo, *Brazilian Tenement,* 9, 22; for the Portuguese original, see Azevedo, *O cortiço.*

33 Lei Municipal No. 10.928, de 8 de janeiro de 1991, "Regulamenta o inciso II do artigo 148 combinado com o inciso *V* do artigo 149 da Lei Orgânica do Município de São Paulo, dispõe sobre as condições de habitação dos cortiços e dá outras providências," Leis Municipais, http://leismunicipa.is /tdgej.

34 Mott et al., "Médicos e médicas em São Paulo," 856–63.

35 Mott et al., "As parteiras eram 'tutte quante' italianas"; and Penteado, *Belènzinho, 1910,* 215.

36 Oro, "Imigrantes calabreses e religiões afro-brasileiras no Rio Grande do Sul."

37 "Saúde Pública," *Correio Paulistano,* February 9, 1892, 1.

38 Ramos, "Indicadores do nível de saúde."

39 São Paulo, Directoria do Serviço Sanitário, *Annuario demographico,* 1912, 12–13.

40 Meyer and Teixeira, Serviço Sanitário do estado de São Paulo, *A gripe epidêmica no Brazil e especialmente em São Paulo,* 3; Penna, *Saneamento do Brasil,* 30; and Mascarenhas, "História da saúde pública no Estado de São Paulo," 5.

41 Blount, "Public Health Movement."

42 Brazil, Directoria Geral de Estatística, "Coeficiente de Natalidade e Mortalidade—Anno 1907, Exposição Nacional de 1908."

43 Seabra, "Meandros dos rios nos meandros do poder," 38.

44 "Planta—São Paulo Chácaras, Sítios e Fazendas, ao Rédor do Centro (Desaparecidas com o Crescer da Cidade)," undated, item number BR_ APESP_IGC_IGG_CAR_I_S_Scan-2014-12-16_08-34-34. Núcleo de Acervo Cartográfico, APESP. For a reproduction of the map, see "Reprodução de planta: São Paulo chácaras, sítios e fazendas, ao rédor do centro (Desaparecidas com o crescer da cidade)," Museu Paulista (USP) collection, public domain, accessed June 28, 2024, https://pt.m.wikipedia.org/wiki

/Ficheiro:Reprodu%C3%A7%C3%A3o_de_Planta_-_S%C3%A3o_Paulo
_Ch%C3%A1caras,_S%C3%ADtios_e_Fazendas,_ao_R%C3%A9dor_do
Centro(Desaparecidas_com_o_Crescer_da_Cidade)_-_1,_Acervo_do
_Museu_Paulista_da_USP.jpg.

45 Mangili, *Bom Retiro*, 157; and Salla, "Produzir para construir," 110.

46 F. Santos et al., "A enchente de 1929 na cidade de São Paulo."

47 Müller, "A área central da cidade," 175.

48 Penteado, *Belènzinho, 1910*, 271n35. The street name Três Rios was official-
    ized in 1916. Acto Prefeito No. 972, de 24 de agosto de 1916, Prefeitura de
    São Paulo, Legislação Municipal, http://legislacao.prefeitura.sp.gov.br/leis
    /ato-gabinete-do-prefeito-972-de-24-de-agosto-de-1916#correlacionadas.

49 São Paulo, Secretaria Municipal da Saúde, Coordenação de Epidemiolo-
    gia e Informação, *Boletim CEInfo Saúde em Dados 2022*, 6; Perillo, "Novos
    caminhos da migração no Estado de São Paulo," 78–79; São Paulo, Secre-
    taria Municipal da Saúde, Coordenação de Epidemiologia e Informação *Bo-
    letim CEInfo Informativo Censo Demográfico* 2012.), https://www.prefeitura
    .sp.gov.br/cidade/secretarias/upload/saude/arquivos/publicacoes/Boletim
    _CEInfo_Censo_02.pdf; "Perfil dos Municípios Paulistas," Fundação
    SEADE, accessed June 28, 2024, https://perfil.seade.gov.br/; and Caldeira,
    Política dos outros.

50 Rede Nossa São Paulo, "População total por distrito." *Mapa da Desigual-
    dade 2022*, 8, accessed June 28, 2024, https://www.nossasaopaulo.org.br
    /wp-content/uploads/2022/11/Mapa-da-Desigualdade-2022_Tabelas.pdf.

51 Dean, *Industrialization of São Paulo*, 49–51, 64.

52 São Paulo, Directoria do Serviço Sanitário, *Annuario demographico*,
    1912, 9.

53 Portnoy, "Rent Strike"; *Correio Paulistano*, April 21, 1882, 4; Sábato and
    Romero, *Los trabajadores de Buenos Aires*; and Yee, "Housing."

54 Marins, *Um lugar para as elites*.

55 Mangili, *Bom Retiro*, 32–33.

56 "Editaes," *Correio Paulistano*, May 25, 1880, 2; and E. Campos, "Nos camin-
    hos da Luz, antigos palacetes da elite paulistana," 32.

57 "A Província de São Paulo," *O Estado de S. Paulo*, October 8, 1880, 3.

58 Lei Municipal No. 414, de 28 de agosto de 1899, Prefeitura de São Paulo,
    Legislação Municipal, https://legislacao.prefeitura.sp.gov.br/leis/lei-414-de
    -28-de-agosto-de-1899/detalhe; and Mangili, *Bom Retiro*, 158–64.

59 "Indicações," *Correio Paulistano*, March 12, 1884, 2; "Rua Helvetia," *Cor-
    reio Paulistano*, May 1, 1884, 2; and "Pareceres de Commissões," *Correio
    Paulistano*, March 10, 1885, 2.

60 "Casamentos livres," *Correio Paulistano*, December 28, 1866, 2.

61 "O dr. Climaco Barbosa," *Jornal da Tarde*, December 29, 1879, 2.

62 "Planta dos Terrenos da Chácara Dulley," 1904, accession number 1-05834-0000-0000, João Baptista de Campos Aguirra Collection, Museu Paulista, São Paulo, https://commons.wikimedia.org/wiki/File:Planta_dos_Terrenos_da_Ch%C3%A1cara_Dulley.jpg.

63 The Salesian order might be termed an "immigrant organization" since it arrived in Brazil from Italy via Uruguay in the late nineteenth century. "Urbanizaçào do Bairro do Bom Retiro: O Loteamento da Chácara Dulley—2," in Projeto IPHAN, *Multiculturalismo em Situação Urbana*. See also Lei Municipal No. 959, de 19 de novembro de 1906, Prefeitura de São Paulo, Legislação Municipal, http://legislacao.prefeitura.sp.gov.br/leis/lei-959-de-19-de-novembro-de-1906/consolidado.

64 Telarolli, "Imigração e epidemias no estado de São Paulo," 275–76.

65 Penteado, *Belènzinho, 1910*, 31.

66 Dean, *Industrialization of São Paulo*.

67 Fausto, *Crime e cotidiano*, 10.

68 Márcia Silva, "O processo de urbanização paulista," 265; and Carvalho, "Novidades clínicas na cirurgia paulista."

69 Such approaches continue to this day. US Centers for Disease Control and Prevention, Division of Global Migration and Quarantine, "Immigrant and Refugee Health," accessed June 28, 2024, https://www.cdc.gov/immigrantrefugeehealth/index.html; and Biehl and Petryna, "Peopling Global Health."

70 Americano, *São Paulo Naquele Tempo*, 15–126.

71 Rodrigues, *Vias públicas*, 154.

72 Maria Elisa Campiotti Bérgami, "Lampião de Gás" (1958). Recorded by Inezita Barroso, accompanied by the Hervê Cordovil Orchestra. The lyrics are available at https://www.luso-poemas.net/modules/news/article.php?storyid=33124.

73 São Paulo, *Relatório de 1904 apresentado à Câmara Municipal de São Paulo pelo prefeito Dr. Antonio da Silva Prado*, 26–28.

74 Penteado, *Belènzinho, 1910*, 235.

75 Rolnik, *A cidade e a lei*, 78. See also Lei Municipal No. 130, de 23 de janeiro de 1895, Prefeitura de São Paulo, Legislação Municipal, https://legislacao.prefeitura.sp.gov.br/leis/lei-130-de-23-de-janeiro-de-1895/consolidado; Decreto Estadual No. 2.141, de 14 de novembro de 1911, Artigo 293, ALESP, https://www.al.sp.gov.br/repositorio/legislacao/decreto/1911/decreto-2141-14.11.1911.html; Secretaria da Segurança Pública do Estado de São Paulo,

Grupo 12G6—Delegacias da Grande São Paulo, 8-Registros de acidente de trabalho da 2ª Delegacia—Bom Retiro (1934–41), Acadepol 738, APESP, http://icaatom.arquivoestado.sp.gov.br/ica-atom/index.php/delegacias-da-grande-sao-paulo-degran;isad.

76   Americano, *São Paulo Naquele Tempo*, 97–98. Sorocaba, a city less than a hundred kilometers from Bom Retiro with an intense textile industry, was also known as the Manchester Paulista. C. Cunha, "O patrimônio cultural da cidade de Sorocaba"; and Herrera, "Manchester Paulista?"

77   Oliva and Fonseca, "O 'modelo São Paulo,'" 33.

78   Dean, "A fábrica São Luiz de Itu."

79   Alfredo Pinto, *A cidade de São Paulo em 1900*, 210.

80   Rago, *Do cabaré ao lar*, 71; "Factos policiaes, operários em parede," *O Commercio de São Paulo*, December 16, 1902, 1; "Factos policiaes, ainda a greve," *O Commercio de São Paulo*, December 18, 1902, 1; and "No Bom Retiro e em Santa Iphigenia," *Correio Paulistano*, May 19, 1912, 7.

81   Miniguccio Cicinderella, "Cartas do Bô Ritiro," *Vida Paulista: Humorismo, Literatura, e Esporte* 2, no. 21 (August 1, 1921), 6; Penteado, *Belènzinho, 1910*, 240–41; and "A manifestação anticlerical do dia 15," *A Lanterna: Folha Anti-Clerical e de Combate*, April 29, 1911, 1.

82   "Vida operaria," *A Lanterna: Folha Anti-Clerical e de Combate*, August 12, 1911, 3; and C. H. Santos, "Sob a luz dos infames."

83   "O povo contra o regimen da fome," *A Lanterna: Folha Anti-Clerical e de Combate*, March 22, 1913, 3; "Contra a carestia da vida e a desocupação," *A Lanterna: Folha Anti-Clerical e de Combate*, March 7, 1914, 3; Blay, *Eu não tenho onde morar*, 134; and Penteado, *Belènzinho, 1910*, 241.

84   "O povo contra a carestia da vida," *A Lanterna: Folha Anti-Clerical e de Combate*, April 19, 1913, 2.

85   "Contra a carestia da vida," *A Lanterna: Folha Anti-Clerical e de Combate*, June 22, 1912, 3; and "O proletariado em revolta afirma o seu direito à vida," *A Plebe: Pela Liberdade e o Anarquismo*, July 21, 1917, 1.

86   Aguiar, "Tecnologias e cuidado em saúde," 106–9. See also Losco and Gemma, "Atenção primária em saúde para imigrantes bolivianos no Brasil."

87   Harvey, "Labor, Capital, and Class Struggle"; and Silvana Silva, "Os bairros do Brás e Bom," 91–113.

88   Marins, "Habitação e vizinhança," 132–33.

89   Americano's list of physiognomic "types" included immigrants, migrants from other parts of Brazil, and Afro-Brazilians. Americano, "Gente que a gente via," in *São Paulo Naquele Tempo*, 318.

90   "Os effeitos dos temporais," *Correio Paulistano*, February 16, 1929, 5.

91   Hacon, *Geo Saúde.*

92   Betoldi, *Relatório sobre o movimento das águas observadas no vale do Tietê e Tamanduatehy durante a enchente de Janeiro de 1887,* 8, 11.

93   *Correio Paulistano,* November 25, 1889, 2.

94   T. Sampaio, "Relatório da Commissão do saneamento das várzeas São Paulo 1890–1891," http://www2.unifesp.br/himaco/enchente_1887.php#; São Paulo. Comissão do Saneamento das Várzeas, Relatório dos estudos para o saneamento e aformoseamento das várzeas.

95   Raffard, *Alguns dias na Paulicéia,* 18–19.

96   Bandeira, *Indústria no estado de São Paulo.* See also Chalhoub, *Cidade febril.*

97   Guimarães, "Os dramas da cidade nos jornais," 328.

98   "Camara Municipal, requerimentos," *Correio Paulistano,* December 13, 1883, 1; and Ortigara, "Cartografia, plantas e projetos históricos," 80.

99   Dertônio, *O bairro do Bom Retiro,* 67.

100   Bosi, *Memória e sociedade,* 108.

101   Alfredo Pinto, *A cidade de São Paulo em 1900,* 16. More than 10 percent of the accidents registered by the Bom Retiro police between 1934 and 1941 involved the Department of Water and Sewers. Secretaria da Segurança Pública do Estado de São Paulo, Grupo 12G6—Delegacias da Grande São Paulo, 8-Registros de acidente de trabalho da 2ª Delegacia—Bom Retiro (1934–41).

102   Leão, *São Paulo em 1920,* 12; and Bertolli Filho, *A gripe espanhola em São Paulo,* 45.

103   Paula, "Os operários pedem passagem!," 4, 146–47.

104   Frehse, *O tempo das ruas na São Paulo de fins do império,* 97.

105   São Paulo, *Mensagem enviada ao Congresso Legislativo a 14 de julho de 1909,* 39; and Greenfield, "Development of the Underdeveloped City," 108–9.

106   "Noticias de Tabuaté," *Correio Paulistano,* March 30, 1890, 1; and "Saúde Pública," *Correio Paulistano,* February 9, 1892, 1.

107   Faerman, "Bairro de Szmul, de Isaac, de Jacob, do *beigale,* do arenque, das dez sinagogas: Ontem, na primeira parte da reportagem, mostramos o Bom Retiro dos italianos," *Jornal da Tarde,* November 24, 1981, 14–15.

108   Dertônio, *O bairro do Bom Retiro,* 34; Hochman, *Sanitation of Brazil;* Finkelman, *Caminhos da saúde pública no Brasil;* Eibenschutz, *Política de saúde;* and Cueto and Palmer, *Medicine and Public Health.*

109   "Notas e notícias, terro dos mosquitos," *Commercio de São Paulo,* January 10, 1908, 2.

110   "No Bom Retiro e em Santa Iphigenia, queixas e reclamações," *Correio Paulistano*, February 13, 1912, 7.

111   Pingel et al., "Committing to Continuity"; C. Silva, "Estudo epidemiológico da dengue no município de São Paulo," 37; Cristiane Bomfim, "Bom Retiro tem maior incidência de dengue," *Jornal da Tarde/O Estado de S. Paulo*, May 5, 2011; and Guilherme Balza, "Oito dos dez bairros com mais mortes por Covid-19 estão no centro 'pobre' de São Paulo," *Portal G1—Globo*, May 27, 2020. In 2020 the district had the highest COVID-19 death rates in the city.

112   Resende and Amed, "O jardim da luz e os desdobramentos da urbanização paulistana," 107.

113   Rodrigues, *Vias públicas*, 48.

114   Penteado, *Belènzinho, 1910*, 236.

115   Americano, *São Paulo Naquele Tempo*, 39.

116   Jorge, "São Paulo das Enchentes, 1890–1940."

117   Rodrigues, *Vias públicas*, 48.

118   Campos, "São Paulo Antigo."

119   J. Pereira, *Defesa dos Bens Dominaes do Município de São Paulo*, 136–38.

120   Alfredo Pinto, *A cidade de São Paulo em 1900*, 27.

121   "Igreja Santa Cruz das Almas dos Enforcados," Arquidiocese de São Paulo, Região Episcopal Sé, Paróquias, Mosteiros, Igrejas Históricas, Oratórios da Região Sé, accessed June 28, 2024, https://arquisp.org.br/regiaose /paroquias/mosteiros-igrejas-historicas-oratorios-da-regiao-se/igreja -santa-cruz-das-almas-dos-enforcados.

122   Projeto de Lei No. 71 /2020, 6 de Março de 2020, "Denomina 'Japão– Liberdade–África' a atual estação Japão-Liberdade do Metrô de São Paulo," ALESP, https://www.al.sp.gov.br/propositura/?id=1000319630; Lei Municipal No. 17954, de 31 de maio de 2023, "Denomina Japão— Liberdade—África a área livre que especifica, localizada no distrito da Liberdade, subprefeitura da Sé, e dá outras providências," Câmara Municipal de São Paulo, https://splegisconsulta.saopaulo.sp.leg.br/Pesquisa /DetalhesDetalhado?COD_MTRA_LEGL=1&COD_PCSS_CMSP=23&ANO _PCSS_CMSP=2020; and Willian Moreira, "Deputado quer mudar novamente o nome da Estação Liberdade do Metrô de São Paulo," *Diário do Transporte*, March 8, 2020, https://diariodotransporte.com.br/2020/03/08 /deputado-quer-mudar-novamente-nome-da-estacao-liberdade-do-metro -de-sao-paulo/.

123   Jéssica Moreira and Dayana Araújo, "Não podemos nomear o Bom Retiro como bairro de um povo só, alertam moradores," *Portal Aprendiz*, April 14, 2017, https://portal.aprendiz.uol.com.br/2017/04/14/nao-podemos

-nomear-o-bom-retiro-como-bairro-de-um-povo-alertam-moradores/; and Casa do Povo, "MOBILIZAÇÃO E FESTEJO PELA DIVERSIDADE CULTURAL E SOCIAL DO BOM RETIRO," October 7, 2021, https://www .facebook.com/casadopovoxxi/videos/1257473124698316.

124 Casa do Povo, accessed June 28, 2024, https://casadopovo.org.br.

125 Lesser, *Welcoming the Undesirables*.

126 Raquel Rolnik, "'Bom Retiro é o Mundo': Projeto Korea Town exclui outros povos e ignora problemas reais," *Labcidade*, November 24, 2022, http:// www.labcidade.fau.usp.br/de-bom-retiro-a-korea-town-projeto-exclui -outros-povos-e-ignora-problemas-reais/.

127 "Mobilização e festejo pela diversidade cultural e social do Bom Retiro," Teatro Popular União e Olho Vivo, Facebook, October 10, 2021, https:// www.facebook.com/casadopovoxxi/videos/1257473124698316.

128 "Hino do Corinthians," *Letras*, accessed June 28, 2024, https://www.letras .mus.br/corinthians/1539059/.

Chapter 2. Bom Retiro Is the World?

Epigraph: Bananére, "A invençó do Brasile," Cartas d'Abax'o Pigues, *O Pirralho* 89, May 3, 1913, 19. Bananére's poem may well have inspired Lamartine Babo's 1934 carnival hit "História do Brasil," whose lyrics also posited that Pedro Cabral had "invented" Brazil. Cukierman, "Who Invented Brazil?"

1 Bananére, "O studenti du Bó Retiro: Poisia Patriotica, (Premiata c'oa medaglia de pratina na insposiçó da Xéca-Slovaca i c'oa medaglia di brigliantina na sposiçó internazionale da Varzea du Carmo)" [The student of Bó Retiro: Patriotic Poem (Awarded the silver medal at the Czechoslovakian Exposition and the shiny medal at the Carmo Flood Plains International Exposition, 1913)], *La divina increnca*, 1924, 17. The original poem was published in *O Pirralho*, February 14, 1913, 13.

2 Del Picchia, *Poesias, 1907/1946*, 195–96.

3 "Variola," *Correio Paulistano*, June 5, 1887, 2.

4 Romero, "Construção da nação e exclusão social," 81.

5 Projeto IPHAN, *Multiculturalismo em situação urbana*, 1.

6 André Klotzel, "O Bom Retiro é o mundo," YouTube, https://www.youtube .com/watch?v=7i7Dlu3vGCY.

7 Americano, "Gente que a gente viu," in *São Paulo Naquele Tempo*, 318.

8 Penteado, *Belènzinho, 1910*, 34–35.

9 Marcos Faerman, "Lembrando os Bons Tempos," *Jornal da Tarde*, November 23, 1981, 14–15; Faerman, "O bairro de Szmul, de Isaac, de Jacob, do beigale, do arenque, das dez sinagogas: Ontem, na primeira parte da

reportagem, mostramos o Bom Retiro dos italianos. Nesta página e na seguinte está outro Bom Retiro—o bairro dos judeus," *Jornal da Tarde*, November 24, 1981, 14–15.

10 Patai, "Minority Status," 52; Fendler, "Others"; Brunger, "Problematizing the Notion of 'Community,'" 245–56; and "A Gazeta no Bom Retiro," *A Gazeta*, February 7, 1914, 2.

11 Ortega y Gasset, "La pedagogía del paisaje," 55. Octavio Paz later wrote, "Tell me how you die and I will tell you who you are." Paz, *Labyrinth of Solitude*, 54.

12 This Google Map shows how geographically close the "ethnic" neighborhoods of São Paulo are: https://maps.app.goo.gl/UNhVNc6odoAyciDp9.

13 Araújo, "Enquistamentos étnicos," 227–46; and El-Dine, "Eugenia e seleção imigratória," 243–52.

14 Moacir Assunção, "Mistura cultural marca Bom Retiro," *Diário Popular*, February 15, 1997.

15 Feldman, "Bom Retiro"; Truzzi, "Etnias em convívio"; Ana Corrêa, "Imigrantes judeus em São Paulo"; and Póvoa, *A territorialização dos judeus na cidade de São Paulo*.

16 J. Borges, "O estrangeiro nos dicionários de língua portuguesa."

17 Karam, *Another Arabesque*.

18 Logan, Zhang, and Alba, "Immigrant Enclaves," 299. See also Portes and Manning, "Immigrant Enclave."

19 Hesse-Wartegg, *Zwischen Anden und Amazonas*, 148.

20 Petrone, "A cidade de São Paulo no século XX," 135–36.

21 Almeida, *Cosmópolis*.

22 Almeida, *Cosmópolis*, 4.

23 São Paulo, *Anuário Demográfico da Seção de Estatísticas Demógrafo-Sanitárias 1907*, 12.

24 Morse, "São Paulo since Independence," 442.

25 Azevedo, *A cidade de São Paulo*, 19.

26 Ministério da Agricultura, Indústria e Comércio, Directoria Geral de Estatística, *Recenseamento do Brazil*: Municipality of São Paulo, "Dados demográficos dos distritos pertencentes às Subprefeituras"; and Bassanezi, "São Paulo do passado—dados demográficos (1836–2020)."

27 Kelsey, "How the Other Nine-Tenths Lived"; and Joseph Leidy, "Mapping Newcomers in Buenos Aires, 1928," *Not Even Past*, September 12, 2016, https://notevenpast.org/13770-2/.

28 Shinohara and Comarú, "Dinâmica Habitacional e Demográfica da Metrópole Paulista."

29 Rede Nossa São Paulo, "Mapa da desigualidade," 2019, https://www
    .nossasaopaulo.org.br/wp-content/uploads/2019/11/Mapa_Desigualdade
    _2019_tabelas.pdf.

30 Fundação Seade, "Perfil dos municípios paulistas: Distrito de Bom Retiro,"
    accessed June 28, 2024, https://www.perfil.seade.gov.br/.

31 Sposati, "Mapa exclusão/inclusão social do município de São Paulo—III
    (2010); Prefeitura Municipal de São Paulo, *DIRETRIZES DE INTERVENÇÃO—
    Quadras 37 e 38—Campos Elíseos,*" 46; Prefeitura de São Paulo, Dados
    Abertos, "Cortiços no Município de São Paulo," accessed June 28, 2024,
    http://dados.prefeitura.sp.gov.br/dataset/corticos; and São Paulo (City),
    Cortiços em São Paulo: Frente e verso (São Paulo: Município de São Paulo,
    Secretaria Municipal do Planejamento, 1986).

32 Sposati, "Mapa exclusão/inclusão social do município de São Paulo—III
    (2010)."

33 Sposati et al., *Mapa da exclusão/inclusão*, 1996; and Sposati, "Mapa ex-
    clusão/inclusão social do município de São Paulo—III (2010)."

34 Lei Municipal No. 11.220, de 20 de maio de 1992, "Institui a divisão
    geográfica da área do Município em Distritos, revoga a Lei n. 10.932, de
    15 de janeiro de 1991, e dá outras providências," Casa Civil do Gabinete do
    Prefeito, Legislação Municipal, accessed June 28, 2024, https://legislacao
    .prefeitura.sp.gov.br/leis/lei-11220-de-20-de-maio-de-1992; Sposati, *Mapa
    da exclusão/inclusão social da cidade de São Paulo 2000*; and Waldman,
    Silva, and Monteiro, "Trajetória das doenças infecciosas."

35 Min, *Caught in the Middle*; Logan, Zhang, and Alba, "Immigrant Enclaves";
    Sánchez, *Boyle Heights*; Andrews, *Blackness in the White Nation*; Ortiz, *Afri-
    can American and Latinx History*; Hou, "Spatial Assimilation"; and Douglas
    Massey, "New Immigration and Ethnicity."

36 Alberto and Hoffnung-Garskof, "'Racial Democracy.'"

37 A dual-language (Portuguese-Japanese) manga that treats this question is
    D'Angelo and Giassetti, *O filho da costureira e o catador de batatas*.

38 Gonçalves and Costa, *Um porto no capitalismo global*, 75–96.

39 Fernandes, *A integração do negro na sociedade de classes*, 41.

40 Rocha, "Saindo das sombras," 146–50.

41 Bernardo, *Memória em branco e negro*, 45–46.

42 Instituto Brasileiro de Geografia e Estatística, Censo 2010, "Brasil 1 por
    1" accessed June 28, 2024, http://mapasinterativos.ibge.gov.br/atlas_ge
    /brasil1por1.html.

43 Rede Nossa São Paulo, "Remuneração média mensal (em R$) do emprego
    formal, por distrito," *Mapa da Desigualdade 2022*, 8, accessed June 28, 2024,

https://www.nossasaopaulo.org.br/wp-content/uploads/2022/11/Mapa-da
-Desigualdade-2022_Tabelas.pdf.

44   Fernandes, *A integração do negro na sociedade de classes*, 38–42; and Elaine
       Muniz Pires, "História dos bairros paulistanos—Bom Retiro," Banco de
       Dados Folha, *Almanaque Folha*, accessed June 28, 2024, http://almanaque
       .folha.uol.com.br/bairros_bom_retiro.htm. A groundbreaking study of Rio
       de Janeiro's Praça Onze/Pequena África is Bitter, "Narrativas de memória e
       performances musicais dos judeus cariocas da 'Pequena África.'" See also
       Skidmore, *Black into White*; Dávila, *Diploma of Whiteness*; Telles, *Race in
       Another America*; and Travassos and Williams, "Concept and Measurement
       of Race."

45   Britt, "Re/Mapping São Paulo's Geographies"; and Guimarães, "Preconceito
       de cor e racismo no Brasil."

46   P. Fontes, *Um nordeste em São Paulo*; and Melo and Fusco, "Migrantes
       nordestinos na região metropolitana de São Paulo."

47   Butler, *Freedoms Given, Freedoms Won*; and Weinstein, *Color of Modernity*.

48   Estado de São Paulo, Diretoria de Serviços Sanitários, *Boletim Mensal de
       Estatística Demógrafo-Sanitária* 8 (January–December 1925): 1–12, and 7
       (January–December 1929): 1–12, cited in Butler, *Freedoms Given, Freedoms
       Won*, 76.

49   *GL'Italiani in San Paulo*, February 28, 1889, 2; Panizzolo, "Italian and
       Italian-Descendant Children," 63–64; and Lei Provincial No. 8, de 15 de fe-
       vereiro de 1884, Artigo 1, ALESP, https://al.sp.gov.br/repositorio/legislacao
       /lei/1884/lei-59-25.04.1884.html.

50   Penteado, *Belènzinho, 1910*, 41. For an examination of the whitening of
       teachers in public schools, see Dávila, *Diploma of Whiteness*.

51   Lowrie, "O elemento negro na população de São Paulo," 57.

52   M. Araújo, "A escolarização de crianças negras paulistas," 142–44.

53   Zylbersztajn, *O filho de Osum*.

54   Pingel, "Primary Care," 44–45; and P. Fontes, *Um nordeste em São Paulo*.

55   Chi, "O Bom Retiro dos coreanos."

56   Universidade Zumbi dos Palmares, "Sobre nós: conheça a Universidade
       Zumbi dos Palmares." Accessed June 28, 2024, https://zumbidospalmares
       .edu.br/sobre-nos/.

57   Putnam, *Radical Moves*, 124–25.

58   Bastide, "A imprensa negra no Estado de São Paulo," 8; and Seigel, *Uneven
       Encounters*.

59   *O Menelick*, January 1, 1916, 3–4; Côrtes, "'Leitoras,'" 170; and F. Santos,
       Aspectos da luta pela cidadania negra.

60   Alberto, *Terms of Inclusion*, 36.

61   Monsma, "Symbolic Conflicts, Deadly Consequences," 1123–52.

62   Fernandes, *A integração do negro na sociedade de classes*. See also Andrews, *Blacks and Whites in São Paulo, Brazil*.

63   Cuti, *E disse o velho militante Jose Correia Leite*, 26, 45.

64   Americano, "Desafios e guerras entre meninos," in *São Paulo Naquele Tempo*, 50.

65   Fernandes, "As 'Trocinhas' do Bom Retiro." See also Cruz, "Gênero e culturas infantis."

66   LABCidade "A verticalização de mercado em São Paulo é branca"; Jorge, *Tietê, o rio que a cidade perdeu*, 47–48; and R. Araújo et al., "São Paulo Urban Heat Islands."

67   Somekh, *A cidade vertical e o urbanismo modernizador*; Toledo, *A capital da vertigem*; Stewart, "Framing the City"; Cwerner, "Helipads, Heliports"; and Caldeira, *City of Walls*.

68   Nakano, "Desenvolvimento territorial e regulação urbanística," 394.

69   Chi, "O Bom Retiro dos coreanos," 53–54.

70   "A Gazeta no Bom Retiro," *A Gazeta*, February 7, 1914, 2.

71   Koulioumba, "Construtores estrangeiros e a produção arquitetônica moderna no Bom Retiro (1950–1970)."

72   Medina, "Apresentação," 9; and Kim, "Nas curvas do rio ídiche," 13.

73   Claire Rigby, "São Paulo's Water Crisis," *Guardian*, April 15, 2015.

74   Mendonça, Veiga e Souza, and Almeida Dutra, "Saúde pública, urbanização e dengue no Brasil."

75   Pimenta Velloso, "Os restos na história," 1958.

Chapter 3. Bad Health in a Good Retreat

1   Fausto, *Crime e cotidiano*, 10.

2   "Tiros de Espingarda—consequencias de álcool," *Correio Paulistano*, August 10, 1914, 4.

3   Secretaria da Segurança Pública do Estado de São Paulo, Registro de ocorrências da Assistência Policial, 1911–40, docs. 018863, 018864, 018865, 018866, and 018867, vol. 13988, all dated August 9, 1914, APESP.

4   "Futebol, E'cos," *A Gazeta*, March 9, 1923, 2; and "Futebol, E'cos," *A Gazeta*, March 17, 1923, 3.

5   Britt, "Spatial Projects of Forgetting."

6   Nakano, "Desigualdades habitacionais," 56.

7 Granada et al., "A pandemia de covid-19 e a mobilidade internacional no Brasil."

8 Hutter, *Imigração italiana em São Paulo*, 118; and Telarolli, "Imigração e epidemias no estado de São Paulo," 270.

9 Blount, "Public Health Movement," 59.

10 Lesser, *Immigration, Ethnicity and National Identity*, 96; Kenzo, *Não há cura sem anúncio*, 33; Telarolli, "Imigração e epidemias no estado de São Paulo," 271; and Aliano, "Brazil through Italian Eyes."

11 Márcia Silva, "O mundo transformado em laboratório," 40.

12 Motta Junior, *Relatorio apresentado ao Senhor Doutor Presidente do Estado de São Paulo*, LII; Shively, "Sanitary Tenements"; and Campbell, "What Tuberculosis Did for Modernism."

13 Vaz, "Dos cortiços às favelas e aos edifícios de apartamentos"; and Silva de Souza, "Cortiços em São Paulo," 43–44.

14 Codigo de Posturas do Municipio de São Paulo, de 6 de outubro de 1886, especially Artigos 1–28, Câmara Municipal de São Paulo, SPLEGIS, https:// www.saopaulo.sp.leg.br/iah/fulltext/leis/LCP-1886.pdf. See also Scarlato, "Estrutura e sobrevivência dos cortiços no bairro Bexiga," 117–27; M. Sampaio, "O cortiço paulistano entre as ciências sociais e política," 130; and Bonduki, "Origens da habitação social no Brasil."

15 "Sondagem preliminar a um estudo sobre a habitação em São Paulo (1947): Estudo contratado pela Escola de Sociologia e Política de São Paulo, coordenado por J. L. Lebret," *Revista do Arquivo Municipal* 139–40 (April–June 1951): 3–48; Lagenest, "Os Cortiços de São Paulo"; M. Sampaio and Pereira, "Habitação em São Paulo," 178; and Pingel, "Primary Care," 73–74.

16 Companhia de Desenvolvimento Habitacional e Urbano do Estado de São Paulo, *Relatório Geral do Programa de atuação em cortiços*, 17.

17 Lucchesi, "Do cortiço às vilas operárias."

18 Bernardo, *Memória em branco e negro*, 58.

19 Lei Municipal No. 1, de 29 de setembro de 1892, Artigo 1b, Prefeitura de São Paulo, Legislação Municipal, http://legislacao.prefeitura.sp.gov.br/leis /lei-1-de-29-de-setembro-de-1892/consolidado.

20 Decreto Estadual No. 264, de 27 de outubro de 1894, "Dá regulamento á Repartição Central de Policia," Leis Estaduais, https://leisestaduais.com.br /sp/decreto-n-264-1894-sao-paulo-da-regulamento-a-reparticao-central -de-policia; and Lei Municipal No. 203, de 27 de fevereiro de 1896, Artigo 1, Prefeitura de São Paulo, Legislação Municipal, http://legislacao.prefeitura .sp.gov.br/leis/lei-203-de-27-de-fevereiro-de-1896/consolidado.

21 Mota, *Tempos cruzados*, 93.

22 Lei Municipal No. 1, de 29 de setembro de 1892, Artigo 1b; Lei Munici-
pal No. 203, de 27 de fevereiro de 1896, Act 2; and Documentos Avulsos,
Polícia e Higiene, 1892–98, Arquivo Histórico Municipal Washington Luís
(AHM), São Paulo.

23 Decreto Estadual No. 2.141, de 14 de novembro de 1911, Artigo 293, ALESP,
https://www.al.sp.gov.br/repositorio/legislacao/decreto/1911/decreto-2141
-14.11.1911.html (the full set of new regulations is in articles 291–99); and
Lemos, "Os primeiros cortiços paulistanos," 15.

24 Blay, *Eu não tenho onde morar*, 95.

25 Decreto Estadual No. 2.141, de 14 de novembro de 1911, Artigo 293.

26 Guzzo, "A habitação popular em São Paulo," 60.

27 Cano, "A cidade dos cortiços."

28 Wilhelm, *São Paulo Metrópole*, 65; and Nakano, "Desenvolvimento territorial e regulação urbanística nas áreas centrais de São Paulo," 397.

29 Walle, *Au Brésil*, 8; and Leite, *Maria Lacerda de Moura*, 18.

30 Dertônio, *O bairro do Bom Retiro*, 17.

31 Gallois and Rosalen, "Direitos indígenas 'diferenciados' e seus efeitos entre
os Wajãpi no Amapá"; Marinelli et al., "Assistência à população indígena";
and Lacerda, Figueira, and Pinto, "Conhecimentos tradicionais dos povos
indígenas da região Pantaneira Sul-Mato-Grossense," 150–58.

32 Cunningham and Black, "Healing the Sick City"; Piccini, *Cortiços na cidade*; and Kowarick and Ant, "One Hundred Years of Overcrowding."

33 "Variola," *Correio Paulistano*, June 5, 1887, 2.

34 *A Provincia de São Paulo*, February 1, 1884, 2.

35 "Mais notas falsas: Auctoridade no forno: Com a bocca na botija," *Correio
Paulistano*, September 13, 1898, 1.

36 Carbone, *Park, Tenement, Slaughterhouse*; M. Jones, "Tuberculosis, Housing"; Garb, "Health, Morality, and Housing"; Gilman, *Difference and Pathology*; and Kraut, *Silent Travelers*.

37 *Relatório da Comissão de Exame e Inspecção das Habitações Operárias
e Cortiços do Districto de Santa Iphygenia, apresentado pelo Intendente
Municipal Cesario Motta Jr.* (São Paulo: Câmara Municipal de São Paulo,
1893), 43–44, quoted in Cordeiro, *Os cortiços de Santa Ifigênia*, 43–44.

38 Bonduki, *Origens da habitação social no Brasil*, 59.

39 Brazil, "Celso Garcia, Indicação 144 of 1905, 24th Sessão Ordinária de 29 de
Julho de 1905," *Anais da Câmara Municipal*, p. 115, https://www.saopaulo.sp
.leg.br/static/atas_anais_cmsp/anadig/Sessoes/Ordinarias/024SO1905.pdf.

40 Peixoto-Mehrtens, *Urban Space and National Identity*, 129; and Jorge, "Rios
e saúde na cidade de São Paulo."

41   Mário de Andrade, "Colloque sentimental," 99–100.

42   Guzzo, "A habitação popular em São Paulo," 63.

43   *Fanfulla*, March 23, 1906, quoted in Kowarick, "Cortiços," 49. See also Trento, "A Itália em guerra."

44   "Bom Retiro," *A Lanterna: Folha Anti-Clerical e de Combate*, March 22, 1913, 3.

45   Cusano, *Italia d'oltre mare*, 117.

46   Arquivo Públic do Estado de São Paulo, Acervo, Instrumentos de Pesquisa, "Fichas de coleta de informações da Comissão de exame e inspeção das habitações operarias e cortiços no Distrito de Santa Efigênia (1893)," accessed June 28, 2024. http://www.arquivoestado.sp.gov.br/site/acervo /repositorio_digital/corticos_ephigenia. See also Cordeiro, *Os cortiços de Santa Ifigênia*, 139.

47   Beiguelman, *Os companheiros de São Paulo*, 88; and Câmara Municipal de São Paulo, "Centro de Memória CMSP—uma história em transformação," accessed June 28, 2024, https://www.saopaulo.sp.leg.br/memoria/.

48   Celso Garcia, Indicação 144 of 1905, p. 115.

49   "Dezenas de famílias despejadas no bairro do Bom Retiro," *A Plebe: Pela Liberdade e o Anarquismo*, September 15, 1947, 1.

50   L. Camargo, "Habitações populares em São Paulo"; Adolpho Pinto, *A transformação e o embellezamento de São Paulo*, 27–29; and Barros, "A habitação e os transportes."

51   Americano, "Os Bondes Eléctricos (1901)," in *São Paulo Naquele Tempo*, 186–87; and Frehse, *O tempo das ruas na São Paulo de fins do império*, 201–3.

52   "Pela cidade," *A Lanterna: Folha Anti-Clerical e de Combate*, June 24, 1911, 2.

53   Passos and Emídio, *Desenhando São Paulo*, 88–91.

54   Penteado, *Belènzinho, 1910*, 34.

55   Mimesse, "O cotidiano da escolarização primária paulistana nos anos iniciais do século XX."

56   Panizzolo, "A escola étnica na cidade de São Paulo e os primeiros tons de uma identidade italiana"; and "A Escola Moderna em S. Paulo," *A Lanterna: Folha Anti-Clerical e de Combate*, February 12, 1910, 2.

57   Romani, *Da Biblioteca Popular à Escola Moderna*, 87–100.

58   "No Bom Retiro," *Correio Paulistano*, April 11, 1911, 5.

59   Cordeiro, "Moradia popular na cidade de São Paulo."

60   Siqueira, "Os hotéis na cidade de São Paulo na primeira década do século XX," 345.

61 C. Santos, *Nem tudo era italiano*, 135–71; and Britt, "'I'll Samba Someplace Else.'"

62 Fantin, "Do interior para os porões, dos porões para as fachadas." In 2016 I co-taught a course for the Centro de Pesquisa e Formação, SESC São Paulo (Center for Research and Training of the Social Service of Commerce, SESC), a nonprofit funded by Brazilian corporate interests, that included a visit to contemporary porões on Rua Glicério. Centro de Pesquisa e Formação, SESC São Paulo, Atividades, Liberdade ao avesso: Novos olhares sobre o bairro paulistano, accessed June 28, 2024, https://centrodepesquisaeformacao.sescsp.org.br/atividade/liberdade-ao-avesso-novos-olhares-sobre-o-bairro-paulistano.

63 Blay, *Eu não tenho onde morar*, 7.

64 "A 'Gazeta' no Bom Retiro," *A Gazeta*, April 5, 1916, 2; and Alfredo Pinto, *A cidade de São Paulo em 1900*, 9.

65 "Michele Anastasi," *Il Pasquino Coloniale*, June 19, 1937, 14.

66 "Michele Anastasi," *Il Pasquino Coloniale*, May 26, 1934, 8.

67 "Premiada Distillaria Italiana," *Correio Paulistano*, January 8, 1936, 10.

68 Instituto Butantan/Museu Emílio Ribas, *História, imigração e saúde*. I visited Vila Michele Anastasi multiple times with one of the community health workers from the Bom Retiro Public Health Clinic, who himself became the subject of an academic study. Steffens and Martins, "Falta um Jorge"; and Rafael Ciscati, "Agentes de saúde estrangeiros atendem uma crescente população imigrante em São Paulo," *O Globo*, January 8, 2018.

69 Caldeira, *City of Walls*, 14.

70 São Paulo, Governo do Estado, SEADE- Fundação Sistema Estadual de Análise de Dados, accessed June 28, 2024, https://www.seade.gov.br/?s=cortico.

71 Prefeitura Municipal de São Paulo, DIRETRIZES DE INTERVENÇÃO—*Quadras 37 e 38—Campos Elíseos*, 46; Blount, "Public Health Movement," 122; Leonardo Guandeline, "Coreanos eram principais clientes de restaurante fechado por vender carne de cachorro em SP," *O Globo*, November 10, 2011; Frúgoli and Spaggiari, "Networks and Territorialities"; "Surto de sarampo em SP faz Paraná entrar em alerta," *Gazeta do Povo* (Curitiba), July 22, 2019; "Vacina, contaminação e surto em SP," *Folha de S. Paulo*, July 24, 2019; and "Vacina reforça xenofobia, e imigrantes pesam medo de Covid-19 e deportação," *Folha de S. Paulo*, December 7, 2020.

72 Maram, "Immigrant and the Brazilian Labor Movement."

73 Lee and Yung, *Angel Island*; Pegler-Gordon, *In Sight of America*; and FitzGerald and Cook-Martín, *Culling the Masses*.

74   Reznik and Fernandes, "Hospedarias de Imigrantes nas Américas," 237; R. Teixeira, "Sob a perspectiva de uma política expansionista," 288; and Kushnir, "Hospedaria Central, o Expurgo na Ilha das Flores."

75   Lei Provincial No. 36, de 21 de fevereiro de 1881, ALESP, https://www.al.sp .gov.br/repositorio/legislacao/lei/1881/lei-36-21.02.1881.html; and Udaeta, *Nem Brás, nem Flores*, 100.

76   Holloway, *Immigrants on the Land*, 36–37.

77   Riis, *How the Other Half Lives*; Diner, Shandler, and Wenger, *Remembering the Lower East Side*; and Dans and Wasserman, *Life on the Lower East Side*.

78   "Secção Livre," *Correio Paulistano*, May 20, 1883, 2.

79   "Sociedade Central de Immigração," *Gazeta de Notícias* (Rio de Janeiro), March 2, 1885, 2.

80   "Immigração," *Correio Paulistano*, February 9, 1882, 1; "Chronologia Paulista," *Correio Paulistano*, May 18, 1882, 2; and "Serviço Provincial de Immigração," *Correio Paulistano*, November 16, 1882, 1.

81   Cruz Paiva e Moura, *Hospedaria de Imigrantes de São Paulo*, 21.

82   Museu da Imigração, Centro de Preservação, Pesquisa e Referência "Ebook do Acervo Digital do Museu da Imigração," 9, https://museudaimigracao .org.br/acervo-e-pesquisa/e-book.

83   "Immigração," *Correio Paulistano*, February 9, 1882, 1; and *Correio Paulistano*, April 16, 1885, 2.

84   "Serviço Provincial de Immigração," *Correio Paulistano*, November 16, 1882, 1; and Udaeta, *Nem Brás, nem Flores*, 107.

85   Hutter, *Imigração italiana em São Paulo*, 80–83.

86   "Immigração provincial," *Correio Paulistano*, April 17, 1885, 2; "Immigrantes," *Correio Paulistano*, May 28, 1885, 2; and L. Teixeira and Almeida, "Os primórdios da vacina antivariólica em São Paulo."

87   "Sociedade de Immigração de S. Paulo," *A Immigração* 2, no. 11 (May– June 1885); and "Serviço Provincial de Immigração," *Correio Paulistano*, November 16, 1882, 1.

88   Márcia Silva, "Concepção de saúde e doença nos debates parlamentares paulistas entre 1830 e 1900," 72–73.

89   Carrega, "As propagandas imigrantistas do Brasil no século XIX."

90   Koseritz, *Imagens do Brasil*, 204–5. The German original, *Bilder aus Brasilien*, was published in 1885, with the first Brazilian edition appearing only sixty years later.

91   Lesser, *Immigration, Ethnicity and National Identity*, 66–70.

92   "Article from *A Germania*," reprinted as "A hospedaria dos imigrantes em S. Paulo," *Gazeta de Notícias* (Rio de Janeiro), March 18, 1885, 2.

93 "A 'hespanhola' em S. Paulo, numerosos casos suspeitos," *O Combate*, November 10, 1918, 1.

94 "Immigração," *Gazeta de Notícias* (Rio de Janeiro), March 9, 1885, 2.

95 "Sociedade Central de Immigração," *Gazeta de Notícias* (Rio de Janeiro), March 21, 1885, 2.

96 Reznik and Fernandes, "Hospedarias de Imigrantes nas Américas," 238; Lei Provincial No. 56, de 21 de março de 1885, "Autoriza o Governo a construir um prédio para Hospedaria de Imigrantes, nas proximidades das linhas férreas do norte e inglesa," ALESP, https://www.al.sp.gov.br/repositorio /legislacao/lei/1885/lei-56-21.03.1885.html; and "Relatório apresentado à Assembléia Legislativa Provincial de São Paulo pelo Presidente da Província barão de Parnahyba, no dia 17 de janeiro de 1887," 123.

97 "Ospedaria degli Imigranti," *GL'Italiani in San Paulo*, February 9, 1889, 2; "Hospedaria dos Imigrantes," *Sentinella da Monarchia: Orgam Conservador*, July 21, 1889, 1; "Repatriação de immigrantes," *Sentinella da Monarchia: Orgam Conservador* , August 7, 1889, 2; "Repatriação de immigrantes," *A Immigração* 6, no. 61 (September 1889): 4; Lesser, *Immigration, Ethnicity and National Identity*, 73–77; and Reale, *Brás, Pinheiros, Jardins*, 19.

98 P. Fontes, *Making of Industrial São Paulo*.

99 Segawa, "Arquitetura de hospedarias de imigrantes."

100 Dean, "Visit to the Hospedaria," unpublished manuscript, May 13, 1963, quoted in Gloria La Cava, *Italians in Brazil*, 59.

101 "Inspectoria geral de hygiene," *Correio Paulistano*, September 4, 1886, 3.

102 Begliomini, "Cadeira no 96—Patrono Ignácio Emílio Achiles Betholdi, 1810–1886"; and Francisco, "A maçonaria e o processo da abolição em São Paulo," 54.

103 L. Camargo, "Viver e morrer em São Paulo," 151.

104 *Almanach Paulista* 1 (1881): 191; Martins, *São Paulo Antigo*, 93; "Camara Municipal, expedientes,"*Correio Paulistano*, November 3, 1888, 2; and E. Campos, "Nos caminhos da Luz, antigos palacetes da elite paulistana," 40.

105 *Folha do Braz*, November 12, 1899, 1; *Relatório da Comissão de Exame e Inspecção das Habitações Operárias e Cortiços do Districto de Santa Iphygenia*, 1893.

106 Alfredo Pinto, *A cidade de São Paulo em 1900*, 97; and Secretaria da Segurança Pública do Estado de São Paulo, Grupo 12G6—Delegacias da Grande São Paulo, 8-Registros de acidente de trabalho da 2ª Delegacia—Bom Retiro (1934–41), Acadepol 738, APESP.

107 The location of the former headquarters of the São Paulo Sewer and Water Distribution Company is at the contemporary Avenida Casper Libero, 605.

108   Riess, "From Pitch to Putt"; and S. Jones, *Sport, Politics.*

109   Americano, "Golfe," in *São Paulo Naquele Tempo*, 300.

110   SPAC: Clube Atlético São Paulo, accessed June 28, 2024, https://www.spac
       .org.br/.

111   "S. Paulo Athletic Club," *Correio Paulistano*, December 8, 1888, 2; and
       Barbosa, *Soccer and Racism*, 14. There is an uninteresting debate about
       the exact date of the game. It was in 1898, says Diego Monteiro Gutierrez.
       Gutierrez, "O Rugby, identidade e processos econômicos no Brasil," 58–59;
       and Mills, *Charles Miller.*

112   "Desastre lamentável," *Correio Paulistano*, October 10, 1878, 3; and "Noti-
       ciario geral, desastre lamentável," *Correio Paulistano*, October 11, 1878, 3.

113   "Bom Retiro," *O Combate*, December 2, 1920, 2.

114   In the center-city districts, Bom Retiro rooted more for Corinthians than
       half the other districts did. Instituto Datafolha, "Pesquisa de torcidas do
       Instituto Datafolha no município de São Paulo em 2008," http://www
       .spfcpedia.com/2009/06/torcidas-na-cidade-de-sao-paulo.html. Subse-
       quent Datafolha research did not ask questions about place of residence.

115   Field notes from home visit with Dr. Jacob of the Bom Retiro Public Health
       Clinic to a residential building on Rua Correia de Melo, May 19, 2016, 8:30
       to 10:30 a.m.

116   Roth, "Mean-Spirited Sport."

117   Prefeitura da Cidade de São Paulo, "Programa Clube Amigo do Refugiado,"
       June 21, 2018, https://www.prefeitura.sp.gov.br/cidade/secretarias/esportes
       /noticias/?p=259185.

118   Lombroso, accessed June 28, 2024, https://www.lombroso.com.br/.

119   Cavaglion, "Was Cesare Lombroso Antisemitic?"; and Alvarez, "A crimi-
       nologia no Brasil ou como tratar desigualmente os desiguais."

120   Dicionário de Ruas: História das Ruas da Cidade de São Paulo, s.v. "Rua Pro-
       fessor Cesare Lombroso," accessed June 28, 2024, https://dicionarioderuas
       .prefeitura.sp.gov.br/historia-da-rua/rua-professor-cesare-lombroso.

121   Zylbersztajn, *O filho de Osum*; and Paula Janovitch, "Prostituição e con-
       finamento em São Paulo: Um percurso pela antiga zona do meretrício do
       Bom Retiro," August 12, 2022, https://www.instagram.com/p/ChKPZp1lb1C
       /. Contemporary sex work around the Luz Railway Station is a frequent
       topic in the press. For just one of many examples, see Leandro Calixto
       and Leonardo Soares, "Estação da Luz vira ponto para dezenas de prosti-
       tutas," *O Estado de S. Paulo*, February 27, 2010, https://www.estadao.com
       .br/noticias/geral,estacao-da-luz-vira-ponto-para-dezenas-de-prostitu-
       tas,517127. On Chinese sex worker arrests, see "Polícia descobre rede de
       prostituição em karaokê de fachada no Bom Retiro," *VEJA São Paulo*, July 3,

2019; Camila Yunes, "Polícia resgata 14 chinesas mantidas como escravas sexuais em karaokê de fachada em São Paulo," *JPNews*, July 4, 2019; and Patrícia Pasquini, "Chinesas viviam como escravas em prostíbulo no Bom Retiro," *Folha de São Paulo*, July 4, 2019.

122 Lesser, *Welcoming the Undesirables*, 31–39.

123 Fonseca, *História da prostituição em São Paulo*, 210.

124 Fonseca, *História da prostituição em São Paulo*, 216.

125 Furlan, "Alguns aspectos da regulamentação da prostituição em São Paulo."

126 Langfur, "Uncertain Refuge."

127 Rechtman, "Itaboca, rua de triste memória."

128 "Rebelião das Meretrizes," *Diário da Noite*, January 1, 1954, 16.

Chapter 4. Enforcing Health

1 Márcia Silva, "Santa Casa de Misericórdia de São Paulo," 398.

2 Tonini, "Saúde da população Síria."

3 "Por lerem a 'Laterna,' dois moços foram explusos da 'Santa' Casa," *A Lanterna: Folha Anti-Clerical e de Combate*, October 3, 1914, 3.

4 *O Estado de S. Paulo*, August 23, 1896, 3; Americano, *São Paulo naquele tempo*, 149; Marcos Silva, "Os Protocolos Italianos," 174–77; and Riccò, "'Il segno di Menelik."

5 Anna Corrêa, *A rebelião de 1924 em São Paulo*.

6 Fausto, "Imigração e participação política," 12.

7 Cohen, *Bombas sobre São Paulo*, 35.

8 Assunção Filho, "1924—DELENDA SÃO PAULO," 57.

9 O. Andrade, *Estética e política*, 161.

10 "Na camara dos deputados," *Correio Paulistano*, December 28, 1928, 3.

11 "Major José Molinaro," *Correio Paulistano*, December 29, 1928, 7.

12 Faerman, "Lembrando os Bons Tempos," *Jornal da Tarde*, November 23, 1981, 14–15.

13 Quoted in João Marcos Carvalho, "Testemunhas falam da guerra de 1924," *Folha de S. Paulo*, July 24, 1994, https://www1.folha.uol.com.br/fsp/1994/7/24/mais!/26.html.

14 Faerman, "Lembrando os Bons Tempos," 14.

15 Lesser, *Negotiating National Identity*, 111–13.

16 Faerman, "Lembrando os Bons Tempos," 15. See also Nastri, "Bom Retiro em capítulos."

17   Mantovani, "O que foi a polícia médica?"; D. Pereira, "Aspectos históricos e atuais da perícia médico legal e suas possibilidades de evolução," 42; Foucault, "Birth of Social Medicine," 134–56; and Rosen, "Cameralism."

18   Decreto Estadual No. 264, de 27 de outubro de 1894, "Dá regulamento à Repartição Central de Polícia," Leis Estaduais, https://leisestaduais.com.br /sp/decreto-n-264-1894-sao-paulo-da-regulamento-a-reparticao-central -de-policia.

19   Decreto Estadual No. 264, de 27 de outubro de 1894, Capítulo IV, Título IX, Dos Médicos, Artigos 28, 29.

20   Lei Federal das Contravenções Penais, Decreto-lei No. 3.688, de 3 de outubro de 1941, Artigo 66, 2, *Jusbrasil*, https://presrepublica.jusbrasil.com.br /legislacao/110062/lei-das-contravencoes-penais-decreto-lei-3688-41.

21   Lei Estadual No. 666, de 16 de março de 1950, "Dispõe sôbre extinção do Pôsto Médico da Assistência Policial, atualmente subordinado à Secretaria da Segurança Pública, a dá outras providências," ALESP, https://www.al.sp .gov.br/repositorio/legislacao/lei/1950/lei-666-16.03.1950.html.

22   Decreto Estadual No. 1.414, de 24 de outubro de 1906. São Paulo, Governo do Estado, *Diário Oficial*, http://dobuscadireta.imprensaoficial.com .br/default.aspx?DataPublicacao=19061025&Caderno=Diario%20 Oficial&NumeroPagina=2519.

23   Rocha, "Saindo das sombras," 101. See also French, *Drowning in Laws*.

24   Lei Estadual No. 1.252, de 14 de setembro de 1911, "Crêa logares de medicos e enfermeiros para o serviço de assistência policial, e define-lhes as atribuições," Leis Estaduais, https://leisestaduais.com.br/sp/lei-ordinaria -n-1252-1911-sao-paulo-crea-logares-de-medicos-e-enfermeiros-para-o -servico-de-assistencia-policial-e-define-lhes-as-attribuicoes; and Maestrini, "Em busca da cidade moderna."

25   *O Estado de S. Paulo*, March 25, 1906, 2; and Processo: Rua dos Italianos 30, Secretaria Geral, Secção de Polícia e Hygiene, Processos de Fiscalização, 1906, box 15, AHM, São Paulo.

26   Carroll, "Medical Police," 465.

27   Stepan, *"Hour of Eugenics"*; and Gudmundson and Wolfe, *Blacks and Blackness*.

28   Brazil, "Discurso de Acylino de Leão em 18 de setembro de 1935," *Anais da Câmara dos Deputados*, 432.

29   Antunes, *Eugenia e imigração*.

30   Candelaria, "Acção do posto de hygiene em policiamento sanitário"; and Matos, "Construindo a paulistanidade."

31   Matos, "Na trama urbana," 133.

32 O. Silva, Prando, and Panhoca, "Os imigrantes e a violência na cidade de São Paulo no início do século 20," 328.

33 "Creança baleada," *Correio Paulistano*, December 25, 1892, 1, 8.

34 "Vida diária, assassinato," *Correio Paulistano*, May 1, 1900, 2, 8.

35 "Tribunal de Justiça, agravos, no. 2669," *O Commercio de São Paulo*, May 15, 1901.

36 "Prefeitura Municipal, requerimentos despachados," *Correio Paulistano*, July 4, 1903, 3.

37 "Senhorio feroz," *Correio Paulistano*, March 12, 1906, 3.

38 Processo, Rua dos Italianos 30, 1906.

39 Lei Estadual No. 1.252, de 14 de setembro de 1911, Artigo 1; Decreto Estadual No. 2.141, de 14 de Novembro de 1911, "Reorganiza o Serviço Sanitário do Estado," Artigos 177, 461, Leis Estaduais, https://leisestaduais.com.br/sp /decreto-n-2141-1911-sao-paulo-reorganiza-o-servico-sanitario-do-estado ?q=Assist%C3%AAncia%20Policial; and Lei Estadual No. 1.342, de 16 de dezembro de 1912, "Reorganiza vários departamentos da Secretaria da Justiça e da Segurança Pública," Artigo 11, Leis Estaduais, https://leisestaduais.com.br /sp/lei-ordinaria-n-1342-1912-sao-paulo-reorganiza-varios-departamentos -da-secretaria-da-justica-e-da-seguranca-publica.

40 Lei Estadual No. 1.252, de 14 de setembro de 1911, Artigo 3: 1 e 2.

41 Hanley, *Public Good*, 14. See also MacDougall, *Activists and Advocates*, 30–31; and R. Carrillo, "Balance epidemiológico argentine."

42 Cosby, "Flowers Grew," 85. See also Weinstein, *Color of Modernity*; and Skidmore, *Black into White*.

43 Débora Nascimento, "Corpos violados."

44 Secretaria da Segurança Pública do Estado de São Paulo, Registro de ocorrências da Assistência Policial, 1911–40, vol. E14015, doc. 36905, November 27, 1916, APESP.

45 "O dia de hontem, *A Gazeta*, November 28, 1916, 5; and "Cobrança de uma divida," *Correio Paulistano*, November 28, 1916, 7.

46 Secretaria da Segurança Pública do Estado de São Paulo, Registro de ocorrências da Assistência Policial, 1911–40, vol. E14015, doc. 36906, November 27, 1916, APESP.

47 See, for example, "Policiamento Sanitário," *Diário Official*, July 3, 1901, 1726– 27, https://www.imprensaoficial.com.br/DO/BuscaDO2001Documento _11_4.aspx?link=%2f1901%2fdiario%2520oficial%2fjulho%2f03%2fpag _1726_0HHHJ78279IN8e5VFP21N8PRRF3.pdf&pagina=1726&data=03 /07/1901&caderno=Di%C3%A1rio%20Oficial&paginaordenacao=101726; and "Policiamento Sanitário," *Diário Official*, May 30, 1902, 1141–42,

https://www.imprensaoficial.com.br/DO/BuscaDO2001Documento_11
_4.aspx?link=%2f1902%2fdiario%2520oficial%2fmaio%2f30%2fpag_1141
_EB1B6KM16VHDTeD62V50IOICV9D.pdf&pagina=1141&data=30/05
/1902&caderno=Di%C3%A1rio%20Oficial&paginaordenacao=101141.

48 Decreto Estadual No. 2.215, de 15 de março de 1912, "Dá regulamento para
o serviço da assistência policial," Titulo II, Direcção da Assistência e modo
de internação, Capitulo II, Da Internação dos Mendigos e Inválidos, Lou-
cos, Doentes e Crianças e processo dos Vadios," Artigos 94–106, ALESP,
https://www.al.sp.gov.br/repositorio/legislacao/decreto/1912/decreto-2215
-15.03.1912.html.

49 Miniguccio Cicinderella, "Cartas do Bô Ritiro," *Vida Paulista: Humorismo,
Literatura, e Esporte* 2, no. 18 (June 16, 1921): 8.

50 Decreto Estadual No. 2.215, de 15 de março de 1912, Titulo 1, Capitulo II,
Da Estação Telegraphica e Telephonica and Capitulo III, Dos Aparelhos
de Avisos, Artigos 24–62.

51 In 2000 the company was purchased by Honeywell. "Our History,"
Gamewell Fire Control Instruments by Honeywell, Internet Archive Way-
back Machine, May 12, 2008, https://web.archive.org/web/20080512201708
/http://www.gamewell-fci.com/history.html. Images of the call boxes used
by the São Paulo police can be found here: Mauricio Xavier, "Memória
Paulistana: Telegrapho Policial," *VEJA São Paulo*, August 19, 2011, https://
vejasp.abril.com.br/cidades/memoria-paulistana-telegrapho-policial/.

52 Xavier, "Memória Paulistana: Telegrapho Policial."

53 The 1912 population figure comes from Directoria Geral de Estatística do
Ministério da Agricultura, Indústria e Commércio, *Anuário estatístico
do Brasil*, 349.

54 Decreto Estadual No. 4.715, de 23 de abril de 1930, Título V, Capítulo 1, Artigo 295, published in *Diário Oficial*, May 7, 1930, 4177, http://dobuscadireta
.imprensaoficial.com.br/default.aspx?DataPublicacao=19300507&Caderno
=Diario%20Oficial&NumeroPagina=4177. The 1930 figure is estimated
from the following sources: Repartição de Estatística e do Archivo do
Estado, *Annuario estatistico de São Paulo*, 71–75; São Paulo, *Anuário estatístico do estado de São Paulo 1940*, 91; and Instituto Nacional de Estatística, *Anuario estatístico do Brasil, Ano II—1936*, 63.

55 Decreto Estadual No. 4.715, de 23 de abril de 1930, Título V, Capítulo 1,
Artigos 297, 298.

56 See advertisment for "Alvorada do Amor" at the Cine S. Bento, *Correio
Paulistano*, May 7, 1930, 16.

57 Oliveira, "Utilização de serviços do Sistema Único de Saúde por beneficiários de planos de saúde Rio de Janeiro."

58   Decreto Estadual No. 5.892, de 25 de abril de 1933, "Dispõe sobre os ser-viços da Assistência Policial," ALESP, https://www.al.sp.gov.br/repositorio /legislacao/decreto/1933/decreto-5892-25.04.1933.html.

59   Arquivo Público do Estado de São Paulo, Secretaria da Segurança Pública do Estado de São Paulo, Grupo 12G3 - Assistência Policial, http://icaatom .arquivoestado.sp.gov.br/ica-atom/index.php/assistencia-policial;isad.

60   Jacino, "O negro no mercado de trabalho," 11–13.

61   Jacino, "O negro no mercado de trabalho," 135–36.

62   Rocha, "Saindo das sombras," 111.

63   Rocha, "Saindo das sombras," 259.

64   Cosby, "Flowers Grew," 3.

65   Cosby, "Flowers Grew," 93.

66   "Bom-Retiro. Cadastro de Prédios Servidos de esgotos pela Repartição Technica de Águas e Esgotos de São Paulo em 1894," Memoria Publica, Item number BR_APESP_IGC_IGG_CAR_I_S_0225_001_006. APESP.

67   "Hygiene," *Correio Paulistano*, October 25, 1894, 1; "Notas do reporter," *Correio Paulistano*, February 17, 1895, 2; "Notas do reporter," *Correio Paulistano*, March 14, 1895, 2; "Intendencia de Obras Municipaes, despachos, *Correio Paulistano*, June 16, 1897, 3; "Intendencia municipal de Polícia e Hygiene," *Correio Paulistano*, October 12, 1897, 3; "Intendencia municipal de Polícia e Hygiene," *Correio Paulistano*, December 22, 1897, 4.

68   Secretaria da Segurança Pública do Estado de São Paulo, Assistência Policial, Registro de ocorrências da Assistência Policial, 1911–40, vol. 14440, doc. 213895, November 6, 1935 (by Dr. Alves Martins); vol. 14457, doc. 228644, April 27, 1936 (by Dr. Prisco); vol. 14490, doc. 253424, February 21, 1937 (by Dr. Eurico); vol. 14497, doc. 258584, April 22, 1937 (by Dr. Rodolpho de Freitas); vol. 14497, doc. 259146, April 29, 1937 (by Dr. Teixeira Leite), APESP.

69   Reinehr, "Silêncios e confrontos."

70   Secretaria da Segurança Pública do Estado de São Paulo, Registro de ocorrências da Assistência Policial, 1911–40, vol. 13958, doc. 1020, February 18, 1912; vol. 14592, doc. 336931, 9 September 1937; vol. 13960, doc. 1635, April 1, 1912; vol. 1397, doc. 11929, November 9, 1913; vol. 14062, doc. 73171, November 30, 1920; vol. 14347, doc. 149655, March 13, 1933; vol. 14382, doc. 170706, August 20, 1933; vol. 14447, doc. 244071, December 29, 1935, APESP.

71   Secretaria da Segurança Pública do Estado de São Paulo, Registro de ocorrências da Assistência Policial, 1911–40, vol. 13969, doc. 7111, January 24, 1919; vol. 14012, doc. 34479, November 2, 1917; vol. 14027, doc. 45331, November 8, 1917; vol. 14252, doc. 92154, August 18, 1930; vol. 14547, doc. 294557, May 10 1938, APESP.

72 Matos, *Cotidiano e cultura.*

73 T. Camargo, "LAVADEIRA PAULISTANA."

74 Ferla, "Corpos estranhos na intimidade do lar," 3.

75 Ferla, "Corpos estranhos na intimidade do lar," 3.

76 Candido, *"De cortiço a cortiço,"* 114; and Antonil, *Cultura e opulência do Brasil,* 34.

77 Higham, *Strangers in the Land,* 310.

78 "O perigo dos automóveis," *Correio Paulistano,* January 19, 1920, 5; and "Sempre os autos!,"*A Gazeta,* January 15, 1923, 1. See also "Chronica das ruas: Os automóveis continuam implacáveis," *A Gazeta,* July 14, 1914, 6; and "Deram-se hontem quatro desastres ocasionados pela imprudência dos chauffeurs," *A Gazeta,* September 4, 1915, 6.

79 "Criminosos presos," *Correio Paulistano,* December 4, 1914, 6.

80 Secretaria da Segurança Pública do Estado de São Paulo, Registro de ocorrências da Assistência Policial, 1911–40, vol. E14160, doc. 45240, February 14, 1928, APESP.

81 Secretaria da Segurança Pública do Estado de São Paulo, Grupo 12G6—Delegacias da Grande São Paulo, 8-Registros de acidente de trabalho da 2ª Delegacia—Bom Retiro (1934–41), Acadepol 738, December 2, 1934, 93, APESP.

82 "No Bom Retiro, Cervejaria Germânia," *Correio Paulistano,* April 16, 1911, 4.

83 Arquivo Público do Estado de São Paulo, Reichert, Registro de Autoridade, APESP, "História," http://icaatom.arquivoestado.sp.gov.br/ica-atom/index .php/irmaos-reichert;isaar. See the advertisement for the Cervejaria Germânia, *Correio Paulistano,* November 14, 1911, 7.

84 Quoted in Faerman, "Oh! Bom Retiro," 306.

85 "Pelo Progresso Nacional F. C.," *A Gazeta,* September 23, 1929, 12.

86 "Queda desastrosa," *Correio Paulistano,* December 29, 1911, 6.

87 Secretaria da Segurança Pública do Estado de São Paulo, Registro de ocorrências da Assistência Policial, 1911–40, vol. E13879, doc. 13384, November 16, 1913, APESP.

88 "Um distribuidor da cerveja 'Polonia' for aggregido por empregados da Cervejaria Germânia," *A Gazeta,* September 28, 1916, 6.

89 Justus and Kassouf, "History of Child Labor"; and Moura, "Infância operária e acidente do trabalho."

90 "Um menor operário esta arriscado a ficar cego,"*A Gazeta,* March 12, 1916, 8; and "Accidente no trabalho," *A Gazeta,* March 11, 1916, 8.

91 "Carroceiro Peverso," *Correio Paulistano,* January 29, 1919, 4.

92   Fundo BR SPAPESP SSP—Secretaria da Segurança Pública do Estado de São Paulo, Grupo 12G6—Delegacias da Grande São Paulo, 8-Registros de acidente de trabalho da 2ª Delegacia—Bom Retiro (1934–41), incident of October 19, 1934, p. 61.

93   *A Tribuna* (Santos), January 30, 1923, 1; Santana, "A difícil transformação."

94   Secretaria da Segurança Pública do Estado de São Paulo, Registro de ocorrências da Assistência Policial, 1911–40, vol. E13979, doc. 13274, November 12, 1913, APESP.

95   Secretaria da Segurança Pública do Estado de São Paulo, Assistência Policial, Registro de ocorrências da Assistência Policial, 1911–40, vol. E13980, doc. 13660, December 1, 1913, APESP.

96   For a discussion of suicide attempts among Afro-Brazilian women, see Cosby, "Flowers Grew," 110–12, 145–46.

97   Secretaria da Segurança Pública do Estado de São Paulo, Registro de ocorrências da Assistência Policial, 1911–40, ocorrência 88168, livro E14080, March 10, 1922, APESP.

98   Secretaria da Segurança Pública do Estado de São Paulo, Registro de ocorrências da Assistência Policial, 1911–40, ocorrência 88585, livro E14080, March 25, 1921, APESP.

99   Secretaria da Segurança Pública do Estado de São Paulo, Assistência Policial, Registro de ocorrências da Assistência Policial, 1911–40, ocorrência 103481, livro E14270, February 18, 1931, APESP.

100 Pingel, "Primary Care," 122.

101 "Restaurantes do Bom Retiro compravam carne de abatedouro de cães, diz polícia," *Portal G1—Globo*, November 12, 2009, https://g1.globo.com /Noticias/SaoPaulo/0,,MUL1376382-5605,00-RESTAURANTES+DO+BO M+RETIRO+COMPRAVAM+CARNE+DE+ABATEDOURO+DE+CAES +DIZ+POLICI.html; "Restaurante vende carne de cachorro e gato em São Paulo," *Guiame*, March 29, 2014, https://guiame.com.br/noticias/sociedade -brasil/restaurantes-do-bom-retiro-compravam-carne-de-abatedouro-de -caes-diz-policia.html; and "Restaurante vende carne de cachorro e gato em São Paulo," *Jusbrasil*, n.d., accessed June 28, 2024, https://www.jusbrasil .com.br/noticias/restaurante-vende-carne-de-cachorro-e-gato-em-sao -paulo/112356557.

102 "Cardápio mostra prato com carne de cachorro," *Folha de S. Paulo*, November 13, 2009, https://www1.folha.uol.com.br/fsp/cotidian/ff1311200902 .htm.

103 Kleber Tomaz, "Suspeito de matar catador com flecha em SP esfaqueou homem em 2013," *Portal G1—Globo*, September 17, 2016, http://g1.globo .com/São-paulo/noticia/2016/09/suspeito-de-matar-catador-com-flecha

-em-sp-esfaqueou-homem-em-2013.html; and Sérgio Quintella, "Justiça marca julgamento de homem que matou carroceiro com flecha," *VEJA São Paulo*, March 19, 2019, https://vejasp.abril.com.br/blog/poder-sp/justica -marca-julgamento-de-homem-que-matou-carroceiro-com-flecha/.

104   Benedito Roberto Barbosa, Juliana L. Avanci, and Luiz T. Kohara, "Pandemia nos cortiços de São Paulo e as mortes (in)visíveis em uma cidade que ninguém quer ver," *Labcidade*, June 22, 2020, https://www.labcidade .fau.usp.br/pandemia-nos-corticos-de-sao-paulo-e-as-mortes-invisiveis -em-uma-cidade-que-ninguem-quer-ver/.

105   Guilherme Balza, "Oito dos dez bairros com mais mortes por Covid-19 estão no centro 'pobre' de São Paulo," *Portal G1—Globo*, May 27, 2020, https://g1.globo.com/sp/sao-paulo/noticia/2020/05/27/oito-dos-dez -bairros-com-mais-mortes-por-covid-19-estao-no-centro-pobre-de-sao -paulo.ghtml.

Chapter 5. A Building Block of Health

1   Stepan, *Eradication*.

2   Powell, "Most Lethal Animal," 525; and Powell, Gloria-Soria, and Kotsakiozi, "Recent History of *Aedes aegypti*," 856.

3   The flyer is reprinted in Fioravanti, *O combate à febre amarela*, 25.

4   Ribas, "Profilaxia da febre amarela," 363–64.

5   Almeida, "República dos invisíveis," 190.

6   Transcripts of the original notes of the experiments can be found in Benchimol and Sá, *Adolpho Lutz—obra completa*, 2:569–631.

7   Blount, "Public Health Movement," 116.

8   Deb Roy, *Malarial Subjects*. In twentieth-century Guatemala the flu was presented as a fire-breathing dragon. Folheto de campanha de saúde, "Gripe," Guatemala, 1956, AMSPER/Instituto Butantan, São Paulo.

9   Murtha, Castro, and Heller, "Perspectiva histórica das primeiras políticas de saneamento e de recurso hídricos no Brasil."

10   Silva Filho, Morais, and Silva, "Doenças de veiculação hídrica."

11   By the end of 2015, cases had been identified in all five regions of the country, with the Brazilian Ministry of Health estimating that between 500,000 and 1.5 million people had been infected. From Brazil, the virus migrated to other parts of the Americas, with outbreaks throughout the region.

12   Lesser and Kitron, "Social Geography of Zika."

13   Eduardo de Masi is currently coordinator of the Health Surveillance and Arbovirus Control Program for the secretary of health of São Paulo

city (Coordenador do Programa Municipal de Vigilância e Controle de Arboviroses da Secretaria Municipal da Saúde de São Paulo) as well as a colleague of mine at the Institute for Advanced Studies at the University of São Paulo.

14   Sposati, "Mapa exclusão/inclusão social do município de São Paulo—III (2010)."

15   Daniel Boa Nova, "O bairro de SP que era conhecido pela violência e hoje abriga um dos maiores eventos de literatura da cidade," *Hypeness*, May 7, 2015, https://www.hypeness.com.br/2015/05/um-dos-maiores-eventos-de -literatura-de-sao-paulo-acontece-no-extremo-sul-da-cidade/; Burdick, *Color of Sound*; and Sugayama, "Ferréz."

16   Município de São Paulo, Subprefeituras e Distritos Municipais, "Domicílios por Faixa de Rendimento, em salários-mínimos," 2010, https://www .prefeitura.sp.gov.br/cidade/secretarias/upload/urbanismo/infocidade /htmls/13_domicilios_por_faixa_de_rendimento_em_sa_2010_233.html.

17   H. Cunha et al., "Water Tank and Swimming Pool Detection"; and Lowe et al., "Dengue Risk in Brazil."

18   Aguiar et al., "Zika and Chikungunya Outbreaks."

19   During COVID-19 some drug traffickers enforced masking policies in the neighborhoods they controlled. Leslie Leitão and Marco Antônio Martins, "Tráfico impõe toque de recolher e uso obrigatório de máscaras em favelas do Rio durante a pandemia," *Portal G1—Globo*, May 8, 2020, https://g1 .globo.com/rj/rio-de-janeiro/noticia/2020/05/08/trafico-impoe-toque-de -recolher-em-favelas-do-rio-durante-a-pandemia.ghtml.

20   R. Araújo et al., "São Paulo Urban Heat Islands," table S2 (Bom Retiro is District 9); and Nataly Costa, "Saiba quais bairros têm maior incidência de dengue na capital," *VEJA São Paulo*, February 10, 2016, https://vejasp .abril.com.br/cidades/bairros-São-paulo-casos-dengue-zika/.

21   Cidade de São Paulo, Subprefeitura Sé, "Contra dengue, Subprefeitura Sé notifica donos de 25 imóveis abandonados," April 27, 2015, https://www .prefeitura.sp.gov.br/cidade/secretarias/subprefeituras/se/noticias/?p=56950.

22   Pingel, "Primary Care."

23   Rede Nossa São Paulo, "Agressões por Intervenção policial," *Mapa da Desigualdade 2022*, 70, accessed June 28, 2024, https://www.nossasaopaulo.org.br/wp -content/uploads/2022/11/Mapa-da-Desigualdade-2022_Tabelas.pdf.

24   Rezende and Heller, *O saneamento no Brasil*, 129.

25   Pande, *Medicine, Race and Liberalism*, 187; and Hussain et al., "Antivaccination Movement."

26   The Oswaldo Cruz Foundation (Fiocruz) became a partner with what is today the Brazilian Ministry of Health. Today Fiocruz has ministry-level

responsibilities, including what in the United States would fall under the National Institutes of Health, the Centers for Disease Control, and a university-based public health school training program. Cantisano, "Refuge from Science."

27   Stepan, "Biology and Degeneration"; and D. Borges, "Puffy, Ugly, Slothful, and Inert."

28   Sant'anna, "Guerra e paz."

29   Meade, "'Civilizing Rio de Janeiro'"; Needell, "Revolta Contra Vacina"; Chalhoub, "Politics of Disease Control"; and Sevcenko, *Revolta da vacina.*

30   María Martín, "Brasil destina 60% das suas Forças Armadas na luta contra um mosquito," *El País* (Brazil), February 13, 2016, https://brasil.elpais.com /brasil/2016/02/13/politica/1455383958_196275.html.

31   Almeida and Dantes, "O serviço sanitário de São Paulo, a saúde pública e a microbiologia."

32   Metro de São Paulo, "Ultrafarma terá seu nome na Estacão Saúde de metro de São Paulo," Associação Nacional dos Transportadores de Passageiros sobre Trilhos—ANPTrilhos, https://anptrilhos.org.br/ultrafarma-tera-seu -nome-na-estacao-saude-do-metro-de-sao-paulo/, March 15, 2022.

33   O'Brien, "If They Are Useful"; Bertolli Filho, *História da saúde pública no Brasil*, 5–15; and Mott and Sanglard, *História da saúde em São Paulo.*

34   Calabi, *História do urbanismo europeu.*

35   *O Archivo Illustrado: Encyclopedia Noticiosa, Scientifica e Litteraria*, June 1920, 122. See also Bruno Brasil, "O Archivo Illustrado: Encyclopedia Noticiosa, Scientifica e Litteraria," August 17, 2015, BNDigital Brasil, Artigos, http://bndigital.bn.gov.br/artigos/o-archivo-illustrado-encyclopedia -noticiosa-scientifica-e-litteraria/.

36   "Planta do terreno annexo a Enfermaria do Bom Retiro," November 18, 1892, Núcleo de Acervo Cartográfico, item number BR_APESP_IGC_IGG_ CAR_I_S_09.02.34, APESP; and "Galerias de Águas Pluviaes e drenagem do Solo Construídas em 1893 e 1894 nos Bairros do Bom Retiro e Sta. Efigenia," accession number 1-06035-0000-0000, João Baptista de Campos Aguirra Collection, Museu Paulista.

37   Laguardia, "A geografia sagrada na expansão urbana de São Paulo até finais do XIX," 1.

38   Landmann-Szwarcwald and Macinko, "Panorama of Health Inequalities."

39   Amoruso, "Spaces of Suffering."

40   Processo: 23881/85; Resolução 50 de 26/08/1985; inscrição nº 239, p. 65, 21/01/1987, accessed June 28, 2024, http://condephaat.sp.gov.br /benstombados/desinfectorio-central/; ipatrimônio, patrimônio cultural brasileiro (beta), "São Paulo—Desinfectório Central," accessed June 28,

2024, https://www.ipatrimonio.org/sao-paulo-desinfectorio-central/#!
/map=38329&loc=-23.514747887206905,-46.666080951690674,14.

41   LaCroix, Casagrande, and Lesser, "Sacred Space of Health."

42   *Diário Oficial do Estado* (São Paulo), October 19, 1979, 103.

43   Howard-Jones, "Robert Koch"; and Neto, *O poder e a peste.*

44   Jorge, *Tietê, o rio que a cidade perdeu.*

45   Segawa, "Arquitetura de hospedarias de imigrantes"; Murphy, *Sick Building Syndrome*; Mott and Sanglard, *História da saúde em São Paulo*; Lopez, *Building American Public Health*; and Kisacky, *Rise of the Modern Hospital.*

46   McCaskey, "Disinfection," 246.

47   Benchimol, *Dos micróbios aos mosquitos*, 291–92.

48   Special Commissioner, "Health Resorts of the Riviera," 203.

49   *Public Health* (London), October 7, 1894, 182. See also Brazil, Commissão, Exposição internacional de borracha de New York, *Brazil, the Land of Rubber*, 81.

50   Instituto Butantan/Museu Emílio Ribas, *História, imigração e saúde no bairro do Bom Retiro.*

51   R. Williams, "Street Pavement Materials and Technology," 211.

52   Alfredo Pinto, *A cidade de São Paulo em 1900*, 102. In 1925 the Central Disinfectory, the Isolation Hospital, transportation services, and the Flying Insect Control Service were administratively placed under the Secretary of the Interior, where they remained through World War II.

53   Begliomini, "Cadeira no 58—Patrono Diogo Teixeira de Faria, 1867–1927."

54   Bassanezi, *São Paulo do passado*, 29.

55   Bassanezi and Cunha. "Um espaço, dois momentos epidêmicos."

56   R. Costa, "Apontamentos para a arquitetura hospitalar no Brasil."

57   J. Silva, "Fotogenia do caos," 90.

58   Decreto Estadual No. 219, de 30 de novembro de 1893, "Regulamento para o serviço geral de desinfecções," São Paulo, Governo do Estado, Diário Oficial, http://dobuscadireta.imprensaoficial.com.br/default.aspx ?DataPublicacao=18931208&Caderno=Diario%20Oficial&NumeroPagina =8801.

59   Mastromauro, "Alguns aspectos da saúde pública e do urbanismo higienista em São Paulo no final do século XIX," 56; and E. Campos, "Hospitais paulistanos."

60   Bertolli Filho, *História da saúde pública no Brasil*, 164.

61   Penteado, *Belènzinho, 1910*, 8.

62   Penteado, *Belènzinho, 1910,* 38.

63   Câmara Municipal de São Paulo, Projeto de Lei No. 3, de January 15, 1910, Joaquim Morra, "Dispõe que a prefeitura mandará transferir para lugar mais conveniente e afastado da cidade, os atuais estabelecimentos da empresa da limpeza pública e particular e, nesse lugar, construirá um forno de incineração de lixo," doc. PL0003-1910, https://www.Saopaulo.sp.leg.br /iah/fulltext/documentoshistoricos/PL0003-1910.pdf.

64   "Saúde Publica," *A Gazeta,* April 21, 1914, 3.

65   Decreto Estadual No. 219, de 30 de novembro de 1893, Capítulo 2, Artigos 10–17.

66   Reichman, *Progress in the Balance,* 110.

67   Alfredo Pinto, *A cidade de São Paulo em 1900,* 102.

68   Americano, "Veículos," 175–78.

69   Cytrynowicz, Cytrynowicz, and Stücker, *Do Lazareto dos Variolosos ao Instituto de Infectologia Emílio Ribas.*

70   Penteado, *Belènzinho, 1910,* 276.

71   T. Rogers, "Laboring Landscapes."

72   R. Machado and Kako, "A cartografia da expansão da cidade de São Paulo no período de 1881 a 2001."

73   Instituto Butantan/Museu Emílio Ribas, *História, imigração e saúde no bairro do Bom Retiro.*

74   Lei Estadual No. 432, de 3 de agosto de 1896, Sobre o Serviço Sanitário do Estado Assembleia Legislativa do Estado de São Paulo, Legislação, Normas, accessed June 28, 2024, https://www.al.sp.gov.br/repositorio/legislacao/lei /1896/lei-432-03.08.1896.html.

75   Rochard, "L'Hygiène en 1889," 1889.

76   "Álbum do Desinféctório Central," ca. 1911, reprinted in J. Silva, "Fotogenia do caos," figs. 23–29.

77   David McMacken, "Republic Trucks Put Alma on the Map," *Morning Sun Lifestyle,* June 13, 1913.

78   Sergio de Simone, "Carros Antigos do Museu de Saúde Pública Emílio Ribas," unpublished research report, AMSPER, February 2016.

79   Wolfe, *Autos and Progress.*

80   "Ministério de Agricultura," *Correio Paulistano,* February 4, 1890, 1.

81   "Câmara Municipal,"*Correio Paulistano,* June 15, 1919, 2; and "Câmara Municipal," *Correio Paulistano,* April 25, 1920, 5.

82   *Álbum Serviço Sanitário do Estado de São Paulo: Algumas instalações do Serviço Sanitário de São Paulo* (São Paulo: Impresso gráfico, 1905); Fundo

Serviço Sanitário de São Paulo, Acervo Instituto Butantan/AMSPER; and Câmara Municipal de São Paulo, Requerimento n°83 de 1920, October 15, 1920; *Annaes da Camara Municipal de São Paulo, 1920* (São Paulo: Typographia Piratininga, 1920), 272, https://www.saopaulo.sp.leg.br/static/atas _anais_cmsp/anadig/Volumes/an1920.pdf.

83 "Mensagem apresentada ao Congresso Legislativo, em 14 de julho de 1919, pelo Dr. Altino Arantes, Presidente do Estado de São Paulo," in *Relatório dos Presidentes dos Estados Brasileiros, Mensagem apresentada ao congresso legislativo em 14 de Julho 1919 pelo Dr. Altino Arantes, Presidente do Estado de São Paulo*, 40, https://memoria.bn.gov.br/DocReader/docreader.aspx ?bib=720526&pesq=.&pagfis=1900.

84 "O primeiro 'Centro de Saúde' fundado no Brasil," *Diário da Noite*, January 25, 1927, 5.

85 São Paulo, Secção de Propaganda e Educação Sanitária, Departamento de Saúde, *Combate à Lepra*, 3.

86 The four units were the Center for the Regulation of Emergency Care (Centro de Regulação de Urgência e Emergência do Estado de São Paulo), the Central Management Office for Health Contracts and Services (Coordenadoria de Gestão de Contratos e Serviços de Saúde), the Rua Tenente Pena Dispensary (Almoxarifado da Unidade Dispensadora Tenente Pena), and the Central Management of Strategic Needs (Coordenadoria de Demandas Estratégicas do SUS).

87 Senne and Urzua, "A constituição do acervo do Museu de Saúde Pública Emílio Ribas," 17.

88 Lei Estadual No. 3.852, de 5 de outubro de 1983, "Dá a denominação de 'Dr Octávio Augusto Rodovalho' ao Centro de Saúde II—Bela Vista, Distrito de Santa Cecília, na Capital," ALESP, https://www.al.sp.gov.br/norma/?id =37775.

89 E. Campos, "Hospitais paulistanos."

Chapter 6. Unliving Rats and Undead Immigrants

Epigraphs: Amado, *A Morte e a Morte de Quincas Berro Dágua*, 1; and Kleber Tomaz and Abrahão de Oliveira, "PM desaparecido é achado morto, nu e amarrado dentro de carroça no Centro de SP; 4 foram presos por suspeita de homicídio," *Portal G1—Globo*, November 19, 2020, https://g1 .globo.com/sp/sao-paulo/noticia/2020/10/19/pm-desaparecido-e-achado -morto-nu-e-amarrado-dentro-de-carroca-no-centro-de-sp-4-foram -presos-por-suspeita-de-homicidio.ghtml.

1 Bertolozzi, "Hacking the Debate"; Reny and Barreto, "Xenophobia"; and Xun and Gilman, *"I Know Who Caused COVID-19."*

2   Rodrigo Tammaro, "População de origem asiática é vítima de violência e preconceito na pandemia," *Jornal da USP*, May 27, 2021, https://jornal.usp .br/?p=419827; Luciana Werner, "Ódio e preconceito contra asiáticos crescem no Brasil e nos EUA: Casos vão da agressão física ao assédio verbal pela internet, mulheres são as mais atingidas," *#Colabora*, May 25, 2020, https://projetocolabora.com.br/ods3/cresce-o-odio-contra-asiaticos/; and Katie Rogers, Lara Jakes, and Ana Swanson, "Trump Defends Using 'Chinese Virus' Label, Ignoring Growing Criticism," *New York Times*, March 18, 2020, https://www.nytimes.com/2020/03/18/us/politics/china -virus.html.

3   Terreros, "Saberes y prácticas médicos durante la revolución"; and Birn, "Perspectivizing Pandemics."

4   Schwarcz and Starling, *A bailarina da morte*. A thoughtful examination of the linkage of the two diseases is Beiner, *Pandemic Re-awakenings*. See also Kind and Cordeiro, "Narrativas sobre a morte"; and Karine Rodrigues, "Da peste bubônica à Covid-19: Por que o Brasil parece marcar passo no combate a epidemias," *Notícias Casa de Oswaldo Cruz*, August, 12 2021, http://www.coc.fiocruz.br/index.php/pt/todas-as-noticias/2014-da-peste -bubonica-a-covid-19-por-que-o-brasil-parece-marcar-passo-no-combate -a-epidemias.html.

5   "Defuntos a muque! Um fugiu do Araçá," *A Capital*, November 30, 1918, 1.

6   "Vaccina contra a 'hespanhola,'" *Gazeta do Povo*, October 1, 1918, 1.

7   Lesser, "Reflexões sobre (codi)nomes e etnicidade em São Paulo."

8   "Uma mulher estrangulada," *Correio Paulistano*, October 4, 1913, 3.

9   "Carnaval," *O Combate*, February 13, 1919, 3; "Denúncia contra introductores de moeda falsa na circulação," *Correio Paulistano,* January 16, 1921, 4.

10   "Os amigos do Rolinha," *O Combate*, November 9, 1921, 4; "Desacato a um agente discal da união," *O Combate*, January 18, 1922, 3. João Turco (the gangster) continued to be a media figure at least through 1926; see "Seção futurista," *O Sacy*, January 15, 1926, 18.

11   *O Estado de S. Paulo*, February 15, 1927, 4.

12   "O caso do João Turco," *O Combate*, November 30, 1918, 1; and *O Estado de S. Paulo*, November 8, 1918, 4.

13   "Defuntos a muque! Um fugiu do Araçá," *A Capital*, November 30, 1918, 1.

14   "O caso do Jõao Turco," *O Combate*, November 30, 1918, 1.

15   "O caso do Jõao Turco," *O Combate*, November 30, 1918, 1.

16   R. Santos, "O Carnaval, a peste e a 'espanhola.'"

17   "Telegramas," *Jornal do Commercio*, August 13, 1899, 1.

18   "Peste bubônica no Porto," *Jornal do Commercio*, August 15, 1899, 3.

19   Dicionário Histórico-Biográfico das Ciências da Saúde no Brasil (1832–1930), s.v. "Andrade, Nuno Ferreira de," https://dichistoriasaude.coc.fiocruz.br/wiki_dicionario/index.php/ANDRADE,_NUNO_FERREIRA_DE.

20   Dilene Nascimento and Silva, "'Não é meu intuito estabelecer polêmica.'"

21   "Arsenal da morte," *A Tribuna* (Santos), October 21, 1899, 1.

22   São Paulo, *Mensagem enviada ao Congresso do Estado, a 7 de abril de 1900*, 144, https://bibliotecadigital.seade.gov.br/view/singlepage/index.php?pubcod=10012822&parte=1.

23   Wyman, *Bubonic Plague*, 8–9.

24   Lemos, "Notícias sôbre a epidemia de peste em Santos (1899)," 90–91.

25   Geddings, "Plague on the Steamship"; and Havelburg, "BRAZIL. Report from Rio de Janeiro—Status of Plague in Santos," 79–81.

26   While a vaccine had existed since 1897, it was hard to import to Brazil. Ribas, Lutz, Oswaldo Cruz, Vital Brazil Mineiro da Campanha, and others began intense work on a Brazilian-produced vaccine that was introduced in 1902. Instituto Butantan, Portal do Butantan, "Início do Século XX: O Butantan e o combate à epidemia de peste bubônica," February 5, 2021, https://butantan.gov.br/noticias/inicio-do-seculo-xx-o-butantan-e-o-combate-a-epidemia-de-peste-bubonica.

27   Cueto, *Return of Epidemics*, 21; and A. Carrillo, "¿Estado de peste o estado de sitio?"

28   Kraut, "Immigration, Ethnicity, and the Pandemic," 125; Spaulding, "Haffkine Prophylactic and Antipest Serum."

29   Mangili, *Bom Retiro, bairro central de São Paulo*, 43–55.

30   Soppelsa, "Losing France's Imperial War on Rats."

31   Serviço Sanitário do Estado de São Paulo, PESTE, 3–11.

32   "Pastéis bubonicos," *A Tribuna* (Santos), October 21, 1899, 2.

33   Rio, "A musa das ruas," 182.

34   "Peste bubônica," *O Commercio de São Paulo*, October 28, 1899, 1.

35   Fonseca et al., "Cartografia digital geo-histórica."

36   "D. Anna Lisboa," *O Commercio de São Paulo*, July 6, 1900, 1.

37   The Medical Police did not yet exist, but post-1911 our analysis of this material showed frequent cases of children being accidentally poisoned in Bom Retiro.

38   For a song that makes that connection, see Premeditando o Breque (Premê), "São Paulo, São Paulo," 1983, Letras, https://www.letras.mus.br/premeditando-breque-preme/381602/.

39   "Ratos," *O Commercio de São Paulo*, October 20, 1899, 1.

40 *Diário Oficial da União (DOU)*, November 8, 1899, sec. 1, 16, https://www
    .jusbrasil.com.br/diarios/1687131/pg-16-secao-1-diario-oficial-da-uniao
    -dou-de-08-11-1899; and advertisement for "Formicidina Paranaense,"
    O Commercio de São Paulo, July 29, 1900, 4.

41 Weber, "Como convencer e curar"; and Armus and Gómez, *Gray Zones of
    Medicine*.

42 "Editaes," *O Commercio de São Paulo*, December 24, 1900, 3; "Edi-
    taes," *O Commercio de São Paulo*, December 28, 1900, 3; and "Serviço
    Sanitário," *O Commercio de São Paulo*, September 16, 1901, 3.

43 Penteado, *Belènzinho, 1910*, 38.

44 A. Lutz, "Algumas observações feitas em dois casos de peste pneumônica
    pelo dr. Adolpho Lutz."

45 "Serviço Sanitário," *Correio Paulistano*, March 20, 1903, 5; and "Serviço
    Sanitário," *Correio Paulistano*, August 26, 1903, 3.

46 Oswaldo Cruz, interview in "Notas," *O Commercio de São Paulo*, Sep-
    tember 17, 1903, 1; and O. Cruz, *Peste pelo Dr. Oswaldo Gonçalves Cruz*,
    32–33.

47 Developed in 2022 by Thomas Rogers, the Rogers Coefficient is based on
    his monetary worldview that "I always use a bottle of beer as my default
    measure for assessing the cost of . . . things." Thomas D. Rogers, email to
    Jeffrey Lesser, March 22, 2022. I used newspaper advertisements to de-
    termine beer prices: *Correio Paulistano*, January 1, 1900, 2; *Correio Pau-
    listano*, January 1, 1900, 6; and *Correio Paulistano*, January 26, 1903, 2.
    Jacob Penteado puts the cost of a bottle of beer in Bom Retiro at three
    hundred reis. Penteado, *Belènzinho, 1910*, 35.

48 "Rabiscos," *O Commercio de São Paulo*, December 16, 1899, 1. See also
    Carlos Fioravanti, "Guerra à peste," *Pesquisa FAPESP* 294 (August 2020).
    https://revistapesquisa.fapesp.br/guerra-a-peste/.

49 Alencar, *O carnaval carioca através da música*.

50 Matheus Silva, "Estratégias públicas no combate à peste bubônica no Rio
    de Janeiro (1900–1906)," 8.

51 Vann, "Of Rats, Rice, and Race."

52 "Rabiscos," *O Commercio de São Paulo*, December 16, 1899, 1.

53 "Glosas," *Lavoura e Commercio*, January 24, 1900, 1.

54 "Glosas," *Lavoura e Commercio*, January 24, 1900, 1.

55 Secretaria de Cultura e Juventude de São Bernardo do Campo, *Biblioteca
    Pública—lugar de conhecimentos, uma história das pandemias*; and Moreira
    and Massarani "(En)canto científico," 303.

56 L. Nascimento and Silva, "De protestos e levantes."

57   Góes, "O Rio de Janeiro aos olhos do cronista popular." A version of the song can be heard at Biblioteca Virtual Oswaldo Cruz, http://oswaldocruz.fiocruz.br/musicas/ (accessed June 28, 2024).

58   "Movimento de doentes do Hospital de Isolamento, 1918. Primeiro caso de caso de gripe espanhola registrado no hospital aparece no dia 15/10/1918," IMG_7047, AMSPER/Instituto Butantan; and "A 'razzia' da peste," *O Combate*, November 27, 1918, 1.

59   Beiner, "Great Flu."

60   Winter, "History, Memory, and the Flu," 26. See also Alonso et al., "1918 Influenza Pandemic," B16; and Massad, Burattini, Coutinho, and Lopez, "The 1918 Influenza Epidemic in the City of São Paulo."

61   *Os Imigrantes*, Rede Bandeirantes, April 27, 1981–November 1, 1982. The telenovela is reprised frequently in Brazil, including in 2022, and it was selected as one of the Bandeirantes networks most classic evening series. The Spanish flu first appeared in episode 97 and then became a reference for the remaining 350 episodes.

62   Bavel et al., "Using Social and Behavioural Science," 462.

63   Kraut, "Immigration, Ethnicity, and the Pandemic," 121; and E. Jones, "'Cooperation in All Human Endeavour.'"

64   Meyer and Teixeira, Serviço Sanitário do Estado de São Paulo, *A gripe epidêmica no Brazil e especialmente em São Paulo*; and Lin, *Statistics*.

65   Barata, "Cem anos de endemias e epidemias"; and Penteado, *Belènzinho, 1910*, 260.

66   Guimbeau, Menon, and Musacchio, "Brazilian Bombshell?," 2. See also Almond, "Is the 1918 Influenza Pandemic Over?"

67   Goulart, "Revisitando a espanhola," 105.

68   Bertucci, "Pesquisa e debates sobre a gripe durante a epidemia de 1918."

69   E. Costa, *Crowns of Glory*.

70   Museu da Imigração de São Paulo, Acervo Digital do Museu da Imigração de São Paulo, accessed June 28, 2024, https://acervodigital.museudaimigracao.org.br/pesquisageral.php?id=nomes&busca=DEMERARA.

71   André Bernardo, "Gripe espanhola: A viagem em que o 'navio da morte' *Demerara* venceu bombardeios alemães e trouxe a doença ao Brasil," BBC News Brasil, November 22, 2020, https://www.bbc.com/portuguese/internacional-54907997; Barreira, *Demerara*.

72   Pereira, "O Brasil é ainda um imenso hospital," Discurso pronunciado pel Prof. Miguel Pereira, por ocasião do regresso do Prof. Aloysio de Castro, da Rep. Argentina, em Outubro de 1916. See also "O Rio é um vasto hospital!," *Gazeta de Notícias* (Rio de Janeiro), October 15, 1918, 1; and Sá, "A voz do Brasil."

73 *Careta*, October 5, 1918.

74 Andrea C. T. Wanderley, "E o ex e futuro presidente do Brasil morreu de gripe . . . a Gripe Espanhola de 1918," *Brasiliana Fotográfica*, March 23, 2020, https://brasilianafotografica.bn.gov.br/?p=18866.

75 Meyer and Teixeira, Serviço Sanitário do Estado de São Paulo, *A gripe epidêmica no Brazil e especialmente em São Paulo*, 4.

76 Alonso et al., "1918 Influenza Pandemic," B17.

77 Secretaria da Segurança Pública do Estado de São Paulo, Registro de ocorrências da Assistência Policial, 1911–40, docs. 53939, 53941, and 53964, vol. E14038, , all dated October 21, 1918, APESP.

78 Secretaria da Segurança Pública do Estado de São Paulo, Registro de ocorrências da Assistência Policial, 1911–40, vol. E14040, docs. 55567–55573, 55593, all dated October 26, 1918, APESP.

79 Duarte, "O Código Sanitário Estadual de 1918 e a Epidemia de Gripe Espanhola."

80 Bertucci, *Influenza, a medicina enferma*, 113. See also Penteado, *Belènzinho, 1910*, 39.

81 "A 'hespanhola': A verdade é que não temos Serviço Sanitário," *O Combate*, November 8, 1918, 1.

82 Brito, "'La dansarina.'" See also Penteado, *Belènzinho, 1910*, 15.

83 *O Estado de S. Paulo*, October 28, 1918, 3.

84 Bertolli Filho, "Estratégias jornalísticas no noticiamento de uma epidemia," 18.

85 Meyer and Teixeira, Serviço Sanitário do Estado de São Paulo, *A gripe epidêmica no Brazil e especialmente em São Paulo*, 111; and Lesser, *Immigration, Ethnicity, and National Identity*, 158.

86 Klengel, "Pandemic Avant-Garde," 5.

87 O. Andrade, *Obras Completas IX: Um Homem Sem Profissão*, 106–7.

88 "A 'hespanhola' em S. Paulo, Confirma-se a notícia que demos da sua existência," *O Combate*, October 16, 1918, 1.

89 Secretaria da Segurança Pública do Estado de São Paulo, Registro de ocorrências da Assistência Policial, 1911–40, docs. 55357, 55786, 55788, 55793, and 55799, vol. E14040, all dated October 26, 1918, APESP. See also C. Silva, "Estudo epidemiológico da dengue no município de São Paulo," 37; Cristiane Bomfim, "Bom Retiro tem maior incidência de dengue," *Jornal da Tarde/O Estado de S. Paulo*, May 5, 2011, https://www.estadao.com.br/saude/bom-retiro-tem-maior-incidencia-de-dengue/; and Guilherme Balza, "Oito dos dez bairros com mais mortes por Covid-19 estão no centro 'pobre' de São Paulo," *Portal G1—Globo*, May 27, 2020, https://g1.globo

.com/sp/sao-paulo/noticia/2020/05/27/oito-dos-dez-bairros-com-mais
-mortes-por-covid-19-estao-no-centro-pobre-de-sao-paulo.ghtml.

90   Serufo et al., "Dengue."

91   "A 'hespanhola' em S. Paulo, numerosos casos suspeitos," *O Combate*, November 10, 1918, 1. See also Schwarcz and Starling, *A bailarina da morte*, 25.

92   Penteado, *Belènzinho, 1910*, 261.

93   "A 'razzia' da peste," *O Combate*, November 27, 1918, 1.

94   Bertolli Filho, *História da saúde pública no Brasil*, 89–95.

95   Meyer and Teixeira, Serviço Sanitário do Estado de São Paulo, *A gripe epidêmica no Brazil e especialmente em São Paulo*, 59–161.

96   Marcos Faerman, "Lembrando os Bons Tempos," *Jornal da Tarde*, November 23, 1981, 14–15. See also Ato Municipal No. 1.278, de 18 de novembro de 1918, "Declara de utilidade pública, para desapropriação judicial, uma área de terreno necessária ao aumento do cemitério do Araçá," Prefeitura de São Paulo, Legislação Municipal, http://legislacao.prefeitura.sp.gov.br/leis/ato-gabinete-do-prefeito-1278-de-18-de-novembro-de-1918; and Museu de Futebol—Centro de Referência do Futebol Brasileiro, "Cemitério do Araçá: Histórias sobre a cidade, o futebol e a morte," *Medium*, June 6, 2017, https://medium.com/museu-do-futebol/cemit%C3%A9rio-do-ara%C3%A7%C3%A1-hist%C3%B3rias-sobre-a-cidade-o-futebol-e-a-morte-c4208c67cdf3.

97   Meyer and Teixeira, Serviço Sanitário do Estado de São Paulo, *A gripe epidêmica no Brazil e especialmente em São Paulo*, 64. See also Dall'Ava and Mota, "A gripe espanhola em Sorocaba."

98   Rago, *Do cabaré ao lar*; Cano, *Raízes da concentração industrial em São Paulo*, 234; Wolfe, *Working Women, Working Men*; B. Campos, "Companheiras em greve"; Venancio, "Lugar de mulher é . . . na fábrica"; and M. Ribeiro, *Condições de trabalho na indústria têxtil paulista (1870–1930)*.

99   Meyer and Teixeira, Serviço Sanitário do Estado de São Paulo, *A gripe epidêmica no Brazil e especialmente em São Paulo*, 64–67, 110.

100 Dimas, *Poisoned Eden*, 15.

101 Sr. Amadeu, quoted in Bosi, *Memória e sociedade*, 130.

102 Bertucci, *Influenza, a medicina enferma*, 178.

103 Bertucci, *Influenza, a medicina enferma*, 181.

104 Palma, "From Asia to the Americas."

105 Hoehn, *O que vendem os hervanários da cidade de S. Paulo*, 153.

106 Sr. Antonio, in Bosi, *Memória e sociedade*, 234.

107 Kenzo, *Não há cura sem anúncio*.

108 *O Estado de S. Paulo*, October 18, 1918, 6.

109   For an analysis of the spread of rumors among African (US) Americans, see Turner, *I Heard It*.

110   Dona Brites, in Bosi, *Memória e sociedade*, 314.

111   "Ecos da 'hespanhola,' os escandolos da Crus Vermelha no Braz," *A Rolha*, December 3, 1918, 13. Bertucci, "A onipresença do medo na influenza de 1918," 464.

112   A. Nascimento, "Tourist Topicality."

113   Lobato, "Fatia de vida."

114   Penteado, *Belènzinho, 1910*, 261.

115   Bosi, "Sr. Amadeu," *Memória e sociedade*, 150.

116   "Loucura tragica: A grippe enlouqueceu uma familia inteira," *O Combate*, December 3, 1918, 1.

117   Bertucci, *Influenza, a medicina enferma*, 120.

118   *O Estado de S. Paulo*, November 12, 1918, 4. See also "A 'influeza hespanhola' em São Paulo,"*O Combate*, November 11, 1918, 3.

119   Bertolli Filho, *História da saúde pública no Brasil*; and Bertucci, *Influenza, a medicina enferma*, 119–25.

120   Honigsbaum, *Great Influenza Pandemics*; Bastiampillai et al., "Pandemics and Social Cohesion," 20; and Bastiampillai et al., "Spanish Flu Pandemic."

121   N. Williams, Thornton, and Young-DeMarco, "Migrant Values and Beliefs"; and Khoudja, "Religious Trajectories of Immigrants."

122   Lesser, *Immigration, Ethnicity and National Identity*, 50–52; Biehl, Mugge, and Goldani, "Books of the Dead Revisited"; and Dreher, *A religião de Jacobina*.

123   Lesser, *Negotiating National Identity*, 135–46.

124   "A 'Hespanhola,' scena commovente,"*O Combate*, November 23, 1918, 5; and Bertolli Filho, "Estratégias jornalísticas no noticiamento de uma epidemia."

125   "A 'Hespanhola,' scena commovente," *O Combate*, November 23, 1918, 5.

126   Lesser, *Discontented Diaspora*.

127   *O Estado de S. Paulo*, December 2, 1918, 3–4.

128   "Enterrado vivo! Scena fantástica occorida com um pedreiro," *O Combate*, December 2, 1918, 1; Bryce, "Los caballeros de beneficencia y las damas organizadoras"; and Lesser, *Welcoming the Undesirables*.

129   "Um pedreiro alemão decapitado pelo prpropria mulher e um filho," *A Gazeta*, December 2, 1918, 3; *O Estado de S. Paulo*, December 2, 1918, 3–4; "Enterrado vivo! Scena fantástica occorida com um pedreiro," *O Combate*,

December 2, 1918, 1; *A Época* (Rio de Janeiro), December 4, 1918, 6; and *Archivo Vermelho: Revista Policial Illustrada*, 1, no. 12 (December 1918), 15–16.

130   "Um homen decapitado," *Correio Paulistano*, April 12, 1919, 5.

131   Reis Filho and Suppia, "Dos cânones sagrados às alegorias profanas," 275; and Hertzman, *After Palmares*.

132   *Spectros*, directed by Douglas Petrie (São Paulo: Moonshot Pictures, 2020); Netflix, February 20, 2020.

133   Bondeson, *Buried Alive*; and Casoy, *Ópera em São Paulo*, 23.

134   *O Estado de S. Paulo*, May 11, 1912, 12; and *O Combate*, January 18, 1922, 1.

135   "Balas d'estalo . . . ," *A Tribuna* (Santos), March 10, 1918, 2.

136   Alves and Pereira, "Necropolítica, drogas e ações governamentais na Cracolândia"; and Silva Júnior and Monteiro, "Os significados da morte e do morrer."

137   "Enterrado vivo! Caso fantástico ocorrido com um pedreiro," *O Combate*, November 29, 1918, 1.

138   Bosi, *Memória e sociedade*; and Bertolli Filho, *História da saúde pública no Brasil*, 282n44.

139   "Enterrado vivo! Caso fantástico ocorrido com um pedreiro," *O Combate*, November 29, 1918, 1.

140   "Enterrado vivo! Caso fantástico ocorrido com um pedreiro. O que disse Eugenio Benzana a 'O Combate," *O Combate*, November 30, 1918, 1; and *A Capital*, November 30, 1918, 1. "Um quasi enterrado vivo, quem sao os responsaveis?," *A Rolha*, December 3, 1918, 4. Thank you to Paulo Castagnet of *Revistas Paulistanas Antigas* for sharing digital copies of *A Rolha* with me.

141   "Enterrado vivo! Scena fantástica ocorrido com um pedreiro," *O Combate*, December 2, 1918, 1.

142   "Um quasi enterrado vivo, quem são os responsaveis?," *A Rolha*, December 3, 1918, 3.

143   R. Pereira, "O prefeito do progresso," 217.

144   Taunay, *História da cidade de São Paulo*, 372.

145   "Enterrado vivo! Scena fantástica ocorrido com um pedreiro. O que nos disse o dr. Alarico Silveira," *O Combate*, December 3, 1918, 1.

146   "Um quasi enterrado vivo, quem são os responsaveis?," *A Rolha*, December 3, 1918, 4; and "Enterrado vivo! Scena fantástica ocorrido com um pedreiro. O que nos disse o dr. Alarico Silveira," *O Combate*, December 3, 1918, 1.

147   Bertolli Filho, *História social da tuberculose e do tuberculoso*, 183.

148   Schneider, *Memória e história (Antoninho Da Rocha Marmo)*, 152–74.

Conclusion

1 Pingel, Llovet, Cosentino, and Lesser, "Committing to Continuity."

2 According to the *New York Times*, on October 5, 2021, the state of Georgia (population 10.62 million) reported 2,694 new cases of COVID-19. "Tracking Coronavirus in Georgia" Latest Map and Case Count," March 23, 2023, https://www.nytimes.com/interactive/2021/us/georgia-covid-cases.html. The state of São Paulo (population 44.04 million) on October 6 reported 1,679 new cases. São Paulo, Governo do Estado, "Seade Coronavirus," November 18, 2023, https://www.seade.gov.br/coronavirus/.

3 Graff Zivin, *Wandering Signifier*, 106–31.

BIBLIOGRAPHY

Archives

Acervo do Museu do Ipiranga, São Paulo
Arquivo do Museu de Saúde Pública Emílio Ribas, São Paulo (AMSPER)
Arquivo Histórico Municipal Washington Luís, São Paulo (AHM)
Arquivo Público do Estado de São Paulo, São Paulo (APESP)
Assembleia Legislativa do Estado de São Paulo (ALESP)
Biblioteca Digital Seade, Fundação Sistema Estadual de Análise de Dados, São Paulo
Clinton Digital Library, Clinton Presidential Library and Museum, Little Rock, Arkansas
Instituto Butantan, Centro de Memória, São Paulo

Newspapers, Journals, Magazines, Bulletins, and Websites

Almanach Paulista (São Paulo), http://bndigital.bn.br/acervo-digital/almanach -paulista/830089
Almanaque Folha (São Paulo)
O Archivo Illustrado: Encyclopedia Noticiosa, Scientifica e Litteraria (São Paulo), https://bndigital.bn.gov.br/acervo-digital/archivo/719102
Archivo Vermelho: Revista Policial Illustrada (Rio de Janeiro), http://bndigital.bn .gov.br/acervo-digital/archivo/347841
A Capital (Rio de Janeiro), http://bndigital.bn.br/acervo-digital/capital/570907
Careta (Rio de Janeiro), http://objdigital.bn.br/acervo_digital/div_periodicos /careta/careta_anos.htm

O Combate (São Paulo), http://bndigital.bn.br/acervo-digital/combate/830453

O Commercio de São Paulo, http://bndigital.bn.br/acervo-digital/commercio-de
-sao-paulo/227900

Correio Braziliense (Rio de Janeiro), https://memoria.bn.gov.br/DocReader
/docmulti.aspx?bib=028274&pesq=

Correio Paulistano (São Paulo), http://bndigital.bn.br/acervo-digital/correio
-paulistano/090972

Diário da Noite (Rio de Janeiro), http://bndigital.bn.br/acervo-digital/diario-noite
/221961

Diário de Commercio (Rio de Janeiro)

Diário do Transporte (São Paulo), https://diariodotransporte.com.br/

Diário Oficial da União (São Paulo), https://www.in.gov.br/servicos/diario-oficial
-da-uniao

Diário Oficial do Estado de São Paulo, https://www.imprensaoficial.com.br/DO
/HomeDO_2_0.aspx#25/06/2024

Diário Oficial do Município (São Paulo)

Diário Popular (São Paulo)

A Época (Rio de Janeiro), http://bndigital.bn.br/acervo-digital/epoca/720100

O Estado de S. Paulo, https://www.estadao.com.br/acervo/

Folha da Manhã (São Paulo), https://acervo.folha.com.br/index.do

Folha de S. Paulo, https://acervo.folha.com.br/index.do

Folha do Braz (São Paulo)

A Gazeta (São Paulo), http://bndigital.bn.br/acervo-digital/gazeta/763900

Gazeta de Notícias (Rio de Janeiro), http://bndigital.bn.br/acervo-digital/gazeta
-noticias/721026

Gazeta do Povo (Curitiba), http://bndigital.bn.gov.br/acervo-digital/gazeta-do
-povo/814253

GL'Italiani in San Paulo, https://memoria.bn.gov.br/DocReader/docreader.aspx
?bib=304395&pesq=&pagfis=1

G1—Globo, https://g1.globo.com/

Guardian (London), https://www.theguardian.com/international

A Immigração: órgão da Sociedade Central de Immigração (São Paulo), http://
bndigital.bn.br/acervo-digital/immigracao/239984

Jornal da Tarde, http://bndigital.bn.br/acervo-digital/jornal-tarde/713120

Jornal da USP (São Paulo), https://jornal.usp.br/

Jornal do Commercio (São Paulo), http://bndigital.bn.gov.br//acervo-digital/Jornal
-do-commercio/713074

JP News (São Paulo), https://jovempan.com.br/jpnews

Jusbrasil (São Paulo), https://www.jusbrasil.com.br

Labcidade (São Paulo), https://www.labcidade.fau.usp.br/

A Lanterna: Folha Anti-Clerical e de Combate (São Paulo), http://bndigital.bn.br
/acervo-digital/lanterna/366153

Lavoura e Commercio (São Paulo), http://bndigital.bn.br/acervo-digital/lavoura
-e-commercio/817333

O Menelick (São Paulo), https://memoria.bn.gov.br/DocReader/docreader.aspx
?bib=844829&pesq=&pagfis=1

Morning Sun Lifestyle (Pittsburgh, KS)

New York Times, https://www.nytimes.com

Not Even Past (Austin, TX)

El País (Brazil), https://elpais.com/noticias/brasil/

Il Pasquino Coloniale (São Paulo), http://bndigital.bn.br/acervo-digital/il-pasquino
/359670

O Pirralho (São Paulo), http://bndigital.bn.br/acervo-digital/pirralho/213101

A Plebe: Pela Liberdade e o Anarquismo (São Paulo), https://www.ufrgs.br/
nphdigital/

A Província de São Paulo, https://www.estadao.com.br/acervo/

Public Health (London)

Revista do Arquivo Municipal (São Paulo), https://www.prefeitura.sp.gov.br/cidade
/secretarias/cultura/arquivo_historico/publicacoes/index.php?p=8312

A Rolha (São Paulo), https://memoria.bn.gov.br/DocReader/docreader.aspx?bib
=212695&pesq=&pagfis=1

O Sacy (São Paulo), http://bndigital.bn.br/acervo-digital/sacy/213233

Sentinella da Monarchia: Orgam Conservador (São Paulo), http://bndigital.bn.gov
.br//acervo-digital/Sentinella-da-Monarchia/305049

A Tribuna (Santos), http://bndigital.bn.gov.br/acervo-digital/tribuna/153931

A Tribuna do Povo: Folha republicana parlamentarista (São Paulo), http://bndigital
.bn.br/acervo-digital/tribuna-do-povo/818437

VEJA *São Paulo*, https://vejasp.abril.com.br/

Vida Paulista: Humorismo, Literatura, e Esporte (São Paulo), https://memoria.bn
.gov.br/DocReader/docreader.aspx?bib=216372&pesq=&pagfis=1

Lesser Research Collective Academic Production

Almeida, Cintia Rodrigues de, Luanna Mendes do Nascimento, Monaliza Caetano
dos Santos, and Vitória Martins Fontes. "As lacunas enquanto escolha: Uma
abordagem panorâmica sobre as fichas da Assistência Médica Policial de São
Paulo e as mulheres do Bom Retiro presentes nessa documentação." Unpublished manuscript, 2020.

Cikopana, Doris. "A Case Study of a São Paulo Health Clinic: Accessibility to Health
Services by Patients Who Do Not Speak Portuguese as a First Language." BA
honors thesis, Emory University, 2018.

Ferla, Luis, Karine Reis Ferreira, Fernando Atique, Andrew G. Britt, Karla Donato
Fook, Jeffrey Lesser, Cristiane Miyasaka, Daniela Musa, Thomas D. Rogers,
and Nandamudi Vijaykumar. "Pauliceia 2.0: Mapeamento colaborativo da

história de São Paulo, 1870–1940." *História, Ciências, Saúde—Manguinhos* 27, no. 4 (October–December 2020): 1207–23.

Ferreira, Karine R., Luis Ferla, Gilberto R. de Queiroz, Nandamudi L. Vijaykumar, Carlos A. Noronha, Rodrigo M. Mariano, Denis Taveira, Gabriel Sansigolo, Orlando Guarnieri, Thomas Rogers, Jeffrey Lesser, Michael Page, Fernando Atique, Daniela Musa, Janaina Y. Santos, Diego S. Morais, Cristiane R. Miyasaka, Cintia R. de Almeida, Luanna G. M. do Nascimento, Jaine A. Diniz, and Monaliza C. dos Santos. "A Platform for Collaborative Historical Research Based on Volunteered Geographical Information." *Journal of Information and Data Management* 9, no. 3 (December 2018): 291–304. https://periodicos.ufmg .br/index.php/jidm/article/view/426.

Fook, Karla Donato, Daniela Leal Musa, Nandamudi Vijaykumar, Rodrigo M. Mariano, Gabriel dos Reis Morais, Raphael Augusto O. Silva, Gabriel Sansigolo, Luciana Rebelo, Luís Antônio Coelho Ferla, Cintia Almeida, Luanna Nascimento, Vitória Martins Fontes da Silva, Monaliza Caetano dos Santos, Aracele Torres, Ângela Pereira, Fernando Atique, Jeffrey Lesser, Thomas D. Roger, Andrew G. Britt, Rafael Laguardia, Ana Maria Alves Barbour, Orlando Guarnier Farias, Ariana Marco, Caróu Dickinson, and Tamires P. Camargo. "Collaborative Historical Platform for Historians: Extended Functionalities in Pauliceia 2.0." In *Proceedings of the 17th International Conference on Web Information Systems and Technologies*, 460–66. SCITEPRESS—Science and Technology Publications, Setúbal, Portugal, 2021. https://www.scitepress.org /Papers/2021/107134/107134.pdf.

Gonzalez, Daniella. "Defining Family Planning in a São Paulo Clinic: Healthcare Providers and Patients' Varied Conceptualizations of 'Planned' and 'Unplanned' Pregnancies." BA honors thesis, Emory University, 2018.

Jin, Sabrina. "New Perspectives on Race and Racism among Brazilians of Asian Descent." BA honors thesis, Emory University, 2022.

Kauko, Sara. "Criollo Entrepreneurialism: Transforming Racial and Class Identities and Social Mobility among Mixed-Race Argentines." PhD diss., Emory University, 2020.

LaCroix, Delphine, Juliana Casagrande, and Jeffrey Lesser. "A Sacred Space of Health." Paper presented at the 25th International Congress of History of Science and Technology. Rio de Janeiro, July 27, 2017.

Llovet, Alexandra. "Stigma Continuity of Leprosy in Brazil, 1924–2018." BA honors thesis, Emory University, 2018.

Miller, Savannah. "A Qualitative Assessment of Water, Sanitation, and Hygiene in an Urban Working-Class Neighborhood of São Paulo, Brazil." Master's thesis, Emory University, 2022.

Pingel, Emily Sweetnam. "Immigrants, Migrants, and Paulistanos: Racialized Geographies of Labor and Health in São Paulo, Brazil." *SSM-Qualitative Research in Health* 2 (December 2022): 1–8. https://doi.org/10.1016/j.ssmqr.2022.100074.

Pingel, Emily Sweetnam. "Primary Care and the Reproduction of Health Inequity in a Central São Paulo Neighborhood." PhD diss., Emory University, 2021.

Pingel, Emily Sweetnam. "Seeing Inside: How Stigma and Recognition Shape Community Health Worker Home Visits in São Paulo, Brazil." *Community Health Equity Research and Policy* 44, no. 3 (2024): 303–13. https://doi.org/10.1177/2752535X221137384.

Pingel, Emily Sweetnam, Alexandra Caridad Llovet, Fernando Cosentino, and Jeffrey Lesser. "Committing to Continuity: Primary Care Practices during COVID-19 in an Urban Brazilian Neighborhood." *Health, Education and Behavior* 48, no. 1 (2021): 29–33. https://doi.org/10.1177/1090198120979609.

Santos, Fabio Alexandre dos, Fernando Atique, Janes Jorge, Luis Ferla, Diego de Souza Morais, Janaina Yamamoto, Maíra Rosin, Ana Carolina Nunes Rocha, Nathalia Burato Nascimento, Orlando Guamier Cardin Farias, Wesley Alves de Moura, Thássia Andrade Moro, and Amanda de Lima Moraes. "A enchente de 1929 na cidade de São Paulo: Memória, história e novas abordagens de pesquisa." *Revista do Arquivo Geral da Cidade do Rio de Janeiro* 8 (2014): 149–66. http://www.rio.rj.gov.br/dlstatic/10112/4204432/4133801/revista_agcrj_oito.pdf.

Shrivastava, Surbhi. "Stratified Surgical Births: Disparities in Cesarean Section Births in São Paulo, Brazil." Paper presented at the Population Association of America (PAA) Annual Meeting, Atlanta, GA, April 9, 2022.

Shrivastava, Surbhi, and Heeju Sohn. "Extricating Individual and Contextual Sources of Racial/Ethnic Disparities in C-Sections in Brazil: A Decomposition Analysis of Live Births from 2019." Poster presented at the Academy Health Annual Research Meeting, Seattle, WA, June 26, 2023.

Other Sources

Aguiar, Breno S., Camila Lorenz, Flávia Virginio, Lincoln Suesdek, and Francisco Chiaravalloti-Neto. "Potential Risks of Zika and Chikungunya Outbreaks in Brazil: A Modelling Study." *International Journal of Infectious Diseases* 70, no. 1 (February 2018): 20–29.

Aguiar, Marcia Ernani de. "Tecnologias e cuidado em saúde: A Estratégia Saúde da Família (ESF) e o caso do imigrante boliviano e coreano no bairro do Bom Retiro—SP." Master's thesis, Universidade de São Paulo, 2013.

Alberto, Paulina L. *Terms of Inclusion: Black Intellectuals in Twentieth-Century Brazil.* Chapel Hill: University of North Carolina Press, 2011.

Alberto, Paulina, and Jesse Hoffnung-Garskof. "'Racial Democracy' and Racial Inclusion: Hemispheric Histories." In *Afro-Latin American Studies: An Introduction*, edited by Alejandro de la Fuente and George Reid Andrews, 264–316. New York: Cambridge University Press, 2018.

Alencar, Edigar. *O carnaval carioca através da música.* Vol. 1. Rio de Janeiro: Livraria Francisco Alves Editora, 1979.

Aliano, David. "Brazil through Italian Eyes: The Debate over Emigration to São Paulo during the 1920s." *Altreitalie* 31 (July–December 2005): 87–107. https://www.altreitalie.it/pubblicazioni/rivista/numeri_arretrati/n_31/altreitalie_31_lugliodicembre_2005.

Almeida, Guilherme de. *Cosmópolis: São Paulo 29 - Oito Reportagens de Guilherme de Almeida.* São Paulo: Companhia Editora Nacional, 1962.

Almeida, Marta de. "República dos invisíveis: Emílio Ribas, microbiologia e saúde pública em São Paulo (1898–1917)." Master's thesis, Universidade de São Paulo, 1998.

Almeida, Marta de, and Maria Amélia M. Dantes. "O serviço sanitário de São Paulo, a saúde pública e a microbiologia." In *Espaços da ciência no Brasil: 1800–1930*, edited by Maria Amélia M. Dantes, 133–55. Rio de Janeiro: Editora Fiocruz, 2001. https://doi.org/10.7476/9786557081570.0007.

Almond, Douglas. "Is the 1918 Influenza Pandemic Over? Long-Term Effects of *In Utero* Influenza Exposure in the Post-1940 U.S. Population." *Journal of Political Economy* 114, no. 4 (August 2006): 672–712.

Alonso, Wladimir J., Francielle C. Nascimento, Rodolfo Acuña-Soto, Cynthia Schuck-Paim, and Mark A. Miller. "The 1918 Influenza Pandemic in Florianopolis: A Subtropical City in Brazil." *Vaccine* 29, suppl. 2 (July 2011): B16–B20.

Alvarez, Marcos César. "A criminologia no Brasil ou como tratar desigualmente os desiguais." *DADOS—Revista de Ciências Sociais* 45, no. 4 (2002): 677–704. https://nev.prp.usp.br/wp-content/uploads/2014/08/down068.pdf.

Alves, Ygor Delgado, and Pedro Paulo Gomes Pereira. "Necropolítica, drogas e ações governamentais na Cracolândia." *Barbarói* 1, no. 60 (December 2021): 204–31. https://online.unisc.br/seer/index.php/barbaroi/article/view/15442.

Amadio, Decio. "Desenho urbano e bairros centrais de São Paulo: Um estudo sobre a formação e transformação do Brás, Bom Retiro e Pari." PhD diss., Universidade de São Paulo, 2005.

Amado, Jorge. *A Morte e a Morte de Quincas Berro Dágua.* 1961. São Paulo: Companhia das Letras, 2008.

Americano, Jorge. "O realejo e os macacos." In *São Paulo Naquele Tempo (1895–1915)*, 155. São Paulo: Carrenho Editorial/Narrativa Um/Carbono, 2004.

Americano, Jorge. "Veículos." In *São Paulo Naquele Tempo (1895–1915)*, 175–78. São Paulo: Carrenho Editorial/Narrativa Um/Carbono, 2004.

Amoruso, Michael. "Spaces of Suffering: Religious Transit in São Paulo's Devotion to Souls." *Journal of the American Academy of Religion* 86, no. 4 (December 2018): 989–1013. https://doi.org/10.1093/jaarel/lfy016.

Andrade, Carlos Drummond de. "Resíduo." In *A Rosa do Povo*, 92–95. Rio de Janeiro: Editora Record, 2000.

Andrade, Mário de. "Colloque sentimental." 1922. In *Poesias completas*, edited by Diléa Zanotto Manfio, 99–100. São Paulo: Editora da Universidade de São Paulo, 1987.

Andrade, Monica Viegas, Augusto Quaresma Coelho, Mauro Xavier Neto, Lucas Resende de Carvalho, Rifat Atun, and Marcia C. Castro. "Brazil's Family Health

Strategy: Factors Associated with Programme Uptake and Coverage Expansion over 15 Years (1998–2012)." *Health Policy and Planning* 33, no. 3 (January 2018): 368–80. https://doi.org/10.1093/heapol/czx189.

Andrade, Oswald de. *Estética e política.* Edited by Maria Eugênia Boaventura. São Paulo: Globo, 1992.

Andrade, Oswald de. *Obras Completas IX: Um Homem Sem Profissão: Memórias e Confissões: Sob as Ordens de Mamãe.* Vol. 1. Rio de Janeiro: Editora Civilização Brasileira, 1976.

Andrews, George Reid. *Blackness in the White Nation: A History of Afro-Uruguay.* Chapel Hill: University of North Carolina Press, 2010.

Andrews, George Reid. *Blacks and Whites in São Paulo, Brazil, 1888–1988.* Madison: University of Wisconsin Press, 1991.

Antonil, André João. *Cultura e opulência do Brasil, por suas drogas e minas* [1711]. Rio de Janeiro: Typ. Im. E Const. De J. Villeneuve e Comp, 1837. https://www.gutenberg.org/cache/epub/70662/pg70662-images.html.

Antunes, Paulo C. de Azevedo. "Eugenia e imigração." PhD diss., Universidade de São Paulo, 1926.

Antunes, Paulo C. de Azevedo. *Eugenia e imigração.* São Paulo: Editora Helios, 1926.

Anzaldúa, Gloria. *Borderlands/La frontera: The New Mestiza.* 4th ed. San Francisco: Aunt Lute Books, 2012.

Araújo, Marcia Luiza Pires de. "A escolarização de crianças negras paulistas (1920–1940)." PhD diss., Universidade de São Paulo, 2013. https://www.teses.usp.br/teses/disponiveis/48/48134/tde-27062013-124505/publico/MARCIA_LUIZA_PIRES_DE_ARAUJO_rev.pdf.

Araújo, Oscar Egídio de. "Enquistamentos étnicos." *Revista do Arquivo Municipal* 6, no. 65 (March 1940): 227–46.

Araújo, Ricardo Vieira, Marcos Roberto Albertini, André Luis Costa-da-Silva, Lincoln Suesdek, Nathália Cristina Soares Franceschi, Nancy Marçal Bastos, Gizelda Katz, et al. "São Paulo Urban Heat Islands Have a Higher Incidence of Dengue Than Other Urban Areas." *Brazilian Journal of Infectious Diseases* 19, no. 2 (March–April 2015): 146–55. https://doi.org/10.1016/j.bjid.2014.10.004.

Armus, Diego, ed. *Disease in the History of Modern Latin America: From Malaria to AIDS.* Durham, NC: Duke University Press, 2013.

Armus, Diego, and Pablo F. Gómez. *The Gray Zones of Medicine: Healers and History in Latin America.* Pittsburgh: University of Pittsburgh Press, 2021.

Assunção Filho, Francisco Moacir. "1924—DELENDA SÃO PAULO: A cidade e a população vítimas das armas de guerra e das disputas políticas." Master's thesis, Pontifícia Universidade Católica de São Paulo, 2014.

Azevedo, Aluísio. *A Brazilian Tenement.* Translated by Harry W. Brown. New York: Robert M. McBride and Company, 1926.

Azevedo, Aluísio. *O cortiço.* Rio de Janeiro: B. L. Garnier, 1890.

Azevedo, Aroldo de. *A cidade de São Paulo: Estudos de geografia urbana.* São Paulo: Companhia Editora Nacional, 1958.

Baeninger, Rosana, and Duval Fernandes. *Atlas temático: Observatório das migrações em São Paulo—Migrações Internacionais*. Campinas: Núcleo de Estudos de População "Elza Berquó", 2017.

Baeninger, Rosana, Natália Belmonte Demétrio, and Jóice de Oliveira Santos Domeniconi. "Espaços das migraçoes transnacionais: Perfil sociodemográfico de imigrantes da África para o Brasil no século XX." *REMHU: Revista Interdisciplinar da Mobilidade Humana* 27, no. 56 (August 2019): 35–60. https://www.scielo.br/j/remhu/a/NTVNKhcQScbJpqHRSn96RQj/?format=pdf&lang=pt.

Ball, Molly. *Navigating Life and Work in Old Republic São Paulo*. Gainesville: University of Florida Press, 2020.

Bananére, Juó. *La divina increnca*. São Paulo: Livraria do Globo, 1924.

Bandeira, Antonio Francisco, Jr. *Indústria no estado de São Paulo em 1901*. São Paulo: Typ. do Diário Official, 1901.

Barata, Rita Barradas. "Cem anos de endemias e epidemias." *Ciência and Saúde Coletiva* 5, no. 2 (2000): 333–45.

Barbosa, Rosana. *Soccer and Racism: The Beginnings of Futebol in São Paulo and Rio de Janeiro, 1895–1933*. London: Anthem, 2022.

Barnett, Elizabeth D., and Patricia F. Walker. "Role of Immigrants and Migrants in Emerging Infectious Diseases." *Medical Clinics of North America*, 92, no. 6 (November 2008): 1447–58.

Barreira, Wagner G. *Demerara*. São Paulo: Editoria Instante, 2020.

Barros, Antônio Souza, Jr. "A habitação e os transportes." *Revista do Arquivo Municipal* 82 (1942): 83–86.

Bassanezi, Maria Silvia C. Beozzo. *São Paulo do passado: Dados Demográficos, 1890*. Campinas: NEPO-Núcleo de Estudos em População/UNICAMP, 1998.

Bassanezi, Maria Silvia C. Beozzo. "São Paulo do passado—dados demográficos (1836–2020)." *Revista Brasileira De Estudos De População* 16, nos. 1–2 (1999): 139–41. https://www.rebep.org.br/revista/article/view/399.

Bassanezi, Maria Silvia C. Beozzo. "Imigração e mortalidade na terra da garoa. São Paulo, final do século XIX e primeiras décadas do século XX." Paper presented at the XIX Encontro Nacional de Estudos Populacionais, São Pedro/SP, November 24–28, 2014. http://www.abep.org.br/publicacoes/index.php/anais/article/download/2101/2057.

Bassanezi, Maria Silvia C. Beozzo, and Maisa Faleiros Cunha. "Um espaço, dois momentos epidêmicos: Surtos de febre amarela (1896–1897) e de gripe (1918–1919) em Campinas, estado de São Paulo." *Revista Brasileira De Estudos De População* 36 (2019): 1–29. https://doi.org/10.20947/S0102-3098a0088.

Bastiampillai, Tarun, Stephen Allison, Jonathan Brailey, Mandy Ma, Sherry Kit Wa Chan, and Jeffrey C. L. Looi. "Pandemics and Social Cohesion: 1918–1920 Influenza Pandemic and the Reduction in US Suicide Rates." *Primary Care Companion for CNS Disorders* 23, no. 3 (April 2021). https://www.psychiatrist.com/pcc/depression/suicide/pandemics-social-cohesion-1918-1920-influenza-pandemic-reduction-us-suicide-rates/.

Bastiampillai, Tarun, Stephen Allison, David Smith, Roger Mulder, and Jeffrey C. L. Looi. "The Spanish Flu Pandemic and Stable New Zealand Suicide Rates: Historical Lessons for COVID-19." *New Zealand Medical Journal* 134, no. 1541 (September 3, 2021): 134–37. https://nzmj.org.nz/journal/vol-134-no-1541 /the-spanish-flu-pandemic-and-stable-new-zealand-suicide-rates-historical -lessons-for-covid-19.

Bastide, Roger. "A imprensa negra no Estado de São Paulo." In *Estudos Afro-Brasileiros*. São Paulo: Perspectiva, 1973.

Bastos, Sênia. "A territorialidade portuguesa na cidade de São Paulo nos anos 1930." In *Entre Mares: O Brasil dos portugueses*, edited by Maria de Nazaré Sarges, Fernando de Sousa, Maria Izilda Matos, Antonio Otaviano Vieira Junior, and Cristina Donza Cancela, 108–18. Belém: Editora Paka-Tatu, 2010.

Bavel, Jay J. Van, Katherine Baicker, Paulo S. Boggio, Valerio Capraro, Aleksandra Cichocka, Mina Cikara, Molly J. Crockett, et al. "Using Social and Behavioural Science to Support COVID-19 Pandemic Response." *Nature Human Behavior* 4 (May 2020): 460–71. https://www.nature.com/articles/s41562-020-0884-z.pdf.

Begliomini, Helio. "Diogo Teixeira de Faria, 1867–1927." Academia de Medicina de São Paulo. Accessed June 28, 2024. https://www.academiamedicinasaopaulo .org.br/membros-academicos/diogo-teixeira-de-faria/.

Begliomini, Helio. "Ignácio Emílio Achiles Betholdi, 1810–1886." Academia de Medicina de São Paulo. Accessed June 28, 2024. https://www.academiamedicinasaopaulo .org.br/membros-academicos/ignacio-emilio-achiles-betholdi/.

Beiguelman, Paula. *Os companheiros de São Paulo*. São Paulo: Símbolo, 1977.

Beiner, Guy. "Introduction: The Great Flu between Remembering and Forgetting." In *Pandemic Re-awakenings: The Forgotten and Unforgotten "Spanish" Flu of 1918–1919*: 1-48. New York: Oxford University Press, 2022.

Beiner, Guy, ed. *Pandemic Re-awakenings: The Forgotten and Unforgotten "Spanish" Flu of 1918–1919*. New York: Oxford University Press, 2022.

Benchimol, Jayme Larry. *Dos micróbios aos mosquitos: Febre amarela e revolução pasteuriana no Brasil*. Rio de Janeiro: Editora Fiocruz/Editora UFRJ, 1999.

Benchimol, Jayme Larry, and Magali Romero Sá, eds. *Adolpho Lutz—obra completa*. Vol. 2, *Febre amarela, malária e protozoologia*. Rio de Janeiro: Editora Fiocruz, 2005. https://www.arca.fiocruz.br/bitstream/handle/icict/15124 /benchimol-Adolpho%20Lutz_Febre%20Amarela.pdf.

Bernardo, Teresinha. *Memória em branco e negro—Olhares sobre São Paulo*. São Paulo: UNESP/EDUC/FAPESP, 1998.

Bertolli Filho, Cláudio. "Estratégias jornalísticas no noticiamento de uma epidemia: A Gripe Espanhola em São Paulo." In *História da saúde: Olhares e veredas*, edited by Yara Nogueira Monteiro, 13–26. São Paulo: Instituto de Saúde, 2010.

Bertolli Filho, Cláudio. *A gripe espanhola em São Paulo, 1918: Epidemia e sociedade*. São Paulo: Paz e Terra, 2003.

Bertolli Filho, Cláudio. *História da saúde pública no Brasil*. São Paulo: Editora Ática, 2002.

Bertolli Filho, Cláudio. *História social da tuberculose e do tuberculoso, 1900–1950.* Rio de Janeiro: Editora Fiocruz, 2001.

Bertolozzi, Thayla Bicalho. "Hacking the Debate: Analyzing Cases in Brazil of Invasion and Racist, Sexist and LGBTQIA+ Phobic Attacks on Participants in Virtual Events during the COVID-19 Pandemic." *Internet and Society* 2, no. 1 (June 2021): 25–53. https://revista.internetlab.org.br/wp-content/uploads/2021/07/Hacking-the-debate-analyzing-cases-in-Brazil-of-invasion-and-racist-sexist-and-lgbtqia-phobic-attacks-on-participants-in-virtual-events-during-the-COVID-19-pandemic.pdf.

Bertucci, Liane Maria. *Influenza, a medicina enferma.* Campinas: Editora UNICAMP, 2004.

Bertucci, Liane Maria. "A onipresença do medo na influenza de 1918." *Varia História* 25, no. 42 (July–December 2009): 457–75.

Bertucci, Liane Maria. "Pesquisa e debates sobre a gripe durante a epidemia de 1918." Paper presented at ANPUH—XXV Simpósio Nacional de História, Fortaleza, Brazil 2009. http://www.snh2011.anpuh.org/resources/anais/anpuhnacional/S.25/ANPUH.S25.0258.pdf.

Betoldi, Luiz Bianchi. *Relatório sobre o movimento das águas observadas no vale do Tietê e Tamanduatehy durante a enchente de Janeiro de 1887.* Accessed June 28, 2024. http://www2.unifesp.br/himaco/enchente_1887.php#.

Biehl, João, Miqueias Mugge, and Ana Maria Goldani. "The Books of the Dead Revisited: Mortality and Morbidity in the German Colonies of Southern Brazil, 1850–1880." *História, Ciências, Saúde—Manguinhos* 25, no. 4 (October–December 2018): 1197–217. https://www.scielo.br/j/hcsm/a/mShV3xh838MzCRkJQwvyNRf/?format=pdf&lang=en.

Biehl, João, and Adriana Petryna. "Peopling Global Health." *Saúde e Sociedade* 23, no. 2 (April–June 2014): 376–89.

Birn, Anne-Emanuelle. "Perspectivizing Pandemics: (How) Do Epidemic Histories Criss-Cross Contexts?" *Journal of Global History* 15, no. 3 (November 2020): 336–49. https://doi.org/10.1017/S1740022820000327.

Birn, Anne-Emanuelle, and Raúl Necochea López, eds. *Peripheral Nerve: Health and Medicine in Cold War Latin America.* Durham, NC: Duke University Press, 2020.

Bitter, Daniel. "Narrativas de memória e performances musicais dos judeus cariocas da 'Pequena África.'" *Antropolítica—Revista Contemporânea de Antropologia,* no. 39 (2015): 121–49. https://periodicos.uff.br/antropolitica/article/view/41734.

Blay, Eva Alterman. *Eu não tenho onde morar: Vilas operárias na cidade de São Paulo.* São Paulo: Nobel, 1985.

Blount, John Allen, III. "The Public Health Movement in Sao Paulo, Brazil: A History of the Sanitary Service, 1892–1918." PhD diss., Tulane University, 1971.

Bomtempo, Denise Cristina, and Kananda Beatriz Pinto Sena. "Migração internacional de africanos para o Brasil e suas territorialidades no estado do Ceará." *Geografares: Revista do Programa de Pós-Graduação e do Departamento*

de *Geografia da Ufes* 1, no. 33 (July–December 2021): 1–21. https://doi.org/10
.47456/geo.v1i33.37140.

Bondeson, Jan. *Buried Alive: The Terrifying History of Our Most Primal Fear.*
New York: W. W. Norton, 2002.

Bonduki, Nabil Georges. *Origens da habitação social no Brasil: Arquitetura moderna, lei do inquilinato e difusão da casa própria.* São Paulo: Estação Liberdade/FAPESP, 1998.

Bonduki, Nabil Georges. "Origens da habitação social no Brasil." *Análise Social* 29, no. 127 (1994): 711–32.

Borges, Dain. "Puffy, Ugly, Slothful, and Inert: Degeneration in Brazilian Social Thought, 1880–1940." *Journal of Latin American Studies* 25, no. 2 (May 1993): 235–56.

Borges, Julie Kellen de Campos. "O estrangeiro nos dicionários de língua portuguesa: Sujeito, língua e espaço." *Polifonia* 22, no. 31 (January–June 2015): 200–221.

Bosi, Ecléa. *Memória e sociedade: Lembranças de velhos.* São Paulo: Companhia das Letras, 1994.

Boudia, Soraya, Angela N. H. Creager, Scott Frickel, Emmanuel Henry, Nathalie Jas, Carsten Reinhardt, and Jody A. Roberts. "Residues: Rethinking Chemical Environments." *Engaging Science, Technology, and Society* 4 (2018), 165–76. https://estsjournal.org/index.php/ests/article/view/245/136.

Brazil. Commissão, Exposição internacional de borracha de New York. *Brazil, the Land of Rubber, at the Third International Rubber and Allied Trades Exhibition.* New York, 1912. https://www.biodiversitylibrary.org/bibliography/57128.

Brazil. Directoria Geral de Estatística. "Coefficiente de Natalidade e Mortalidade—Anno 1907, Exposição Nacional de 1908." *Boletim Comemorativo da Exposição Nacional de 1908.* Rio de Janeiro: Typographia da Estatistica, 1909, 88–89. https://biblioteca.ibge.gov.br/visualizacao/livros/liv25380.pdf.

Brazil. Directoria Geral de Estatística do Ministério da Agricultura, Indústria e Commércio. *Anuário estatístico do Brasil (1908–1912).* Vol. 1, *Territorio e população, população do Brazil por municípios e estados (1907–1912).* Rio de Janeiro: Typographia da Estatistica, 1916. https://seculoxx.ibge.gov.br/images/seculoxx/arquivos_download/populacao/1908_12/populacao1908_12v1_082_a_116.pdf.

Brazil. Império do Brasil. *Recenseamento do Brazil em 1872.* Rio de Janeiro: Typ. G. Leuzinger, 1874. https://biblioteca.ibge.gov.br/visualizacao/monografias/GEBIS%20-%20RJ/Recenseamento_do_Brazil_1872/Imperio%20do%20Brazil%201872.pdf.

Brazil. Instituto Brasileiro de Geografia e Estatística, Centro de Documentação e Disseminação de Informações. *Brasil: 500 anos de povoamento.* Rio de Janeiro: IBGE, 2007.

Brazil. "Discurso de Acylino de Leão em 18 de setembro de 1935." In *Anais da Câmara dos Deputados: Sessões de 16 a 24 de setembro de 1935* 17:432. Rio de Janeiro: A Noite, 1935.

Brazil. Ministério da Agricultura, Indústria e Commércio, Directoria Geral de Estatística. *Recenseamento do Brazil—realizado em 1 de setembro de 1920.* Vol. 4, pt. 4. Rio de Janeiro: Typ. Da Estatística, 1922.

Brito, Nara Azevedo. "'La dansarina': A gripe espanhola e o cotidiano na cidade do Rio de Janeiro." *História, Ciências, Saúde—Manguinhos* 4, no. 1 (June 1997): 11–30. https://www.scielo.br/j/hcsm/a/xsvqJXhWnJRwKBJxsxLfH6v/.

Britt, Andrew. "'I'll Samba Someplace Else': Constructing Identity and Neighborhood in São Paulo, 1930s–1980s." PhD diss., Emory University, 2018.

Britt, Andrew. "Re/Mapping São Paulo's Geographies of African Descent." *Items: Insights from the Social Sciences.* February 25, 2020. https://items.ssrc .org/layered-metropolis/re-mapping-sao-paulos-geographies-of-african -descent/.

Britt, Andrew. "Spatial Projects of Forgetting: Razing the Remedies Church and Museum to the Enslaved in São Paulo's 'Black Zone,' 1930s–1940s." *Journal of Latin American Studies* 54, no. 4 (August 2022): 561–92.

Browning, Matthew H. E. M., and Alessandro Rigolon. "Do Income, Race and Ethnicity, and Sprawl Influence the Greenspace-Human Health Link in City-Level Analyses? Findings from 496 Cities in the United States." *International Journal of Environmental Research and Public Health* 15, no. 7 (May 2018): 1–22. https://www.mdpi.com/1660-4601/15/7/1541.

Brunger, Fern. "Problematizing the Notion of 'Community' in Research Ethics." In *Populations and Genetics: Legal and Socio-Ethical Perspectives,* edited by Bartha Maria Knoppers, 245–56. Boston: Martinus Nijhoff, 2003.

Bryce, Benjamin. "Los caballeros de beneficencia y las damas organizadoras: El Hospital Alemán y la idea de comunidad en Buenos Aires, 1880–1930." *Estudios Migratorios Latinoamericanos* 25, no. 70 (June 2011): 79–107. https://www .academia.edu/1845750/Bryce_-_Hospital_Aleman São Paulo.

Buechler, Simone. "Sweating It in the Brazilian Garment Industry: Korean and Bolivian Immigrants and Global Economic Forces in São Paulo." *Latin American Perspectives* 31, no. 3 (May 2004): 99–119.

Burdick, John. *The Color of Sound: Race, Religion, and Music in Brazil.* New York: New York University Press, 2013.

Butler, Kim D. *Freedoms Given, Freedoms Won: Afro-Brazilians in Post-abolition São Paulo and Salvador.* New Brunswick, NJ: Rutgers University Press, 1998.

Caggiano, Sergio. "Inmigrantes en la ciudad Buenos Aires: Demarcaciones y recorridos." *Desarrollo Económico* 54, no. 212 (May–August 2014): 105–29.

Calabi, Donatella. *História do urbanismo europeu: Questões, instrumentos, casos exemplares.* São Paulo: Perspectiva, 2012.

Caldeira, Teresa. *City of Walls: Crime, Segregation, and Citizenship in São Paulo.* Berkeley: University of California Press, 2001.

Caldeira, Teresa. *A política dos outros—o cotidiano dos moradores da periferia e o que pensam do poder e dos poderosos.* São Paulo: Brasiliense, 1984.

Camargo, Luís Soares de. "Habitações populares em São Paulo: precedentes." *Informativo Arquivo Histórico Municipal* 4, no. 19 (July–August 2008). http://www.arquiamigos.org.br/info/info19/i-manu.htm.

Camargo, Luís Soares de. "Viver e morrer em São Paulo: A vida, a morte e as doenças na cidade de São Paulo no século XIX." Master's thesis, Pontifícia Universidade Católica de São Paulo, 2007. https://repositorio.pucsp.br/jspui/handle/handle/13020.

Camargo, Tamires Pereira. "LAVADEIRA PAULISTANA: Uma personagem da história do cotidiano de São Paulo (1890–1910)." *Projeto de Pesquisa.* Universidade Federal do Estado de São Paulo, Escola de Filosofia, Letras e Ciências Humanas, 2023.

Campbell, Margaret. "What Tuberculosis Did for Modernism: The Influence of a Curative Environment on Modernist Design and Architecture." *Medical History* 49, no. 4 (October 2005): 463–88. https://doi.org/10.1017/s0025727300009169.

Campos, Beatriz Luedemann. "Companheiras em greve: O movimento paredista da União das Costureiras em junho de 1919." *Revista Angelus Novus* 12, no. 17 (2021): 1–19. https://doi.org/10.11606/issn.2179-5487.v12i17p189595.

Campos, Eudes. "Hospitais paulistanos: Do século XVI ao XIX." *Informativo Arquivo Histórico de São Paulo* 6, no. 29 (April/June 2011). http://www.arquiamigos.org.br/info/info29/i-estudos3.htm.

Campos, Eudes. "Nos caminhos da Luz, antigos palacetes da elite paulistana." *Anais do Museu Paulista* 13, no. 1 (January–June 2005): 11–57. https://doi.org/10.1590/S0101-47142005000100002.

Campos, Eudes. "São Paulo Antigo: Plantas da Cidade." *Informativo Arquivo Histórico Municipal* 4, no. 20 (September/October 2008). http://www.arquiamigos.org.br/info/info20/i-intro.htm.

Candelaria, Jayme. "Acção do posto de hygiene em policiamento sanitario." In *Terceiro Congresso Brasileiro de Hygiene, São Paulo, 1926,* edited by Congresso Brasileiro de Hygiene, 373–80. São Paulo: São Paulo Editora, 1929.

Candido, Antonio. *"De cortiço a cortiço": O discurso e a cidade.* São Paulo: Duas Cidades, 1993.

Cano, Jefferson. "A cidade dos cortiços: Os trabalhadores e o poder público em São Paulo no final do século XIX." In *Trabalhadores na cidade: Cotidiano e cultura no Rio de Janeiro e em São Paulo, séculos XIX e XX,* edited by Elciene Azevedo, Jefferson Cano, Sidney Chalhoub, and Maria Clementina Pereira Cunha, 221–50. Campinas: Editora da Unicamp, 2009.

Cano, Wilson. *Raízes da concentração industrial em São Paulo.* 1977. 5th ed. Campinas: Universidade Estadual de Campinas, Instituto de Economia, 2007.

Cantisano, Pedro Jimenez. "Refuge from Science: The Practice and Politics of Rights in Brazil's Vaccine Revolt." *Hispanic American Historical Review* 102, no. 4 (November 2022): 611–42. https://doi.org/10.1215/00182168-10025421.

Carbone, Antonio. *Park, Tenement, Slaughterhouse: Elite Imaginaries of Buenos Aires, 1852–1880*. Chicago: University of Chicago Press, 2022.

Caritas: Arquidiocesana de São Paulo and United Nations High Commission on Refugees. *Mapa de Georreferenciamento de Pessoas em Situação de Refúgio Atendidas pela Caritas Arquidiocesana de São Paulo*. 2020. https://www.acnur.org/portugues /wp-content/uploads/2022/07/MAPA-DE-GEORREFERENCIAMENTO-DE -PESSOAS-EM-SITUACAO-DE-REFUGIO-ATENDIDAS-PELA-CARITAS -ARQUIDIOCESANA-DE-SAO-PAULO_2020.pdf.

Carrega, Arthur Daltin. "As propagandas imigrantistas do Brasil no século XIX: O caso da Sociedade Central de Imigração." *Patrimônio e Memória (Assis)* 15, no. 2 (July—December 2019): 154–74. https://pem.assis.unesp.br/index.php /pem/article/download/1065/1103.

Carrillo, Ana María. "¿Estado de peste o estado de sitio? Sinaloa y Baja California, 1902–1903." *Historia Mexicana* 54, no. 4 (April–June 2005): 1049–103.

Carrillo, Ramón. "Balance epidemiológico argentino." Speech at the Second Conference of Epidemiology and Endemic Diseases, October 6, 1947. Republished in *Política sanitaria argentina [1949]*, 139–47. Remedios de Escalada: Universidad Nacional de Lanús, 2018. http://isco.unla.edu.ar/edunla/cuadernos /catalog/view/2/15/19-2.

Carroll, Patrick E. "Medical Police and the History of Public Health." *Medical History* 46, no. 4 (October 2002): 461–94.

Carvalho, Arnaldo Vieira de. "Novidades clínicas na cirurgia paulista." *Revista Médica de São Paulo* 4, no. 20 (October 30, 1901): 355–61. https://memoria .bn.gov.br/DocReader/docreader.aspx?bib=229334&pasta=ano%20191&pesq =&pagfis=2084.

Castro, Marcia C., Adriano Massuda, Gisele Almeida, Naercio Aquino Menezes-Filho, Monica Viegas Andrade, Kenya Valéria Micaela de Souza Noronha, Rudi Rocha, et al. "Brazil's Unified Health System: The First 30 Years and Prospects for the Future." *Lancet* 394, no. 10195 (July 2019): 345–56. https://doi.org/10 .1016/S0140-6736(19)31243-7.

Casoy, Sergio. *Ópera em São Paulo 1952–2005*. São Paulo: Edusp, 2007.

Cavaglion, Gabriel. "Was Cesare Lombroso Antisemitic?" *Journal for the Study of Antisemitism* 3, no. 2 (December 2011): 647–55.

Césaro, Filipe Seefeldt de. "Uma etnografia da mobilidade internacional de senegaleses em Porto Alegre (RS, Brasil) e Atlanta (GA, Estados Unidos)." PhD diss., Universidade Federal do Rio Grande do Sul, 2023.

Chalhoub, Sidney. *Cidade febril: Cortiços e epidemias na Corte imperial*. São Paulo: Companhia das Letras, 1996.

Chalhoub, Sidney. "The Politics of Disease Control: Yellow Fever and Race in Nineteenth Century Rio de Janeiro." *Journal of Latin American Studies* 25, no. 3 (October 1993): 441–63. https://doi.org/10.1017/S0022216X00006623.

Chi, Jung Yun. "O Bom Retiro dos coreanos: Descrição de um enclave étnico." Master's thesis, Universidade de São Paulo, 2016.

Cidade de São Paulo. "Imigrantes na cidade de São Paulo: Cinco anos de atendimento do Centro de Referência de Atendimento para Imigrantes—CRAI." *Informes Urbanos*, no. 41 (December 2019). https://www.prefeitura.sp.gov.br/cidade /secretarias/upload/Informes_Urbanos/41_IU_IMIGRANTES_final.pdf.

Cococi, Alexandre Mariano and L. Fructuoso Costa. *Planta guia da cidade de São Paulo*. São Paulo: Companhia Lithographica Hartmann Reichenbach, 1913.

Cohen, Ilka Stern. *Bombas sobre São Paulo: A revolução de 1924*. São Paulo: Editora UNESP, 2006.

Colgrove, James. *Epidemic City: The Politics of Public Health in New York*. New York: Russell Sage Foundation, 2011.

Companhia de Desenvolvimento Habitacional e Urbano do Estado de São Paulo. *Relatório Geral do Programa de atuação em cortiços*. São Paulo: Governo do Estado de São Paulo, 2010. https://www.cdhu.sp.gov.br/documents/20143/37069 /RelatorioGeralProgramaCorticos.pdf/cef12342-5419-23a0-bf8c-95360484fe86.

Constantino, Núncia Santoro de. *Italiano na cidade: A imigração itálica nas cidades brasileiras*. Passo Fundo: Editora da UPF, 2000.

Cordeiro, Simone, ed. *Os cortiços de Santa Ifigênia: Sanitarismo e urbanização, 1893*. São Paulo: Arquivo Público do Estado de São Paulo, Imprensa Oficial, 2010.

Cordeiro, Simone Lucena. "Moradia popular na cidade de São Paulo (1930–1940)— projetos e ambições." *Revista Histórica* 1 (April 2005): 2–14. http://www .historica.arquivoestado.sp.gov.br/materias/anteriores/edica001/materia03/.

Corrêa, Ana Cláudia Pinto. "Imigrantes judeus em São Paulo: A reinvenção do cotidiano no Bom Retiro (1930–2000)." PhD diss., Pontifícia Universidade Católica de São Paulo, 2007. https://tede2.pucsp.br/bitstream/handle/13023/1 /ANA%20CLAUDIA%20PINTO%20CORREA.pdf.

Corrêa, Anna Maria Martinez. *A rebelião de 1924 em São Paulo*. São Paulo: Hucitec, 1976.

Cortinois, Andrea A., and Anne-Emanuelle Birn. "What's Technology Got to Do with It? Power, Politics, and Health Equity beyond Technological Triumphalism." *Global Policy* 12, no. 56 (July 2021): 75–79. https://doi.org/10.1111/1758-5899.12982.

Côrtes, Giovana Xavier da Conceição. "'Leitoras,' gênero, raça, imagem e discurso em O Menelik (São Paulo, 1915-1916)." *Afro-Asia* 46 (2012): 163–91. https:// periodicos.ufba.br/index.php/afroasia/article/view/21265/13847.

Cosby, Katherine Ann. "Flowers Grew out of the Asphalt: Black Women's Territories in São Paulo, 1871–1930." PhD diss., University of California, 2021. https://escholarship.org/content/qt10n452m7/qt10n452m7_noSplash_e13b7 519cfca22b471cc747f772cfe39.pdf.

Costa, Emília Viotti da. *Crowns of Glory, Tears of Blood: The Demerara Slave Rebellion of 1823*. New York: Oxford University Press, 1994.

Costa, Renato Gama-Rosa. "Apontamentos para a arquitetura hospitalar no Brasil: Entre o tradicional e o moderno." *História, Ciências, Saúde—Manguinhos* 18, no. 1 (December 2011): 53–66.

Cruz, Andrea Uzal, Elaine Lagonegro Santana Martinho, Ésio Pessoa Caracas de Souza, Fernando Costa de Carvalho Cosentino, Jéssica Fernanda de Lima

Mendes, and Raquel Costa Candido. "Estudo de análise—UBS Bom Retiro." Final project, Curso de Especialização em Administração Hospitalar e de Sistemas de Saúde (Specialization in Hospital Administration and Health Systems), Fundação Getúlio Vargas, 2022.

Cruz, Oswaldo. *Peste pelo Dr. Oswaldo Gonçalves Cruz.* Rio de Janeiro: Typ. Bernard Freres, 1906. https://www.obrasraras.fiocruz.br/media.details.php ?mediaID=217.

Cruz, Tânia Mara. "Gênero e culturas infantis os clubinhos da escola e as trocinhas do Bom Retiro." *Educação e Pesquisa* 38, no. 1 (2012): 63–78.

Cruz Paiva, Odair da, and Soraya Moura. *Hospedaria de Imigrantes de São Paulo.* São Paulo: Paz e Terra, 2008.

Cueto, Marcos. *The Return of Epidemics: Health and Society in Peru during the Twentieth Century.* Aldershot, UK: Ashgate, 2001.

Cueto, Marcos, and Steven Palmer. *Medicine and Public Health: A History.* New York: Cambridge University Press, 2014.

Cukierman, Henrique. "Who Invented Brazil?" In *Beyond Imported Magic: Essays on Science, Technology, and Society in Latin America,* edited by Eden Medina, Ivan da Costa Marques, and Christina Holmes, 27–45. Cambridge, MA: MIT Press, 2014.

Cunha, Claudia dos Reis. "O patrimonio cultural da cidade de Sorocaba: Análise de uma trajetória." Master's thesis, Universidade de São Paulo, 2005.

Cunha, Higor Souza, Brenda Santana Sclauser, Pedro Fonseca Wildemberg, Eduardo Augusto Militão Fernandes, Jefersson Alex dos Santos, Mariana de Oliveira Lage, Camila Lorenz, Gerson Laurindo Barbosa, José Alberto Quintanilha, and Francisco Chiaravalloti-Neto. "Water Tank and Swimming Pool Detection Based on Remote Sensing and Deep Learning: Relationship with Socioeconomic Level and Applications in Dengue Control." *PLoS ONE* 16, no. 12 (December 2021): e0258681. https://journals.plos.org/plosone/article ?id=10.1371/journal.pone.0258681.

Cunningham, Erin, and Joel E. Black. "Healing the Sick City: Local Guides, Visiting Nurses, and Vernaculars of Pain on New York's Lower East Side." *Journal of Urban History* 48, no. 2 (March 2022): 285–301. https://doi.org/10.1177 /0096144220946318.

Cusano, Alfredo, *Italia d'oltre mare: Impresioni e ricordi de mei cinque anni di Brasile.* Milan: Stablimento tipográfico E. Reggiani, 1911.

Cuti, [Luiz Silva]. *E disse o velho militante José Correia Leite.* 19th ed. rev. São Paulo: Noovha América, 2007.

Cwerner, Saulo. "Helipads, Heliports and Urban Air Space: Governing the Contested Infrastructure of Helicopter Travel." In *Aeromobilities,* edited by Saulo Cwerner, Sven Kesselring, and John Urry, 225–46. London: Routledge, 2008.

Cymbalista, Renato, and Kazuo Nakano. "São Paulo, Brazil: A Need for Stronger Policy Advocacy." In *International Migrants and the City,* edited by Marcelo Balbo, 211–34. Venice: UN-HABITAT/Università Iuav di Venezia, 2005.

Cytrynowicz, Monica Musatti, Roney Cytrynowicz, and Ananda Stücker. *Do Lazareto dos Variolosos ao Instituto de Infectologia Emílio Ribas: 130 anos de história da saúde pública no Brasil*. São Paulo: Narrativa Um, 2010.

D'Angelo, Bruno, and Ricardo Giassetti. *O filho da costureira e o catador de batatas*. São Paulo: Editora JBC, 2008.

Dall'Ava, João Paulo, and André Mota. "A gripe espanhola em Sorocaba e o caso da fábrica Santa Rosália, 1918: Contribuições da história local ao estudo das epidemias no Brasil." *História Ciência e Saúde—Manguinhos* 24, no. 2 (April–June 2017): 429–46. https://doi.org/10.1590/s0104-59702017000200007.

Dans, Peter, and Suzanne Wasserman. *Life on the Lower East Side: Photographs by Rebecca Lepkoff, 1937–1950*. Princeton, NJ: Princeton Architectural Press, 2010.

Dávila, Jerry. *Diploma of Whiteness: Race and Social Policy in Brazil, 1917–1945*. Durham, NC: Duke University Press, 2003.

Dean, Warren. "A fábrica São Luiz de Itu: Um estudo de arqueologia industrial." *Anais de História—Assis* 8 (1976): 9–25.

Dean, Warren. *The Industrialization of São Paulo, 1800–1945*. Austin: University of Texas Press, 1969.

Dean, Warren. "Visit to the Hospedaria." Unpublished manuscript of May 13, 1963. Quoted in Gloria La Cava, *Italians in Brazil: The Post–World War II Experience*, 59 (table 7). New York: Peter Lang, 1999.

Deb Roy, Rohan. *Malarial Subjects: Empire, Medicine and Nonhumans in British India, 1820–1909*. Cambridge: Cambridge University Press, 2017.

Del Picchia, Menotti. *Poesias, 1907/1946*. São Paulo: Martins, 1958.

Dertônio, Hilário. *O bairro do Bom Retiro*. São Paulo: Prefeitura Municipal, Secretaria de Educação e Cultura, Departamento de Cultura São Paulo, 1971.

De Simone, Sergio. "Carros Antigos do Museu de Saúde Pública Emílio Ribas." Unpublished research report, Museu de Saúde Pública Emílio Ribas, February 2016.

Dimas, Carlos S. *Poisoned Eden: Cholera Epidemics, State-Building, and the Problem of Public Health in Tucumán, Argentina, 1865–1908*. Lincoln: University of Nebraska Press, 2022.

Diner, Hasia R., Jeffrey Shandler, and Beth S. Wenger. *Remembering the Lower East Side: American Jewish Reflections*. Bloomington: Indiana University Press, 2000.

Directoria do Serviço Sanitário. *Annuario demographico: Secção de estatística demographo-sanitaria: Anno XIX—1912*. São Paulo: Typographia Brasil de Rothschild, 1913. https://bibliotecadigital.seade.gov.br/view/singlepage/index.php?pubcod=10011015&parte=1.

Dreher, Martin N. *A religião de Jacobina*. São Leopoldo: Editora Oikos, 2012.

Duarte, Ivomar Gomes. "O Código Sanitário Estadual de 1918 e a Epidemia de Gripe Espanhola." *Cadernos de História da Ciência—Instituto Butantan* 5, no. 1 (January–July 2009): 55–73.

Dwork, Deborah. "Health Conditions of Immigrant Jews on the Lower East Side of New York: 1880–1914." *Medical History* 25 (1981): 1–40. https://www.ncbi.nlm .nih.gov/pmc/articles/PMC1138984/pdf/medhisto0092-0005.pdf.

Eibenschutz, Catalina, ed. *Política de saúde: O público e o privado.* Rio de Janeiro: Editora Fiocruz, 1996.

Faerman, Marcos. "Oh! Bom Retiro." 1981. In *A arte da reportagem,* edited by Igor Fuser, 1:305–28. São Paulo: Scritta, 1996.

Fantin, Jader Tadeu. "Do interior para os porões, dos porões para as fachadas: Os japoneses no bairro da Liberdade em São Paulo." ACTA *Geográfica* 9, no. 20 (May–August 2015): 72–95. https://doi.org/10.18227/2177-4307.acta .v9i20.2240.

Farias, Cynthia Moura Louzada, Ligia Giovanella, Adauto Emmerich Oliveira, and Edson Theodoro dos Santos Neto. "Tempo de espera e absenteísmo na atenção especializada: Um desafio para os sistemas universais de saúde." *Saúde em Debate* 43, no. 5 (December 2019): 190–204. https://doi.org/10.1590/0103 -11042019S516.

Farmer, Paul. *Pathologies of Power: Health, Human Rights, and the New War on the Poor.* Berkeley: University of California Press, 2004.

Fausto, Boris. *Crime e cotidiano: A criminalidade em São Paulo, 1880–1924.* São Paulo: Brasiliense, 1984.

Fausto, Boris. "Imigração e participação política no Estado de São Paulo, durante a Primeira República." Paper presented at the XVII Encontro Anual da AN-POCS, Caxambu, MG. Seminário Temático: Os imigrantes e a política no Brasil (October 22–25 1993): 1–22. https://biblioteca.sophia.com.br/terminal/9666 /acervo/detalhe/10835?guid=48acb158a88d84c0f5e3&returnUrl=%2fterminal %2f9666%2fresultado%2flistar%3fguid%3d48acb158a88d84c0f5e3%26quanti dadePaginas%3d1%26codigoRegistro%3d10835%2310835&i=1.

Fee, Elizabeth, and Liping Bu. "Origins of Public Health Nursing: The Henry Street Visiting Nurse Service." *American Journal of Public Health* 100, no. 7 (July 2010): 1206–7.

Feldman, Sarah. "Bom Retiro: Bairro múltiplo, identidade étnica mutante." *Anais do XV Enanpur* 15, no. 1 (2013). https://anais.anpur.org.br/index.php /anaisenanpur/article/view/370.

Fendler, Lynn. "Others and the Problem of Community." *Curriculum Inquiry* 36, no. 3 (2006): 303–26.

Ferla, Luis Antonio Coelho. "Corpos estranhos na intimidade do lar: As empregadas domésticas no Brasil da primeira metade do século XX." *Anais do XXVI Simpósio Nacional de História,* edited by Marieta de Moraes Ferreira, 1–13. Associação Nacional de História: São Paulo, 2011. https://anpuh.org.br /uploads/anais-simposios/pdf/2019-01/1548856588_120e611a09d80d8033e77 fa00608509e.pdf.

Fernandes, Florestan. *A integração do negro na sociedade de classes.* São Paulo: Dominus, 1965.

Fernandes, Florestan. "As 'Trocinhas' do Bom Retiro." *Pro-Posições* 15, no. 1 (2016): 229–50. Accessed June 28, 2024. https://periodicos.sbu.unicamp.br/ojs/index .php/proposic/article/view/8643855.

Fernandez, Raffaella. *A poética de resíduos de Carolina Maria de Jesus.* São Paulo: Aetia Editorial, 2019.

Ferrari, Rosa Hassan de, Anthony Ocepek, Rachel Travis, and Ariel C. Armony. "Migration and Urban Development in São Paulo." *Ethnic and Racial Studies* 46, no. 11 (2023): 2446–66. https://doi.org/10.1080/01419870.2023.2174809.

Ferraz, Luiz Marcelo Robalinho, and Isaltina Maria de Azevedo Mello Gomes. "A construção discursiva sobre a dengue na mídia." *Revista Brasileira De Epidemiologia* 15, no. 1 (March 2012): 63–74. https://doi.org/10.1590/S1415 -790X2012000100006.

Ferreira, Irma Teresinha Rodrigues Neves, Maria Amélia de Sousa Mascena Veras, and Rubens Antonio Silva. "Participação da população no controle da dengue: uma análise da sensibilidade dos planos de saúde de municípios do Estado de São Paulo, Brasil." *Cadernos De Saúde Pública* 25, no. 12 (December 2009): 2683–94. https://doi.org/10.1590/S0102-311X2009001200015.

Ferrero, Gina Lombroso. *Nell'America meridionale (Brasile-Uruguay-Argentina).* Milan: Fratelli Treves, 1908.

Figueiredo, Luiz Tadeu Moraes. "Dengue in Brazil." *Revista Da Sociedade Brasileira De Medicina Tropical* 45, no. 3 (March 2012): 285. https://doi.org/10.1590/S0037 -86822012000300001.

Finkelman, Jacobo, ed. *Caminhos da saúde pública no Brasil.* Rio de Janeiro: Editora Fiocruz, 2002.

Fioravanti, Carlos Henrique. *O combate à febre amarela no Estado de São Paulo: história, desafios e inovações.* São Paulo: São Paulo—Secretaria da Saúde, Coordenadoria de Controle de Doenças, Centro de Vigilância Epidemiológica, 2018.

FitzGerald, David Scott, and David Cook-Martín. *Culling the Masses: The Democratic Origins of Racist Immigration Policy in the Americas.* Cambridge, MA: Harvard University Press, 2014.

Fonseca, Fernanda Padovesi, Eduardo Dutenkefer, Luciano Zoboli, and Jaime Tadeu Oliva. "Cartografia digital geo-histórica: Mobilidade urbana de São Paulo de 1877 a 1930." *Revista do Instituto de Estudos Brasileiros*, no. 64 (2016): 131–66. https://doi.org/10.11606/issn.2316-901X.v0i64p131–166.

Fonseca, Guido. *História da prostituição em São Paulo.* São Paulo: Resenha Universitária, 1982.

Fontes, Maria Aparecida. "Paisagens impermanentes . . . Espaço urbano nas narrativas brasileiras de imigração." In *Literatura e (i)migração no Brasil/ Literature and (Im)migration in Brazil,* edited by Waïl S. Hassan and Rogerio Lima, 370–96. Rio de Janeiro: Edições Makunaima, 2020.

Fontes, Paulo. *Migration and the Making of Industrial São Paulo.* Durham, NC: Duke University Press, 2016.

Fontes, Paulo. *Um nordeste em São Paulo: Trabalhadores migrantes em São Miguel Paulista (1945–66)*. Rio de Janeiro: Ed. FGV, 2008.

Formiga, Dayana de Oliveira, Charles Aparecido Silva Melo, and Ana Beatriz Rodrigues de Paula. "O pensamento eugênico e a imigração no Brasil (1929–1930)." *Intelligere* 7, no. 22 (September 2019): 75–96. https://www.revistas.usp.br/revistaintelligere/article/view/142881.

Foucault, Michel. "The Birth of Social Medicine." In *Power*, edited by J. D. Faubion, 134–56. New York: New Press, 2000.

Francisco, Renata Ribeiro. "A maçonaria e o processo da abolição em São Paulo." PhD diss., Universidade de São Paulo, 2018.

Frehse, Fraya. *O tempo das ruas na São Paulo de fins do império*. São Paulo: Edusp, 2017.

Freire, Alipio, Izias Almada, and J. A. de Granville Ponce, eds. *Tiradentes, um presidio da ditadura: Memorias de presos políticos*. São Paulo: Scipione, 1997.

French, John D. *Drowning in Laws: Labor Law and Brazilian Political Culture*. Chapel Hill: University of North Carolina Press, 2004. Published in Portuguese as *Afogados em leis: A CLT e a cultura política dos trabalhadores brasileiros*, translated by Paulo Fontes (São Paulo: Editora Fundação Perseu Abramo, 2001).

Frúgoli, Heitor, Jr., and Enrico Spaggiari. "Networks and Territorialities: An Ethnographic Approach to the So-Called Cracolândia ['Crackland'] in São Paulo." *Vibrant: Virtual Brazilian Anthropology* 8, no. 2 (December 2011): 550–79.

Furlan, Elvira Aguiar Borges. "Alguns aspectos da regulamentação da prostituição em São Paulo." Bachelor's thesis, Pontifícia Universidade Católica, 1955.

Gallois, Dominique Tilkin, and Juliana Rosalen. "Direitos indígenas 'diferenciados' e seus efeitos entre os Wajãpi no Amapá." *REA* 4, no. 2 (June 2016): 33–41. https://www.academia.edu/34860224/DIREITOS_IND%C3%8DGENAS_DIFERENCIADOS_E_SEUS_EFEITOS_ENTRE_OS_WAJ%C3%83PI_NO_AMAP%C3%81.

Galvão, Patrícia. *Parque industrial*. 1933. Rio de Janeiro: José Olympio, 2006.

Gandhi, Ajay. "Catch Me If You Can: Monkey Capture in Delhi." *Ethnography* 13, no. 1 (2012): 43–56.

Garb, Margaret. "Health, Morality, and Housing: The 'Tenement Problem' in Chicago." *American Journal of Public Health* 93, no. 9 (September 2003): 1420–30. https://doi.org/10.2105/ajph.93.9.1420.

Geddings, H. D. "Plague on the Steamship J. W. Taylor at New York Quarantine." *Public Health Reports* 14, no. 49 (December 8, 1899): 2165–67.

Georges, Isabel P. H., and Yumi Garcia dos Santos. "Olhares cruzados: Relações de cuidado, classe e gênero." *Tempo Social* 26, no. 1 (June 2014): 47–60. https://doi.org/10.1590/S0103-20702014000100004.

Gilman, Sander. *Difference and Pathology: Stereotypes of Sexuality, Race and Madness*. Ithaca, NY: Cornell University Press, 1985.

Gonçalves, Guilherme Leite, and Sérgio Costa. *Um porto no capitalismo global*. São Paulo: Boitempo, 2020.

Góes, Fred. "O Rio de Janeiro aos olhos do cronista popular." *Revista Z Cultural* 3, no. 2 (2015). http://revistazcultural.pacc.ufrj.br/o-rio-de-janeiro-aos-olhos -do-cronista-popular-de-fred-goes-2/.

Gordillo, Gastón R. *Rubble: The Afterlife of Destruction.* Durham, NC: Duke University Press, 2014.

Goulart, Adriana da Costa. "Revisitando a espanhola: A gripe pandêmica de 1918 no Rio de Janeiro." *História, Ciências, Saúde—Manguinhos* 12, no. 1 (January–April 2005): 101–42.

Graff Zivin, Erin. *The Wandering Signifier: Rhetoric of Jewishness in the Latin American Imaginary.* Durham, NC: Duke University Press, 2008.

Graham, Stephen, and Colin McFarlane, eds. *Infrastructural Lives: Urban Infrastructure in Context.* London: Routledge, 2015.

Granada, Daniel, Cássio Silveira, Silvia Regina Viodres Inoue, Regina Yoshie Matsue, and Denise Martin. "A pandemia de covid-19 e a mobilidade internacional no Brasil: Desafios para a saúde e proteção social de migrantes internacionais em tempos de incertezas." *História Ciência e Saúde—Manguinhos* 30, suppl. 1 (2023): 1–18. https://doi.org/10.1590/S0104-59702023000100033.

Green, Nancy. *Ready-to-Wear and Ready-to-Work: A Century of Industry and Immigrants in Paris and New York.* Durham, NC: Duke University Press, 1997.

Greenfield, Gerald Michael. "The Development of the Underdeveloped City: Public Sanitation in São Paulo, Brazil, 1885–1913." *Luso-Brazilian Review* 17, no. 1 (Summer 1980): 107–18.

Gregg, Jessica L. *Virtually Virgins: Sexual Strategies and Cervical Cancer in Recife, Brazil.* Stanford, CA: Stanford University Press, 2003.

Gudmundson, Lowell, and Justin Wolfe. *Blacks and Blackness in Central America: Between Race and Place.* Durham, NC: Duke University Press, 2010.

Guimarães, Antonio Sérgio. "Preconceito de cor e racismo no Brasil." *Revista De Antropologia* 47, no. 1 (2004): 9–43. https://doi.org/10.1590/S0034 -77012004000100001.

Guimarães, Nadya Araujo, and Helena Hirata, eds. *Care and Care Workers: A Latin American Perspective.* New York: Springer: 2021.

Guimarães, Valéria. "Os dramas da cidade nos jornais de São Paulo na passagem para o século XX." *Revista Brasileira De História* 27, no. 53 (January 2007): 323–49. https://doi.org/10.1590/S0102-01882007000100014.

Guimbeau, Amanda, Nidhiya Menon, and Aldo Musacchio. "The Brazilian Bombshell? The Long-Term Impact of the 1918 Influenza Pandemic the South American Way." National Bureau of Economic Research Working Paper 26929, April 2020. http://www.nber.org/papers/w26929.

Gutierrez, Diego Monteiro. "O Rugby, identidade e processos econômicos no Brasil." Master's thesis, Universidade de São Paulo, 2016.

Guzzo, Maria Auxiliadora Dias. "A habitação popular em São Paulo, 1890–1940." *Revista do Arquivo Municipal* 205 (January 2014): 59–79.

Hacon, Sandra. *Geo Saúde: Cidade de São Paulo*. Rio de Janeiro: ENSP/Fiocruz, 2008. https://www.prefeitura.sp.gov.br/cidade/secretarias/upload/arquivos /secretarias/meio_ambiente/publicacoes/0010/geo_Saude_SP.pdf.

Havelburg, W. "BRAZIL. Report from Rio de Janeiro-Status of Plague in Santos." *Public Health Reports* 15, no. 2 (1900): 79–81. http://www.jstor.org/stable/41452398.

Hamburger, Cao, dir. *O ano em que meus pais saíram de férias*. Lereby Produções/ Gullane Filmes/Globo Filmes/Miravista Pictures, 2006.

Hanley, Anne G. *The Public Good and the Brazilian State: Municipal Finance and Public Services in São Paulo, 1822–1930*. Chicago: University of Chicago Press, 2018.

Harvey, David. "Labor, Capital, and Class Struggle around the Built Environment in Advanced Capitalist Societies." *Politics and Society* 6, no. 3 (September 1976): 265–95. https://doi.org/10.1177/003232927600600301.

Hayward, Richard. "Gamarra, Lima, Peru: An International Workshop." *Urban Design International* 3 (March 1998): 43–52.

Heathcott, Joseph. "Infrastructure Designs: Dreaming and Building Worlds." In *The Routledge Handbook of Infrastructure Design: Global Perspectives from Architectural History*, edited by Joseph Heathcott, 1–16. New York: Routledge, 2022.

Herrera, Henrique Martines. "Manchester Paulista? Formação de classe e lutas de trabalhadores e trabalhadoras têxteis em Sorocaba, 1890–1930." Master's thesis, Universidade Federal de São Paulo, 2018. https://repositorio.unifesp.br/items /24c51277-a92d-400a-8c26-a8f063ad0f66.

Hertzman, Marc A. *After Palmares: Diaspora, Inheritance, and the Afterlives of Zumbi*. Durham, NC: Duke University Press, 2024.

Hesse-Wartegg, Ernst. *Zwischen Anden und Amazonas: Reisen in Brasilien, Argentinien, Paraguay, Uruguay*. Berlin: Union Deutsche Verlagsgesellschaft, 1915.

Higham, John. *Strangers in the Land: Patterns of American Nativism, 1860–1925*. New Brunswick, NJ: Rutgers University Press, 1955.

Hochman, Gilberto. "A gripe asiática vem aí! Crônica de uma pandemia antes de sua chegada (Brasil 1957)." *Revista Ciencias de la Salud* 19 (July 2021): 1–22. https://revistas.urosario.edu.co/index.php/revsalud/article/view/10599.

Hochman, Gilberto. *The Sanitation of Brazil: Nation, State, and Public Health, 1889-1930*. Champaign: University of Illinois Press, 2016.

Hochman, Gilberto, and Anne-Emanuelle Birn. "Pandemias e epidemias em perspectiva histórica: Uma introdução." *Topoi* 22, no. 48 (September–December 2021): 577–87. https://doi.org/10.1590/2237-101X02204801.

Hoehn, F. C. *O que vendem os hervanários da cidade de S. Paulo*. São Paulo: Casa Duprat, 1920.

Holloway, Thomas H. *Immigrants on the Land: Coffee and Society in São Paulo, 1886–1934*. Chapel Hill: University of North Carolina Press, 1980.

Honigsbaum, Mark. *A History of the Great Influenza Pandemics: Death, Panic, and Hysteria, 1830–1920*. London: I. B. Taurus, 2014.

Hou, Feng. "Spatial Assimilation of Racial Minorities in Canada's Immigrant Gateway Cities." *Urban Studies* 43, no. 7 (June 2006): 1191–213. http://www .jstor.org/stable/43201630.

Howard-Jones, Norman. "Robert Koch and the Cholera Vibrio: A Centenary." *British Medical Journal* 288, no. 6414 (February 4, 1984): 379–81. https://www .ncbi.nlm.nih.gov/pmc/articles/PMC1444283/pdf/bmjcred00486-0049.pdf.

Hussain, Azhar, Syed Ali, Madiha Ahmed, and Sheharyar Hussain. "The Anti-vaccination Movement: A Regression in Modern Medicine." *Cureus* 10, no. 7 (July 2018): 2–8. https://www.ncbi.nlm.nih.gov/pmc/articles/PMC6122668/.

Hutter, Lucy Maffei. *Imigração italiana em São Paulo (1880–1889): Os primeiros contactos do imigrante com o Brasil.* São Paulo: Universidade de São Paulo, Instituto de Estudos Brasileiros, 1972.

Instituto Butantan/Museu Emílio Ribas. *História, imigração e saúde no bairro do Bom Retiro.* São Paulo: Instituto Butantan, 2016. https://repositorio.butantan .gov.br/bitstream/butantan/3399/1/livreto_museu_emilio_ribas_02.pdf.

Instituto Nacional de Estatística. *Anuario Estatístico do Brasil, Ano II—1936.* Rio de Janeiro: Tip. do Departamento de Estatística e Publicidade, 1936. https://bibliotecadigital.seade.gov.br/view/singlepage/index.php?pubcod =10020581&parte=1.

Jacino, Ramatis. "O negro no mercado de trabalho em São Paulo pós-abolição, 1912/1920." PhD diss., Universidade de São Paulo, 1912.

James, Wesley, Chunrong Jia, and Satish Kedia. "Uneven Magnitude of Dispari-ties in Cancer Risks from Air Toxics." *International Journal of Environmental Research and Public Health* 9, no. 12 (December 2012): 4365–85. https://doi .org/10.3390/ijerph9124365.

Jensen, Katherine. *The Color of Asylum: The Racial Politics of Safe Haven in Brazil.* Chicago: University of Chicago Press, 2023.

Jesus, Carolina Maria de. *Quarto de despejo: Diário de uma favelada.* São Paulo: Francisco Alves, 1960.

Jones, Esyllt W. "'Co-operation in All Human Endeavour': Quarantine and Im-migrant Disease Vectors in the 1918–1919 Influenza Pandemic in Winnipeg." *Canadian Bulletin of Medical History/Bulletin canadien d'histoire de la méde-cine* 22, no. 1 (Spring 2005): 57–82. https://www.utpjournals.press/doi/pdf/10 .3138/cbmh.22.1.57.

Jones, Margaret. "Tuberculosis, Housing and the Colonial State: Hong Kong, 1900–1950." *Modern Asian Studies* 37, no. 3 (June 2003): 653–82.

Jones, Stephen G. *Sport, Politics and the Working Class: Organised Labour and Sport in Inter-war Britain.* Manchester: Manchester University Press, 1992.

Jorge, Janes. "Rios e saúde na cidade de São Paulo, 1890–1940." *História e Perspec-tivas, Uberlândia* 25, no. 47 (July-December 2012): 103–24.

Jorge, Janes. "São Paulo das enchentes, 1890–1940." *Revista Histórica Online* 47 (April 2011): 1-7. https://www.arquivoestado.sp.gov.br/uploads/publicacoes /revistas/historica47.pdf.

Jorge, Janes. *Tietê, o rio que a cidade perdeu: São Paulo, 1890–1940*. São Paulo: Alameda Editorial, 2006.

Justus, Marcelo, and Ana Lucia Kassouf. "The History of Child Labor in Brazil." In *The World of Child Labor: An Historical and Regional Survey*, edited by Hugh D. Hindman, 361–64. New York: M. E. Sharpe, 2009.

Kang, Sam, Denise Razzouk, Jair Jesus de Mari, and Itiro Shirakawa. "The Mental Health of Korean Immigrants in São Paulo, Brazil." *Cadernos de Saúde Pública* 4, no. 25 (April 2009): 819–26.

Karam, John Tofik. *Another Arabesque: Syrian-Lebanese Ethnicity in Neoliberal Brazil*. Philadelphia: Temple University Press, 2007.

Keefer, Phil, Carlos Scartascini, and Razvan Vlaicu. "Shortchanging the Future: The Short-Term Bias of Politics." In *Better Spending for Better Lives: How Latin America and the Caribbean Can Do More with Less*, edited by Alejandro Izquierdo, Carola Pessino, and Guillermo Vuletin, 325–58. Mexico City: Inter-American Development Bank, 2018. https://publications.iadb.org/publications /english/document/Better-Spending-for-Better-Lives-How-Latin-America -and-the-Caribbean-Can-Do-More-with-Less.pdf.

Kelsey, Allison Elizabeth. "How the Other Nine-Tenths Lived: Interpreting the Working Class Experience in Philadelphia, 1870–1900." Master's thesis, University of Pennsylvania, 1997. https://repository.upenn.edu/cgi/viewcontent .cgi?article=1332&context=hp_theses.

Kenzo, Gabriel. *Não há cura sem anúncio: Ciência, Medicina e Propaganda—São Paulo, 1930–1939*. São Paulo: Annablume, 2021.

Khoudja, Yassine. "Religious Trajectories of Immigrants in the First Years after Migration." *Journal for the Scientific Study of Religion* 61, no. 2 (June 2022): 507–29.

Kidambi, Prashant. "'An Infection of Locality': Plague, Pythogenesis, and the Poor in Bombay, c. 1896–1905." *Urban History* 31, no. 2 (2004): 249–67.

Kim, Marcos Seil, "Nas curvas do rio ídiche." In *Paulicéia Prometida*, edited by Cremilda Medina, 13–21. São Paulo: CJE/USP/ECA, 1990.

Kind, Luciana, and Rosineide Cordeiro. "Narrativas sobre a morte: A gripe espanhola e a Covid 19 no Brasil." *Psicologia e Sociedade* 32 (September 2020): 1–19. https://www.scielo.br/j/psoc/a/LdMLvxpDHBYgLqt8fC5SZRp/?lang=pt.

Kisacky, Jeanne. *Rise of the Modern Hospital: An Architectural History of Health and Healing, 1870–1940*. Pittsburgh, PA: University of Pittsburgh Press, 2016.

Klengel, Susanne. "Pandemic Avant-Garde: Urban Coexistence in Mário de Andrade's Pauliceia Desvairada (1922) after the Spanish Flu." Mecila Working Paper Series 30. São Paulo: The Maria Sibylla Merian International Centre for Advanced Studies in the Humanities and Social Sciences Conviviality-Inequality in Latin America, 2020. https://doi.org/10.46877/klengel.2020.30.

Koselleck, Reinhart. *Sediments of Time: On Possible Histories*. Translated and edited by Sean Franzel and Stefan-Ludwig Hoffmann. Stanford, CA: Stanford University Press, 2018.

Koseritz, Karl von. *Imagens do Brasil*. São Paulo: Livraria Martins Editora, 1972.

Koulioumba, Stamatia. "Construtores estrangeiros e a produção arquitetônica moderna no Bom Retiro (1950–1970)." In *São Paulo, os estrangeiros e a construção das cidades*, edited by Ana Lúcia Lanna, Fernanda Peixoto, José de Lira, and Maria Ruth de Sampaio, 261–86. São Paulo: Alameda Editorial, 2011.

Kowarick, Lúcio. "Cortiços: A humilhação e a subalternidade." *Tempo Social* 25, no. 2 (November 2013): 49–77.

Kowarick, Lúcio, and Clara Ant. "One Hundred Years of Overcrowding: Slum Tenements in the City." In *Social Struggles and the City: The Case of São Paulo*, edited by Lúcio Kowarick, 60–76. New York: Monthly Review Press, 1994.

Kraut, Alan M. "Immigration, Ethnicity, and the Pandemic." *Public Health Reports* 125, suppl. 3 (April 2010): 123–33. https://www.ncbi.nlm.nih.gov/pmc/articles /PMC2862341/.

Kraut, Alan M. *Silent Travelers: Germs, Genes, and the "Immigrant Menace."* Baltimore: Johns Hopkins University Press, 1994.

Kropf, Simone Petraglia, and Gilberto Hochman. "From the Beginnings: Debates on the History of Science in Brazil." *Hispanic American Historical Review* 91, no. 3 (August 2011): 391–408.

Kropf, Simone Petraglia, and Gilberto Hochman. "Science, Health, and Development: Chagas Disease in Brazil, 1943–1962." *Parassitologia* 47, no. 3 (December 2005): 379–86.

Kushnir, Beatriz. "Hospedaria Central, o Expurgo na Ilha das Flores." In *As doenças e os medos sociais*, edited by Yara Nogueira Monteiro and Maria Luiza Tucci Carneiro, 159–74. São Paulo: Editora FAP-UNIFESP, 2013.

LABCidade. "A verticalização de mercado em São Paulo é branca." USP/FAU— Faculdade de Arquitetura e Urbanismo. 6 de dezembro de 2021. http://www .labcidade.fau.usp.br/a-verticalizacao-de-mercado-em-sao-paulo-e-branca/.

Lacerda, Léia Teixeira, Kátia Cristina Nascimento Figueira, and Maria Leda Pinto. "Conhecimentos tradicionais dos povos indígenas da região Pantaneira Sul-Mato-Grossense sobre a prevenção das infecções sexualmente transmissíveis." *Geofronter* 3, no. 4 (November 2018): 150–58. https://periodicosonline.uems .br/index.php/GEOF/index.

Laguardia, Rafael Martins de Oliveira. "A geografia sagrada na expansão urbana de São Paulo até finais do XIX: Uma leitura em SIG Histórico." Paper presented at ANPUH 31st Simpósio Nacional de História, ST 141—SIG Histórico e a virada espacial na História, Rio de Janeiro, July 20, 2021. https://www.snh2021.anpuh .org/resources/anais/8/snh2021/1628549342_ARQUIVO_1eddffda1d178b6c784 80621cf883f34.pdf.

Lagenest, Baruel H. D. "Os Cortiços de São Paulo." *Revista Anhembi* 48, no. 139 (1962): 5–17.

Landmann-Szwarcwald, Celia, and James Macinko. "A Panorama of Health Inequalities in Brazil." *International Journal for Equity in Health* 15, no. 1 (2016): 174. https://equityhealthj.biomedcentral.com/articles/10.1186/s12939 -016-0462-1.

Langfur, Hal. "Uncertain Refuge: Frontier Formation and the Origins of the Botocudo War in Late Colonial Brazil." *Hispanic American Historical Review* 82, no. 2 (May 2002): 215–56.

Leão, Antônio Carneiro. *São Paulo em 1920*. São Paulo: Annuario Americano, 1920.

Lee, Erika, and Judy Yung. *Angel Island: Immigrant Gateway to America*. New York: Oxford University Press, 2012.

Leite, Miriam Lifchitz Moreira. *Maria Lacerda de Moura: Uma feminista utópica*. São Paulo: Editora Atica, 1984.

Lemos, Carlos. "Os primeiros cortiços paulistanos." In *Habitação e cidade*, edited by Maria Ruth Amaral de Sampaio, 15–28. São Paulo: FAU-USP, FAPESP, 1998.

Lemos, Fernando Cerqueira. "Notícias sobre a epidemia de peste em Santos (1899)." *Revista do Instituto Adolfo Lutz* 17, nos. 1–2 (February 1957): 71–150. https://doi.org/10.53393/rial.1957.v17.33315.

Lesser, Jeffrey. *A Discontented Diaspora: Japanese-Brazilians and the Meanings of Ethnic Militancy, 1960–1980*. Durham, NC: Duke University Press, 2007. Revised Brazilian edition: *Uma diáspora descontente: Os Nipo-Brasileiros e os significados da militância Étnica, 1960–1980*. São Paulo: Editora Paz e Terra, 2008.

Lesser, Jeffrey. *Immigration, Ethnicity and National Identity in Brazil*. New York: Cambridge University Press, 2013. Revised Brazilian edition: *A invenção da Brasilidade: Identidade nacional, etnicidade e políticas de imigração*. São Paulo: Editora UNESP, 2015.

Lesser, Jeffrey. *Negotiating National Identity: Immigrants, Minorities and the Struggle for Ethnicity in Brazil*. Durham, NC: Duke University Press, 1999. Revised Brazilian edition: *Negociando a identidade nacional: Imigrantes, minorias e a luta pela etnicidade no Brasil*. São Paulo: Editora UNESP, 2001.

Lesser, Jeffrey. "Reflexões sobre (codi)nomes e etnicidade em São Paulo." *Revista de Antropologia* 51, no. 1 (January 2008): 267–83.

Lesser, Jeffrey. *Welcoming the Undesirables: Brazil and the Jewish Question*. Berkeley: University of California Press, 1994. Revised Brazilian edition: *O Brasil e a questão judaica: Imigração, diplomacia e preconceito*. Rio de Janeiro: Imago Editora, 1995.

Lesser, Jeffrey, and Uriel Kitron. "The Social Geography of Zika in Brazil." *NACLA Report on the Americas* 48, no. 2 (July 2016): 123–29. Published in Portuguese as "A geografia social do Zika no Brasil," *Estudos Avançados* 30, no. 88 (September–December 2016): 167–75, https://www.scielo.br/j/ea/a/QMfVJpGDpwKybkbMQzXFN9y/?lang=pt.

Lévi-Strauss, Claude. *A World on the Wane*. New York: Criterion Books, 1961.

Levy, Maria Stella Ferreira. "O papel da migração internacional na evolução da população brasileira (1872 a 1972)." *Revista de Saúde Pública* 8, suppl. (June 1974): 49–90. https://doi.org/10.1590/S0034-89101974000500003.

Lin, Yi-Tang. *Statistics and the Language of Global Health: Institutions and Experts in China, Taiwan and the World, 1917–1960*. Cambridge: Cambridge University Press, 2022.

Link, Bruce, and Jo Phelan. "Social Conditions as Fundamental Causes of Health Inequalities." In *Handbook of Medical Sociology*, edited by Chloe E. Bird, Peter Conrad, and Allen M. Fremont, 3–17. 6th ed. Nashville, TN: Vanderbilt University Press, 2010.

Lisboa, Karen. "Insalubridade, doenças e imigração." *História, Ciências, Saúde—Manguinhos* 20, no. 1 (March 2013): 119–39.

Lobato, Monteiro. "Fatia de vida." In *Negrinha (contos)*. São Paulo: Revista do Brasil, 1920.

Logan, John, Wenquan Zhang, and Richard Alba. "Immigrant Enclaves and Ethnic Communities in New York and Los Angeles." *American Sociological Review* 67, no. 2 (April 2002): 299–322.

Losco, Luiza Nogueira, and Sandra Francisca Bezerra Gemma. "Atenção primária em saúde para imigrantes bolivianos no Brasil." *Interface* 25 (September 2021): 1–14. https://www.scielo.br/j/icse/a/VPvkQXHrXqCFsWm8rfSWZcQ/?format =pdf&lang=pt.

Lotta, Gabriela Spanghero. *Burocracia e implementação de políticas de saúde: Os agentes comunitários na Estratégia Saúde da Família*. Rio de Janeiro: Editora Fiocruz, 2015.

Lopez, Russell. *Building American Public Health: Urban Planning, Architecture, and the Quest for Better Health in the United States*. New York: Palgrave Macmillan, 2012.

Low, Michael Christopher. "Empire and the Hajj: Pilgrims, Plagues, and Pan-Islam under British Surveillance, 1865–1908." *International Journal of Middle East Studies* 40, no. 2 (May 2008): 269–90. http://www.jstor.org/stable/30069613.

Lowe, Rachel, Sophie A. Lee, Kathleen M. O'Reilly, Oliver J. Brady, Leonardo Bastos, Gabriel Carrasco-Escobar, Rafael de Castro Catão, et al. "Combined Effects of Hydrometeorological Hazards and Urbanisation on Dengue Risk in Brazil: A Spatiotemporal Modelling Study." *Lancet Planetary Health* 5, no. 4 (April 2021): 209–19. https://doi.org/10.1016/S2542-5196(20)30292-8.

Lowrie, Samuel Harmon. "O elemento negro na população de São Paulo." *Revista do Arquivo Municipal* 48 (June 1938): 5–56.

Lucchesi, Bianca Melzi D. "Do cortiço às vilas operárias: Políticas públicas e a construção do cotidiano nos quintais paulistanos." Paper presented at ANPUH, 2018. https://www.encontro2018.sp.anpuh.org/resources/anais/8/1531745890 _ARQUIVO_Docorticoasvilasoperariaspoliticaspublicaseaconstrucaodocoti dianonosquintaispaulistanos_BiancaLucchesi.pdf.

Lutz, Adolpho. "Algumas observações feitas em dois casos de peste pneumonica pelo dr. Adolpho Lutz." *Revista Médica de São Paulo, Jornal Pratico de Medicina, Cirurgia e Hygiene* 3, no. 3 (March 1900): 54–56.

MacDougall, Heather Anne. *Activists and Advocates: Toronto's Health Department, 1883–1983*. Toronto: Dundurn, 1990.

Machado, Marta Rodriguez de Assis, and Raquel Pimenta. "Authoritarian Zones within Democracy: Rule of Law in Contemporary Brazil." *Verfassung in Recht und Übersee* 55, no. 4 (January 2022): 441–58.

Machado, Reinaldo Paul Pérez, and Iara Sakitani Kako. "A cartografia da expansão da cidade de São Paulo no período de 1881 a 2001." In *Cartógrafos para toda a terra: Produção e circulação do saber cartográfico ibero-americano: Agentes e contextos*, edited by Francisco Roque de Oliveira, 2:623–40. Lisbon: Biblioteca Nacional de Portugal—Centro de Estudos Geográficos da Universidade de Lisboa—Centro de História d'Aquém e d'Além-Mar da Universidade Nova de Lisboa e da Universidade dos Açores, 2015. https://doi.org/10.13140/RG.2.1.4960.9045.

Maestrini, Karla Aparecida. "Em busca da cidade moderna: As ações de saúde, de higiene e as intervenções urbanas em São Paulo durante a gestão de Antonio da Silva Prado (1899–1910)." Master's thesis, Pontifícia Universidade Católica de São Paulo, 2015. https://sapientia.pucsp.br/bitstream/handle/12877/1/Karla%20Aparecida%20Maestrini.pdf.

Magnani, José Guilherme. "Rua, símbolo e suporte da experiência urbana." *Os Urbanitas: Revista Digital de Antropologia Urbana* 1, no. 0 (October 2003). https://nau.fflch.usp.br/files/upload/paginas/rua_simbolo%20e%20suporte%20da%20experiencia%20-%20magnani_0.pdf.

Malta, Deborah Carvalho, Adauto Martins Soares Filho, Isabella Vitral Pinto, Maria Cecília de Souza Minayo, Cheila Marina Lima, Ísis Eloah Machado, Renato Azeredo Teixeira, et al. "Association between Firearms and Mortality in Brazil, 1990 to 2017: A Global Burden of Disease Brazil Study." *Population Health Metrics* 18, suppl. 1 (2020): 1–14. https://pophealthmetrics.biomedcentral.com/articles/10.1186/s12963-020-00222-3.

Mandelbaum, Henoch Gabriel, and Marísia Margarida Santiago Buitoni. "Territorializations, Transformations, and Chinese Community Life in Liberdade Neighborhood's 'Oriental Quarter' in the City of São Paulo, Brazil." In *Studies on Chinese Migrations: Brazil, China and Mozambique*, edited by André Bueno and Daniel Veras, 147–87. Rio de Janeiro: Projeto Orientalismo/UERJ, 2021.

Mangili, Liziane Peres. *Bom Retiro, bairro central de São Paulo: Transformações e permanências, 1930–1954.* São Paulo: Alameda Editorial, 2011.

Mantovani, Rafael. "O que foi a polícia médica?" *História, Ciências, Saúde—Manguinhos* 25, no. 2 (April–June 2018): 409–27.

Maram, Sheldon L. "The Immigrant and the Brazilian Labor Movement, 1890–1920." In *Essays concerning the Socioeconomic History of Brazil and Portuguese India*, edited by Dauril Alden and Warren Dean, 178–210. Gainesville: University Presses of Florida, 1977.

Marcus, Greil. *Lipstick Traces: A Secret History of the 20th Century.* Cambridge, MA: Harvard University Press, 1990.

Marinelli, Natália Pereira, Deiane Ferreira Nascimento, Alana Ilmara Pereira Costa, Maria Belén Salazar Posso, and Layana Pachêco Araújo. "Assistência à população indígena: Dificuldades encontradas por enfermeiros." *Revista Univap* 18, no. 32 (December 2012): 52–65. https://revista.univap.br/index.php/revistaunivap/article/download/93/106/854.

Marins, Paulo César Garcez. "Habitação e vizinhança: Limites da privacidade no surgimento das metrópoles brasileiras." In *História da vida privada no Brasil: 3*, edited by Nicolau Sevcenko, 131–214. São Paulo: Companhia das Letras, 1998.

Marins, Paulo Cesar Garcez. *Um lugar para as elites: Os Campos Elísios de Glette e Nothmann no imaginário urbano de São Paulo*. São Paulo: Alameda Editorial, 2011.

Markel, Howard, and Alexandra Stern. "The Foreignness of Germs: The Persistent Association of Immigrants and Disease in American Society." *Milbank Quarterly* 80, no. 4 (December 2002): 757–88.

Martes, Ana, and Sarah Faleiros. "Acesso dos imigrantes bolivianos aos serviços públicos de saúde na cidade de São Paulo." *Saúde Social* 22, no. 2 (June 2013): 351–64.

Martin, Denise, Alejandro Goldberg, and Cássio Silveira. "Imigração, refúgio e saúde." *Saúde e Sociedade* 27, no. 1 (January–March 2018): 26–36.

Martinez, Vanessa, Naomi K. Komatsu, Sumie M. De Figueredo, and Eliseu A. Waldman. "Equity in Health: Tuberculosis in the Bolivian Immigrant Community of São Paulo, Brazil." *Tropical Medicine and International Health* 17, no. 11 (August 2012): 1417–24. https://doi.org/10.1111/j.1365-3156.2012.03074.x.

Martins, Antônio Egydio. *São Paulo Antigo (1554 a 1910)*. Rio de Janeiro: Livr. Francisco Alves e C.; São Paulo: Typ. do Diário Official, 1911–12.

Mascarenhas, Rodolfo dos Santos. "História da saúde pública no Estado de São Paulo." *Revista de Saúde Pública* 40, no. 1 (February 2006): 3–19.

Massad, Eduardo, Marcelo Nascimento Burattini, Francisco Antonio Bezerra Coutinho, and Luiz Fernandes Lopez. "The 1918 Influenza Epidemic in the City of São Paulo, Brazil." *Medical Hypothesis* 68, no. 2 (2007): 442–45.

Massey, Doreen. "Double Articulation: A Place in the World." In *Displacements: Cultural Identities in Question*, edited by Angelika Bammer, 110–22. Bloomington: Indiana University Press, 1994.

Massey, Douglas S. "The New Immigration and Ethnicity in the United States." *Population and Development Review* 21, no. 3 (September 1995): 631–52. http://www.u.arizona.edu/~jag/POL596A/massyimmigeth.pdf.

Mastromauro, Giovana Carla. "Alguns aspectos da saúde pública e do urbanismo higienista em São Paulo no final do século XIX." *Cadernos de História da Ciência—Instituto Butantan* 6, no. 22 (July–December 2010): 45–63.

Mateus, Cayo Renan Alves. "Memórias de uma prisão: O Presídio Tiradentes entre a tênue linha do lembrar e do esquecer." *Revista Discente Ofícios de Clio, Pelotas* 6, no. 11 (July–December 2021): 140–54.

Matos, Maria Izilda Santos de. "Construindo a paulistaneidade: As representações do feminino e do masculino no discurso médico-eugênico, São Paulo (1890–1930)." *História Revista* 1, no. 1 (January–June 1996): 125–45.

Matos, Maria Izilda Santos de. *Cotidiano e cultura: História, cidade e trabalho*. Bauru: Editora da Universidade do Sagrado Coração, 2002.

Matos, Maria Izilda Santos de. "Na trama urbana: Do público, do privado e do íntimo." *Projeto História* 13 (January/June 1996): 129–49.

McCaskey, G. W. "Disinfection during and after the Acute Infectious Diseases." *Sanitary News* 16, no. 346 (September 1890): 245–247. https://www.google.com.br/books/edition/Sanitary_News/NpnmAAAAMAAJ?hl=en&gbpv=1&dq=%22disinfectory%22&pg=PA247&printsec=frontcover.

Meade, Teresa. "'Civilizing Rio de Janeiro': The Public Health Campaign and the Riot of 1904." *Journal of Social History* 20, no. 2 (Winter 1986): 301–22. https://doi.org/10.1353/jsh/20.2.301.

Medici, Ademir. "Asseio corporal. Combate à raiva. Noções sobre nutrição. Estamos em 1958 . . ." *Diário do Grande ABC*, February 10, 2022. https://www.dgabc.com.br/Noticia/3829719/asseio-corporal-combate-a-raiva-nocoes-sobre-nutricao-estamos-em-1958.

Medina, Cremilda. "Apresentação." In *Paulicéia Prometida*, edited by Cremilda Medina, 9. São Paulo: CJE/USP/ECA, 1990.

Mele, Christopher. *Selling the Lower East Side: Culture, Real Estate, and Resistance in New York City*. Minneapolis: University of Minnesota Press, 2000.

Melo, Maria das Neves Medeiros de, and Wilson Fusco. "Migrantes nordestinos na região metropolitana de São Paulo." *Confins: Revue franco-brésilienne de géographie / Revista franco-brasilera de geografia* 40 (2019): 1–18. https://journals.openedition.org/confins/19451.

Mendonça, Veiga, Francisco de Assis, Adilson Veiga e Souza, and Denecir de Almeida Dutra. "Saúde pública, urbanização e dengue no Brasil." *Sociedade & Natureza* 21, no. 3 (December 2009): 257–69. https://doi.org/10.1590/S1982-45132009000300003.

Meyer, Carlos Luiz, and Joaquim Rabello Teixeira, Serviço Sanitário do Estado de São Paulo. *A gripe epidêmica no Brazil e especialmente em São Paulo—dados e informações*. São Paulo: Casa Duprat, 1920.

Miéville, China. *The City and the City*. New York: Macmillan, 2009.

Mills, John. *Charles Miller: O pai do futebol brasileiro*. São Paulo: Panda Books, 2005.

Mimesse, Eliane. "O cotidiano da escolarização primária paulistana nos anos iniciais do século XX." Paper presented at the XXVIII Simpósio Nacional de História, Florianópolis, July 27–31, 2015. http://www.snh2015.anpuh.org/resources/anais/39/1423244994_ARQUIVO_texto.pdf.

Min, Pyong Gap. *Caught in the Middle: Korean Communities in New York And Los Angeles*. Berkeley: University of California Press, 1996.

Miranda, Nicanor. "Ensaio de um método de investigação do nível social de São Paulo pela distribuição da profissão dos pais dos alunos das escolas primárias públicas." *Revista do Arquivo Municipal* 2, no. 23 (May 1938), 189–207. https://www.prefeitura.sp.gov.br/cidade/secretarias/cultura/arquivo_historico/publicacoes/index.php?p=8312.

Moimaz, Suzely Adas Saliba, Jeidson Antônio Morais Marques, Orlando Saliba, Cléa Adas Saliba Garbin, Lívia Guimarães Zina, and Nemre Adas Saliba. "Satisfação e percepção do usuário do SUS sobre o serviço público de saúde." *Physis: Revista de Saúde Coletiva* 20, no. 4 (December 2010): 1419–40. https://doi.org/10.1590/S0103-73312010000400019.

Monmonier, Mark. *How to Lie with Maps.* Chicago: University of Chicago Press, 1991.

Monsma, Karl. "Symbolic Conflicts, Deadly Consequences: Fights between Italians and Blacks in Western São Paulo, 1888–1914." *Journal of Social History* 39, no. 4 (Summer 2006): 1123–52. https://doi.org/10.1353/jsh.2006.0049.

Monteyne, David. *For the Temporary Accommodation of Settlers: Architecture and Immigrant Reception in Canada, 1870–1930.* Montreal: McGill-Queen's University Press, 2021.

Moreira, Ildeu de Castro, and Luisa Massarani. "(En)canto científico: Temas de ciência em letras da música popular brasileira." *História, Ciências, Saúde—Manguinhos* 13, suppl. 1 (October 2006): 291–307. https://www.scielo.br/j/hcsm/a/vphm6KLWvSbmQkrmPBmkVQh/abstract/?lang=pt.

Morse, Richard M. "São Paulo since Independence: A Cultural Interpretation." *Hispanic American Historical Review* 34, no. 4 (November 1954): 419–44. https://doi.org/10.1215/00182168-34.4.419.

Moszczyńska, Joanna M. *A memória da destruição na escrita judaico-brasileira depois de 1985: Por uma literatura pós-Holocausto emergente no Brasil.* Berlin: Peter Lang, 2022.

Mota, Andre. *Tempos cruzados: A saúde coletiva no estado de São Paulo, 1920–1980.* São Paulo: Hucitec Editora, 2020.

Mota, Andre. *Tropeços da medicina bandeirante: Medicina paulista entre 1892–1920.* São Paulo: Edusp, 2005.

Mott, Maria Lucia, Maria Aparecida Muniz, Olga Sofia Fabergé Alves, Karla Maestrini, and Tais dos Santos. "As parteiras eram 'tutte quante' italianas (São Paulo, 1870–1920)." *História: Questões e Debates* 47, no. 2 (December 2007): 65–94. https://revistas.ufpr.br/historia/article/view/12111.

Mott, Maria Lucia, Maria Aparecida Muniz, Olga Sofia Fabergé Alves, Karla Maestrini, and Tais dos Santos. "Médicos e médicas em São Paulo e os Livros de Registros do Serviço de Fiscalização do Exercício Profissional (1892–1932)." *Ciência e Saúde Coletiva* 13, no. 3 (June 2008): 853–68. https://www.scielo.br/j/csc/a/jFZsddJRDzCGv4fGvB3r9NG/?lang=pt#.

Mott, Maria Lucia, and Gisele Sanglard, eds. *História da saúde em São Paulo: Instituições e patrimônio arquitetônico (1808–1958).* Rio de Janeiro: Editora Fiocruz/Editora Manole, 2011.

Motta Júnior, Cesário. *Relatorio apresentado ao Senhor Doutor Presidente do Estado de São Paulo pelo Dr. Cesário Motta Júnior, secretario d'Estado dos Negocios do Interior em 28 de Março de 1894.* São Paulo: Vanorden, 1894.

Moura, Esmeralda Blanco Bolsonaro de. "Infância operária e acidente do trabalho em São Paulo." In *História da criança no Brasil,* edited by Mary Del Priore, 112–29. São Paulo: Contexto, 1991.

Müller, Nice Lecocq. "A área central da cidade." In *A cidade de São Paulo: Estudos de geografia urbana*, vol. 3, *Aspectos da metrópole paulista*, edited by Aroldo de Azevedo, 121–82. São Paulo: Companhia Editora Nacional, 1958.

Murphy, Michelle. *Sick Building Syndrome and the Problem of Uncertainty: Environmental Politics, Technoscience, and Women Workers.* Durham, NC: Duke University Press, 2006.

Murtha, Ney Albert, José Esteban Castro, and Léouma Heller. "Uma perspectiva histórica das primeiras políticas de saneamento e de recurso hídricos no Brasil." *Ambiente e Sociedade* 18, no. 3 (July–September 2015): 193–210. https://doi .org/10.1590/1809-4422ASOC1047V1832015.

Museu da Imigração, Centro de Preservação, Pesquisa e Referência. *Ebook - Acervo Digital do Museu da Imigração.* São Paulo: Museu da Imigração, 2018. https:// museudaimigracao.org.br/acervo-e-pesquisa/e-book.

Nakano, Anderson Kazuo. "Desenvolvimento territorial e regulação urbanística nas áreas centrais de São Paulo." In *Caminhos para o centro: Estratégias de desenvolvimento para a região central de São Paulo*, by Empresa Municipal de Urbanização, photography by Cristiano Mascaro, 381–420. São Paulo: Prefeitura Municipal de São Paulo (PMSP), Centro Brasileiro de Análise e Planejamento (CEBRAP) e Centro de Estudos da Metrópole (CEM), 2004.

Nakano, Anderson Kazuo. "Desigualdades habitacionais no 'repovoamento' do centro expandido do município de São Paulo." *Cadernos Metropolitanos* 20, no. 41 (January–April 2018): 53–74. https://doi.org/10.1590/2236-9996.2018-4103.

Nascimento, Alan Faber do. "The Tourist Topicality of the Case of the Spanish Flu in the City of Rio de Janeiro (September 1918–March 1919)." *Revista Brasileira de Pesquisa em Turismo, São Paulo* 14, no. 3 (September–December 2020): 176–88.

Nascimento, Débora Souza do. "Corpos violados: Crimes de defloramento na cidade de São Paulo, 1900–1932." PhD diss., Pontifícia Universidade Católica de São Paulo, 2019.

Nascimento, Dilene Raimundo do, and Matheus Alves Duarte da Silva. "'Não é meu intuito estabelecer polêmica': A chegada da peste ao Brasil, análise de uma controvérsia, 1899." *História, Ciências, Saúde—Manguinhos* 20, suppl. 1 (November 2013): 1271–85. https://www.scielo.br/j/hcsm/a /fZQjpmc9MqKZs6DKYbkmVGK/abstract/?lang=pt.

Nascimento, Luciana Marino do, and Francisco Bento da Silva. "De protestos e levantes: As revoltas da vacina e da chibata na música popular." *Recorte— Revista Eletrônica* 9, no. 2 (2012): 1–16. http://periodicos.unincor.br/index.php /recorte/article/view/620.

Nastri, Pedro. "Bom Retiro em capítulos—parte III. Conversa de Dona Alcina com o pai. Final da história da família Thomas." In São Paulo Minha Cidade, *Leia as histórias: Nossos bairros, nossas vidas.* São Paulo: São Paulo Turismo, 2009. https://saopaulominhacidade.com.br/?p=2657https://saopaulominhacidade .com.br/?p=2657.

Needell, Jeffrey D. "The Revolta Contra Vacina of 1904: The Revolt against 'Modernization' in Belle-Époque Rio de Janeiro." *Hispanic American Historical Review* 67, no. 2 (May 1987): 233–69. https://doi.org/10.2307/2515023.

Nemi, Ana. "Charity and Philanthropy in the History of Brazilian Hospitals." In *The Political Economy of the Hospital in History*, edited by Martin Gorsky, Margarita Vilar-Rodríguez, and Jerònia Pons-Pons, 61–94. Queensgate, England: University of Huddersfield Press, 2020.

Neto, Lira. *O poder e a peste: A vida de Rodolfo Teófilo*. Fortaleza: Editora Fundação Demócrito Rocha, 1999.

O'Brien, Elizabeth. "If They Are Useful, Why Expel Them? Las Hermanas de la Caridad and Religious Medical Authority in Mexico City Hospitals, 1861–1874." *Mexican Studies/Estudios Mexicanos* 33, no. 3 (Fall 2017): 417–42. https:// www.academia.edu/35985076/If_They_Are_Useful_Why_Expel_Them_Las _Hermanas_de_la_Caridad_and_Religious_Medical_Authority_in_Mexico _City_Hospitals_1861_1874.

Oliva, Jaime Tadeu, and Fernanda Padovesi Fonseca. "O 'modelo São Paulo': Uma descompactação antiurbanidade na gênese da metrópole." *Revista Do Instituto De Estudos Brasileiros* 65 (September 2016): 20–56. https://doi.org/10.11606 /issn.2316-901X.v0i65p20-56.

Oliveira, Celina Maria Ferro de. "Utilização de serviços do Sistema Único de Saúde por beneficiários de planos de saúde Rio de Janeiro." Master's thesis, Escola Nacional de Saúde Pública Sergio Arouca, 2009. https://bvsms.saude.gov.br /bvs/publicacoes/premio2009/celina_maria.pdf.

Oro, Ari Pedro. "Imigrantes calabreses e religiões afro-brasileiras no Rio Grande do Sul." *Estudos Ibero-Americanos* 14, no. 1 (December 1988): 73–85. https:// revistaseletronicas.pucrs.br/ojs/index.php/iberoamericana/article/view/30429.

Ortega y Gasset, José. "La Pedagogía del paisaje." [1906]. *Obras completas, Vol. 1*, 53–57. Madrid: Alianza Editorial-Revista de Occidente, 1983.

Ortigara, Yuri Vilas Boas. "Cartografia, plantas e projetos históricos de obras hidráulicas no Arquivo Público do Estado de São Paulo." PhD diss., Universidade de São Paulo, 2017.

Ortiz, Paul. *An African American and Latinx History of the United States*. Boston: Beacon Press, 2018.

Palma, Patricia. "From Asia to the Americas: Chinese Medicine in Latin America and the Caribbean (1840-1930)." *Monde(s)* 20, no. 2 (July 2021): 29–48. https:// www.cairn-int.info/article-E_MOND1_212_0029-from-asia-to-the-americas -chinese-medicine-in-latin-america-and-the-caribbean-1840-1930.htm.

Pande, Ishita. *Medicine, Race and Liberalism in British Bengal: Symptoms of Empire*. New York: Routledge, 2010.

Panizzolo, Claudia. "The Daily Life of Italian and Italian-Descendant Children in Tenements, Work and School (São Paulo, Late 19th and Early 20th Century)." *Espacio, Tiempo y Educación* 8, no. 1 (January-June 2021): 53–71. https://doi .org/10.14516/ete.365.

Panizzolo, Claudia. "A escola étnica na cidade de São Paulo e os primeiros tons de uma identidade italiana (1887–1912)." *História da Educação* 24 (January 2020): 1–31. https://www.scielo.br/j/heduc/a/vpjfnQ4ssDFhdPYR4wMTxSQ/?format =pdf&lang=pt.

Pardue, Derek. "I Only Know the Mosquito Bites: Religious Occupations and Contingent Relationships in São Paulo, Brazil." *Contemporary Brazilian Cities, Culture, and Resistance, Hispanic Issues On Line*, no. 28 (2022): 162–83.

Park, Kyeyoung. "The 'Foxes' Outfoxed: Contestations between Koreans and Jews in South American Textile Industries." *Dialectical Anthropology* 38, no. 1 (March 2014): 17–39.

Passos, Maria Lúcia Perrone, and Teresa Emídio. *Desenhando São Paulo: Mapas e literatura, 1877–1954*. São Paulo: Editora Senac, Imprensa Oficial do Estado de São Paulo, 2009.

Patai, Daphne. "Minority Status and the Stigma of 'Surplus Visibility.'" *Chronicle of Higher Education* 38, no. 10 (October 1991): A52.

Paula, Amir El Hakim de. "Os operários pedem passagem! A geografia do operário na cidade de São Paulo (1900-1917)." Master's thesis: Universidade de São Paulo, 2005.

Paz, Octavio. *The Labyrinth of Solitude: Life and Thought in Mexico*. Translated by Lysander Kemp. New York: Grove, 1961.

Pegler-Gordon, Anna. *In Sight of America: Photography and the Development of U.S. Immigration Policy*. Berkeley: University of California Press, 2009.

Peixoto-Mehrtens, Cristina. *Urban Space and National Identity in Early Twentieth Century São Paulo, Brazil: Crafting Modernity*. New York: Palgrave Macmillan, 2010.

Penna, Belisário. *Saneamento do Brasil: Sanear o Brasil é povoá-lo; é enriquecê-lo; o moralizá-lo*. 2nd ed. Rio de Janeiro: Typ. Jacintho Ribeiro dos Santos, 1923.

Penteado, Jacob. *Belènzinho, 1910: Retrato de uma época*. [1962]. São Paulo: Carrenho Editorial/Narrativa Um, 2003.

Pereira, Daniel de Menezes. "Aspectos históricos e atuais da perícia médico legal e suas possibilidades de evolução." Master's thesis, Universidade de São Paulo, 2013. https://www.teses.usp.br/teses/disponiveis/2/2136/tde-17122013-081615 /publico/Daniel_de_Menezes_Pereira_Dissertacao_Mestrado_Pericia_Medico _Legal_Final_18jan2013.pdf.

Pereira, João Octaviano de Lima. Administração Pires do Rio. *Defesa dos Bens Dominaes do Município de São Paulo, 1927–1928: Relatório Apresentado pelo Dr. João Octaviano de Lima Pereira, Chefe do Serviço*. São Paulo: Empreza Graphica Limitada, 1928.

Pereira, Miguel. "O Brasil é ainda um imenso hospital"—Discurso pronunciado pelo professor Miguel Pereira por ocasião do regresso do professor Aloysio de Castro, da República Argentina, em outubro de 1916. *Revista de Medicina* 7, no. 21 (1916): 3–7.

Pereira, Robson Mendonça. "O prefeito do progresso: Modernização da cidade de São Paulo na administração de Washington Luís (1914–1919)." PhD diss.,

Universidade Estadual Paulista "Júlio de Mesquita Filho," Franca, 2005. https://repositorio.unesp.br/bitstream/handle/11449/103092/pereira_rm_dr_fran.pdf?sequence=1.

Perillo, Sonia Regina. "Novos caminhos da migração no Estado de São Paulo." *São Paulo em Perspectiva* 10, no. 2 (April–June 1996): 73–82.

Peters, Mario. *Apartments for Workers: Social Housing, Segregation, and Stigmatization in Urban Brazil.* Baden-Baden: Nomos, 2018.

Petrone, Pasquale. "A cidade de São Paulo no século XX," *Revista de História, São Paulo* 10, no. 21–22 (1955): 127–70.

Piccini, Andrea. *Cortiços na cidade: Conceito e preconceito na reestruturação do centro urbano de São Paulo.* São Paulo: Annablume, 1999.

Pimenta Velloso, Marta, "Os restos na história: Percepções sobre resíduos." *Ciência & Saúde Coletiva* 13, no. 6 (November–December, 2008): 1953–64.

Pingel, Emily Sweetnam. "Immigrants, Migrants, and Paulistanos: Racialized Geographies of Labor and Health in São Paulo, Brazil." *SSM—Qualitative Research in Health* 2 (December 2022). https://doi.org/10.1016/j.ssmqr.2022.100074.

Pingel, Emily Sweetnam. "Primary Care and the Reproduction of Health Inequity in a Central São Paulo Neighborhood." PhD diss., Emory University, 2021.

Pingel, Emily Sweetnam, Alexandra Caridad Llovet, and Fernando Cosentino. "Committing to Continuity: Primary Care Practices during COVID-19 in an Urban Brazilian Neighborhood." *Health, Education and Behavior* 48, no. 1 (January 2021): 29–33. https://doi.org/10.1177/1090198120979609.

Pinto, Adolpho. *A transformação e o embellezamento de São Paulo.* São Paulo: Cardozo Filho, 1912. https://docvirt.com/docreader.net/DocReader.aspx?bib=livrossp&Pesq=Bom%20Retiro&pagfis=18091.

Pinto, Alfredo Moreira. *A cidade de São Paulo em 1900: Impressões de viagem.* Rio de Janeiro: Imprensa Nacional, 1900. http://docvirt.com/docreader.net/DocReader.aspx?bib=livrossp&pagfis=8261.

Piza, Douglas de Toledo. "Chinese Migration and Changes in Brazilian Society." In *How China Is Transforming Brazil*, edited by Mariana Hase Ueta, Mathias Alencastro, and Rosana Pinheiro-Machado, 41–58. Singapore: Palgrave Macmillan, 2023.

Portelli, Alessandro. "Uchronic Dreams: Working Class Memory and Possible Worlds." *Oral History* 16, no. 2 (Autumn 1988): 46–56. https://www.jstor.org/stable/40179011.

Portes, Alejandro and Robert Manning, "The Immigrant Enclave: Theory and Empirical Examples." In *Competitive Ethnic Relations*, edited by Susan Olzak and Joane Nagel, 47–68. Orlando: Academic Press, 1986.

Portnoy, Eddy. "Rent Strike: A Dramatization of the Lower East Side Rent Strikes of 1908." *Jewish Currents*, Fall 2020. https://jewishcurrents.org/issue/fall-2020.

Póvoa, Carlos Alberto. *A territorialização dos judeus na cidade de São Paulo.* São Paulo: Editora Humanitas, 2010.

Powell, Jeffrey R. "New Contender for Most Lethal Animal." *Nature* 540 (2016): 525.

Powell, Jeffrey R., Andrea Gloria-Soria, and Panayiota Kotsakiozi. "Recent History of *Aedes aegypti*: Vector Genomics and Epidemiology Records." *BioScience* 68, no. 11 (November 2018): 854–60. https://doi.org/10.1093/biosci/biy119.

Prefeitura Municipal de São Paulo. DIRETRIZES DE INTERVENÇÃO—*Quadras 37 e 38—Campos Elíseos*. June 2018. https://www.prefeitura.sp.gov.br/cidade/secretarias/upload/habitacao/180612_Diretrizes_de_Intervencao_Quadras37e38.pdf.

Projeto IPHAN. *Multiculturalismo em situação urbana, inventário de referências culturais do Bom Retiro*. São Paulo: 9a Superintendência Regional do Instituto do Patrimônio Histórico e Artístico Nacional em São Paulo, Departamento de Patrimônio Histórico da Secretaria da Cultura da Prefeitura do Município de São Paulo, 2005.

Putnam, Lara. *Radical Moves: Caribbean Migrants and the Politics of Race in the Jazz Age*. Chapel Hill: University of North Carolina Press, 2003.

Raffard, Henrique. *Alguns dias na Paulicéia*. São Paulo: Academia Paulista de Letras, 1977.

Rago, Margareth. *Do cabaré ao lar: A utopia da cidade disciplinar e a resistência anarquista: Brasil 1890–1930*. São Paulo: Paz e Terra, 2014.

Ramos, Reinaldo. "Indicadores do nível de saúde: Sua aplicação no município de São Paulo (1894–1959)." PhD diss., Universidade de São Paulo, 1962.

Reale, Ebe. *Brás, Pinheiros, Jardins: Três bairros, três mundos*. São Paulo: Livraria Pioneira Editora, 1982.

Rechtman, Enio. "Itaboca, rua de triste memória: imigrantes judeus no bairro do Bom Retiro e o confinamento da zona do meretrício (1940 a 1953)." Master's thesis, Universidade de São Paulo, 2015.

Rede Nossa São Paulo, *Mapa da Desigualdade 2022*. Accessed June 28, 2024. https://www.nossasaopaulo.org.br/wp-content/uploads/2022/11/Mapa-da-Desigualdade-2022_Tabelas.pdf.

Reibscheid, Samuel. "Plétzale. Marco Zero." In *Breve fantasia*. São Paulo: Scritta, 1995.

Reichman, Daniel R. *Progress in the Balance: Mythologies of Development in Santos, Brazil*. Ithaca, NY: Cornell University Press, 2023.

Reinehr, Jaciane Pimentel Milanezi. "Silêncios e confrontos: A saúde da população negra em burocracias do Sistema Único de Saúde (SUS)." PhD diss., Universidade Federal do Rio de Janeiro, 2019.

Reis Filho, Lúcio, and Alfredo Suppia. "Dos cânones sagrados às alegorias profanas: A Laicização do Zumbi no Cinema." MNEME—*Revista de Humanidades* 11, no. 29 (January–July 2011): 272–85. https://periodicos.ufrn.br/mneme/article/download/1013/969/3758.

Reny, Tyler T., and Matt A. Barreto. "Xenophobia in the Time of Pandemic: Othering, Anti-Asian Attitudes, and COVID-19." *Politics, Groups, and Identities* 10, no. 2 (2022): 209–32.

Repartição de Estatística e do Arquivo do Estado. *Annuario estatistico de São Paulo (Brasil) 1922 a 1926.* São Paulo: Casa Vanorden, 1929. https://bibliotecadigital .seade.gov.br/view/singlepage/index.php?pubcod=10011079&parte=1.

Resende, Maurício Rodrigues de, and Jussara Parada Amed. "O jardim da luz e os desdobramentos da urbanização paulistana." *Revista PIBIC* 5, no. 6 (2011): 99–110. https://edisciplinas.usp.br/pluginfile.php/4296200/mod_resource/content/1 /jardim%20da%20luz%20mauricio.pdf.

Rezende, Sonaly Cristina, and Léo Heller. *O saneamento no Brasil: Políticas e interfaces.* Belo Horizonte: Universidade Federal de Minas Gerais, 2008.

Reznik, Luís, and Rui Aniceto Nascimento Fernandes. "Hospedarias de Imigrantes nas Américas: A criação da hospedaria da Ilha das Flores." *História (São Paulo)* 33, no. 1 (January/June 2014): 234–53.

Ribas, Emílio. "Profilaxia da febre amarela: Memória apresentada ao 5o Congresso Brasileiro de Medicina e Cirurgia. Rio de Janeiro." *O Brazil Médico* 17, no. 37 (October 1903): 363–64. https://www.obrasraras.fiocruz.br/media.details.php ?mediaID=167.

Ribeiro, Ednaldo Aparecido. "Confiança política na America Latina: Evolução recente de determinante individuais." *Revista de Sociologia e Política (Curitiba)* 19, no. 39 (June 2011): 167–82.

Ribeiro, Maria Alice Rosa. *Condições de trabalho na indústria têxtil paulista (1870–1930).* Campinas: Editora da UNICAMP; Hucitec, 1988.

Ribeiro, Maria Alice Rosa. "O engenheiro e o inquérito: as habitações operárias no Distrito de Santa Ifigênia, São Paulo, 1893." *Cadernos De História Da Ciência* 11, no. 2, 130–69. https://doi.org/10.47692/cadhistcienc.2015.v11 .33895.

Riccò, Giulia. "'Il segno di Menelik': Enrico Corradini, the *Protocolos*, and the Restaging of Adwa in São Paulo." *Italian Culture* 41, no. 1 (February 2023): 6–24. https://doi.org/10.1080/01614622.2023.2167325.

Riess, Steven A. "From Pitch to Putt: Sport and Class in Anglo-American Sport." *Journal of Sport History* 21, no. 2 (Summer 1994): 138–84.

Riis, Jacob. *How the Other Half Lives: Studies among the Tenements of New York.* New York: Charles Scribner's Sons, 1890.

Rio, João do (Paulo Barreto). "A musa das ruas." In *A alma encantadora das ruas* [1910], 173–86. Rio de Janeiro: Prefeitura da Cidade do Rio de Janeiro, Secretaria Municipal de Cultura, 1995. https://www.rio.rj.gov.br/dlstatic/10112 /4204210/4101365/alma_encant_ruas.pdf.

Rocha, Fábio Dantas. "Saindo das sombras: Classe e raça na São Paulo pós-abolição (1887–1930)." Master's thesis, Universidade Federal de São Paulo, 2018.

Rochard, Jules. "L'Hygiène en 1889." *Revue des Deux Mondes* 96, no. 1 (November 1889): 54–85.

Rodrigues, Gustavo Partezani. *Vias públicas: Tipo e construção em São Paulo (1898-1945).* São Paulo: Imprensa Oficial do Estado de São Paulo, 2010.

Rodriguez, Julia. "Inoculating against Barbarism? State Medicine and Immigrant Policy in Turn-of-the-Century Argentina." *Science in Context* 19, no. 3 (September 2006): 357–80. https://doi.org/10.1017/s0269889706000974.

Rogers, Thomas D. "Laboring Landscapes: The Environmental, Racial, and Class Worldview of the Brazilian Northeast's Sugar Elite, 1880s–1930s." *Luso-Brazilian Review* 46, no. 2 (December 2009): 22–53.

Rolnik, Raquel. *A cidade e a lei: Legislação, política urbana e territórios na cidade de São Paulo.* São Paulo: Studio Nobel: FAPESP, 1997.

Romani, Carlo. *Da Biblioteca Popular à Escola Moderna: Breve história da ciência e educação libertária na América do Sul.* Vol. 1. São Paulo: Educação Libertária, 2006.

Romero, Mariza. "Construção da nação e exclusão social: São Paulo-Brasil (1889-1930)." *Amérique Latine Histoire et Mémoire. Les Cahiers ALHIM* 29 (2015): 79–100. http://journals.openedition.org/alhim/5258.

Rosen, George. "Cameralism and the Concept of Medical Police." *Bulletin of the History of Medicine* 27, no. 1 (January–February 1953): 21–42.

Roth, Joshua. "A Mean-Spirited Sport: Japanese Brazilian Croquet in São Paulo's Public Spaces." *Anthropological Quarterly* 79, no. 4 (Fall 2006): 609–32.

Sá, Dominichi Miranda de. "A voz do Brasil: Miguel Pereira e o discurso sobre o 'imenso hospital.'" *História, Ciências, Saúde—Manguinhos* 16, suppl. 1 (July 2009): 333–48. https://www.scielo.br/j/hcsm/a/jhCVgqYXYJyF85D4FZJJp6P/#.

Sábato, Hilda, and Luis Alberto Romero. *Los trabajadores de Buenos Aires: La experiencia del mercado, 1850–1880.* Buenos Aires: Sudamericana, 1992.

Salgado, Plínio. *O estrangeiro (Crônica da vida paulista).* 1926. 4th ed. São Paulo: Edições Panorama, 1948.

Salla, Natália Maria. "Produzir para construir: A indústria cerâmica paulistana no período da Primeira República (1889–1930)." Master's thesis, Universidade de São Paulo, 2014.

Sampaio, Maria Ruth Amaral de. "O cortiço paulistano entre as ciências sociais e política." *Revista do IEB* 44 (February 2007): 125–40. https://www.revistas.usp.br/rieb/article/download/34565/37303/0.

Sampaio, Maria Ruth Amaral de, and Paulo Cesar Xavier Pereira, "Habitação em São Paulo." *Estudos Avançados* 17, no. 48 (2003): 167–83.

Sánchez, George. *Boyle Heights: How a Los Angeles Neighborhood Became the Future of American Democracy.* Berkeley: University of California Press, 2022.

Santana, Márcio Santos de. "A difícil transformação: Os industriais e a oposição ao Código de Menores de 1927." *Dimensões* 30 (November 2013): 315–34.

Sant'anna, Denise Bernuzzi de. "Guerra e paz: Alguns cenários da vida hospitalar." In *História da Saúde em São Paulo: Instituições e patrimônio arquitetônico (1808–1958),* edited by Maria Lucia Mott and Gisele Sanglar, 1–24. Rio de Janeiro: Editora Fiocruz /Editora Manole, 2011.

Santos, Carlos Henrique Neres dos. "Sob a luz dos infames: Anticlericalismo nas imagens do jornal A Lanterna—folha anticlerical de combate (São Paulo, 1909-1916)." Master's thesis, Universidade Estadual Paulista, 2019.

Santos, Carlos José Ferreira dos. *Nem tudo era italiano: São Paulo e pobreza, 1890-1915*. São Paulo: Annablume, 2008.

Santos, Edirlei Machado dos, and Débora Isane Ratner Kirschbaum. "A trajetória histórica da visita domiciliária no Brasil: Uma revisão bibliográfica." *Revista Eletrônica de Enfermagem* 10, no. 1 (November 2008): 220-27. https://doi.org /10.5216/ree.v10i1.8014.

Santos, Fabio Alexandre dos, Fernando Atique, Janes Jorge, Luis Ferla, Diego de Souza Morais, Janaina Yamamoto, Maíra Rosin, et al. "A enchente de 1929 na cidade de São Paulo: Memória, história e novas abordagens de pesquisa." *Revista do Arquivo Geral da Cidade do Rio de Janeiro* 8 (2014): 149-66. http://www .rio.rj.gov.br/dlstatic/10112/4204432/4133801/revista_agcrj_oito.pdf.

Santos, Fernando de Oliveira dos. *Aspectos da luta pela cidadania negra na cidade de São Paulo (1891-1930)*. São Paulo: Dialética, 2020.

Santos, Milton. *A natureza do espaço: Técnica e tempo, razão e emoção*. São Paulo: Editora da Universidade de São Paulo, 2006.

Santos, Ricardo Augusto dos. "O Carnaval, a peste e a 'espanhola.'" *História, Ciências, Saúde—Manguinhos* 13, no. 1 (January–March 2006): 129-58.

São Paulo (City). *Annaes da Camara Municipal de São Paulo, 1920*. São Paulo: Typographia Piratininga, 1920.

São Paulo (State). *Anuário demográfico da Seção de Estatísticas Demógrafo-Sanitárias 1907*. São Paulo: Serviço Sanitário do Estado de São Paulo, 1907. https://bibliotecadigital.seade.gov.br/view/listarPublicacao.php?lista =0&opcao=8&busca=1&tipoFiltro=periodo&filtro=%271907%27&descFiltro =1907&listarConteudo=Cole%C3%A7%C3%B5es%20%C2%BB%20 Anu%C3%A1rio%20de%20Estat%C3%ADstica%20Dem%C3%B3grafo -Sanit%C3%A1ria.

São Paulo (State). *Annuario demographico: Secção de estatistica demographo-sanitaria 1913*. São Paulo: Serviço Sanitário do Estado de São Paulo, 1913. https://bibliotecadigital.seade.gov.br/view/singlepage/index.php?pubcod =10011016&parte=1.

São Paulo (City). Câmara Municipal de São Paulo. "Celso Garcia, Indicação 144 of 1905, 24th Sessão Ordinária de 29 de Julho de 1905." In *Anais da Câmara Municipal: Legislatura de 1905*, 111. São Paulo: Edição da Câmara Municipal de São Paulo, 1905.

São Paulo (City). Câmara Municipal de São Paulo. *Relatório da Comissão de Exame e Inspecção das Habitações Operárias e Cortiços do Districto de Santa Iphygenia, apresentado pelo Intendente Municipal Cesario Motta Jr.* São Paulo: Câmara Municipal de São Paulo, 1893. http://www.arquivoestado.sp.gov.br/site/acervo /repositorio_digital/corticos_ephigenia.

São Paulo (State). Comissão do Saneamento das Várzeas. *Relatório dos estudos para o saneamento e aformoseamento das várzeas adjacentes a cidade de São Paulo apresentado ao Presidente do Estado Dr Américo Brasiliense de Almeida Mello, pela comissão para este fim em 1890 pelo então governador Dr. Prudente*

José de Moraes e Barros. São Paulo: Comissão do Saneamento das Várzeas, 1891. http://www2.unifesp.br/himaco/enchente_1887.php.

São Paulo (City). *Cortiços em São Paulo: Frente e verso.* São Paulo: Município de São Paulo, Secretaria Municipal do Planejamento, 1986.

São Paulo (State). Departamento Estadual de Estatística. *Anuário estatístico do estado de São Paulo 1940.* São Paulo: Tipografia Brasil, 1940. https://bibliotecadigital .seade.gov.br/view/singlepage/index.php?pubcod=10011085&parte=1.

São Paulo (State). Directoria do Serviço Sanitário, *Boletim Mensal de Estatística Demógrafo-Sanitária.* São Paulo: Directoria do Serviço Sanitario. Volumes between 1894 and 1929 available at https://bibliotecadigital.seade.gov.br/view /listarPublicacao.php.

São Paulo (State). *Mensagem enviada ao Congresso do Estado, a 7 de abril de 1900, pelo Dr. Fernando Prestes de Albuquerque, Presidente do Estado.* São Paulo: Typographia do Diário Oficial, 1900. https://bibliotecadigital.seade.gov.br/view /singlepage/index.php?pubcod=10012822&parte=1.

São Paulo (State). *Mensagem enviada ao Congresso Legislativo a 14 de julho de 1909 pelo Dr. M. J. de Albuquerque Lins.* São Paulo: Duprat, 1909.

São Paulo (Province): *Relatório apresentado à Assembléia Legislativa Provincial de São Paulo pelo Presidente da Província barão de Parnahyba, no dia 17 de janeiro de 1887.* São Paulo: Typ. A Vapor de Jorge Seckler & Comp., 1887.

São Paulo (City). *Relatório de 1904 apresentado a Câmara Municipal de São Paulo pelo prefeito Dr. Antonio da Silva Prado.* São Paulo: Typographia Vanorden & Co., 1905.

São Paulo (State). *Relatório dos Presidentes dos Estados Brasileiros, Mensagem apresentada ao congresso legislativo em 14 de Julho 1919 pelo Dr. Altino Arantes, Presidente do Estado de São Paulo.* Rio de Janeiro: Typographia do "Jornal do Commercio" de Rodrigues and Co., 1919.

São Paulo (State). Secção de Propaganda e Educação Sanitária, Departamento de Saúde. *Combate à Lepra.* São Paulo: Imprensa Oficial do Estado, 1957.

São Paulo. Secretaria Municipal da Saúde, Coordenação de Epidemiologia e Informação. *Boletim CEInfo Saúde em Dados* 21:21 (July 2022). https://www .prefeitura.sp.gov.br/cidade/secretarias/upload/saude/arquivos/ceinfo/capas _publicacoes/Boletim_CEInfo_Dados_2022.pdf#page=8.

São Paulo. Serviço Sanitário do Estado de São Paulo. *Desinfectório Central de São Paulo.* São Paulo: Vanorden, 1905.

São Paulo. Serviço Sanitário do Estado de São Paulo. *PESTE: Matança dos Ratos.* São Paulo: Escola Typographica Salesiana, 1899. https://revistapesquisa.fapesp .br/wp-content/uploads/2020/07/Folheto-Peste.pdf.

Scarlato, Francisco. "Estrutura e sobrevivencia dos cortiços no bairro Bexiga." *Revista do Departamento de Geografia* 9 (7 November 2011): 117–27. http://www .revistas.usp.br/rdg/article/view/53697.

Schneider, Marília. *Memória e história (Antoninho Da Rocha Marmo).* São Paulo: T. A. Queiroz, 2001.

Schwarcz, Lilia Moritz, and Heloisa Murgel Starling. *A bailarina da morte: A gripe espanhola no Brasil*. São Paulo: Companhia das Letras, 2020.

Scranton, Philip, B., ed. *Silk City: Studies on the Paterson Silk Industry, 1860–1940*. Newark: New Jersey Historical Society, 1985.

Seabra, Odette Carvalho de Lima. "Os meandros dos rios nos meandros do poder: Tietê e Pinheiros; Valorização dos rios e das várzeas na cidade de São Paulo." PhD diss., Universidade de São Paulo, 1987.

Secretaria de Cultura e Juventude de São Bernardo do Campo. *Biblioteca Pública— Lugar de conhecimentos, Uma história das pandemias. Parte 9: Rato Bum Bum Tam Tam*. https://www.saobernardo.sp.gov.br/web/cultura/-biblioteca-publica -lugar-de-conhecimentos-uma-historia-das-pandemias-parte-9-rato-bum-bum -tam-tam.

Segawa, Hugo. "Arquitetura de hospedarias de imigrantes." *Revista do Instituto de Estudos Brasileiros* 30 (December 1989): 23–42.

Seigel, Micol. *Uneven Encounters: Making Race and Nation in Brazil and the United States*. Durham, NC: Duke University Press, 2009.

Senne, Catia Alves de, and Flávia Andréa Machado Urzua. "A constituição do acervo do Museu de Saúde Pública Emílio Ribas: Subsídios para a análise de sua trajetória institucional." *Cadernos de História da Ciência—Instituto Butantan* 6, no. 2 (July–December 2010): 7–25.

Serufo, José Carlos, Andréa Marcia Souza, Valéria Aparecida Tavares, Marcos Cézar Jammal, and Josimar Gerônimo Silva. "Dengue in the South-Eastern Region of Brazil: Historical Analysis and Epidemiology." *Revista de Saúde Pública* 27, no. 3 (June 1993): 157–67.

Sevcenko, Nicolau. *A revolta da vacina: Mentes insanas em corpos rebeldes*. São Paulo: Editora UNESP, 2018.

Shah, Nayan. *Contagious Divides: Epidemics and Race in San Francisco's Chinatown*. Berkeley: University of California Press, 2001.

Shear, Matthew. "When the Virus Came for the American Dream." *New York Times Magazine*. November 2, 2020. https://www.nytimes.com/2020/11/02/magazine/ covid-business-atlanta.html.

Shinohara, Denise Yoneya, and Francisco de Assis Comarú. "Dinâmica Habitacional e Demográfica da Metrópole Paulista: Caracterização e análises preliminares." PPLA: Seminário Política, Território e Desenvolvimento, 2009, Curitiba.

Shively, Henry L. "Sanitary Tenements for Tuberculous Families." *British Journal of Tuberculosis* 3, no. 3 (July 1909): 193–96.

Shmulevitsh, Shlomo. מענטשן־פרעסער, *Mentshn-Fresser ("People Devourer"), a Pandemic Ballad by Shlomo Shmulevitsh*. New York: Hebrew Publishing Company, 1916.

Shu, Chang-sheng. *Chinese Migration to Brazil: History, Mobility and Identities*. Newcastle upon Tyne: Cambridge Scholars, 2023.

Shu, Chang-seng, and Pan Tiashu. "Studies on Chinese Migration to Brazil: Present State and Future Tendencies." In *Studies on Chinese Migrations: Brazil,*

China and Mozambique, edited by André Bueno and Daniel Veras, 189–223. Rio de Janeiro: Projeto Orientalismo/UERJ, 2021.

Silva, Cleudo Menezes. "Estudo epidemiológico da dengue no município de São Paulo." Master's thesis, Universidade de São Paulo, 2015. https://www.teses.usp.br/teses/disponiveis/99/99131/tde-25112016-095542/publico/CLEUDOFINAL.pdf.

Silva, James Roberto. "Fotogenia do caos: Fotografia e instituições de saúde em São Paulo (1880–1920)." Master's thesis, Universidade de São Paulo, 1998.

Silva, Márcia Regina Barros da. "Concepção de saúde e doença nos debates parlamentares paulistas entre 1830 e 1900." In *História da saúde em São Paulo: Instituições e patrimônio arquitetônico (1808–1958)*, edited by Maria Lucia Mott and Gisele Sanglard, 64–73. Rio de Janeiro: Editora Fiocruz /Editora Manole, 2011.

Silva, Márcia Regina Barros da. "História da assistência hospitalar em São Paulo: A subvenção do Estado às misericórdias paulistas." *História, Ciências, Saúde—Manguinhos* 26 (December 2019): 79–108. https://doi.org/10.1590/S0104 -59702019000500005.

Silva, Márcia Regina Barros da. *O laboratório e a república: Saúde pública, ensino médico e produção de conhecimento em São Paulo, 1891–1933*. Rio de Janeiro: Editora Fiocruz, 2014.

Silva, Márcia Regina Barros da. "O mundo transformado em laboratório: Ensino médico e produção de conhecimento em São Paulo de 1891 a 1933." PhD diss., Universidade de São Paulo, 2003.

Silva, Márcia Regina Barros da. "O processo de urbanização paulista: A medicina e o crescimento da cidade moderna." *Revista Brasileira de História* 27, no. 53 (June 2007): 243–66.

Silva, Márcia Regina Barros da. "Santa Casa de Misericórdia de São Paulo: Saúde e assistência se tornam públicas (1875–1910)." *Varia História* 26, no. 44 (July–December 2010): 395–420. https://doi.org/10.1590/S0104-87752010000200004.

Silva, Marcos Rafael. "Os Protocolos Italianos—1892–1897." PhD diss., Universidade de São Paulo, 2018.

Silva, Matheus Alves Duarte da. "Estratégias públicas no combate à peste bubônica no Rio de Janeiro (1900–1906)." Paper presented at XIV Encontro da ANPUH-Rio, Rio de Janeiro, Brazil, June 19–23, 2010. http://snh2011.anpuh.org/resources /anais/8/1276725973_ARQUIVO_resumodaAnpuh.pdf.

Silva, Olga Maria Panhoca da, Rodrigo A. Prando, and Luiz Panhoca. "Os imigrantes e a violência na cidade de São Paulo no início do século 20." *Salusvita (Bauru)* 27, no. 3 (2007): 317–36. https://secure.unisagrado.edu.br/static /biblioteca/salusvita/salusvita_v26_n3_2007_art_04.pdf.

Silva, Sidney Antonio da. *Costurando sonhos: trajetória de um grupo de imigrantes bolivianos em São Paulo*. São Paulo: Paulinas, 1997.

Silva, Silvana Cristina da. "Os bairros do Brás e Bom Retiro e a metrópole informacional." *Boletim Goiano de Geografia* 35, no. 1 (January–April 2015): 91–113.

Silva de Souza, Thais Cristina. "Cortiços em São Paulo: Programas/Vistorias/Relatos." Master's thesis: Universidade São Paulo, 2011.

Silva Filho, Antonio Cardoso, Rafael Dantas de Morais, and Janaina Barbosa da Silva. "Doenças de veiculação hídrica: Dados epidemiológicos, condições de abastecimento e armazenamento da água em Massaranduba/PB." *Geoambiente On-line*, no. 20 (June 2013): 1–14. https://doi.org/10.5216/revgeoamb.v0i20.26089.

Silva Junior, Fernando José Guedes da, and Claudete Ferreira de Souza Monteiro. "Os significados da morte e do morrer: A perspectiva de usuários de crack." *Revista Latino-Americana de Enfermagem* 20, no. 2 (March–April 2012): 378–83. https://www.scielo.br/j/rlae/a/mtZGdp4vhKtrdq4pWw5rMnb/?format=pdf&lang=pt.

Silveira, Cássio, Alejandro Goldberg, Tatiane Barbosa da Silva, Mara Helena de Andrea Gomes, and Denise Martin. "O lugar dos trabalhadores de saúde nas pesquisas sobre processos migratórios internacionais e saúde." *Cadernos de Saúde Pública* 32, no. 10 (October 2016): e00063916. https://doi.org/10.1590/0102-311X00063916.

Siqueira, Lucilia. "Os hotéis na cidade de São Paulo na primeira década do século XX: Diversidade no tamanho, na localização e nos serviços." *Revista Brasileira de História* 32, no. 63 (2012): 345–63. https://www.scielo.br/j/rbh/a/7BMfs3sTcLXcXC97KCYqRfd/?lang=pt.

Skidmore, Thomas E. *Black into White: Race and Nationality in Brazilian Thought*. New York: Oxford University Press, 1974.

Somekh, Nadia. *A cidade vertical e o urbanismo modernizador*. São Paulo: Mackenzie, 2014.

Sontag, Susan. *Illness as a Metaphor*. New York: Farrar, Straus and Giroux, 1977.

Soppelsa, Peter. "Losing France's Imperial War on Rats." *Journal of the Western Society for French History* 47 (2021): 67–87. http://hdl.handle.net/2027/spo.0642292.0047.006.

Spaulding, O. L. "Haffkine Prophylactic and Antipest Serum." *Public Health Reports (1896-1970)* 15, no. 35 (August 1900): 2135–42.

Special Commissioner. "The Health Resorts of the Riviera." *Medical Record: A Weekly Journal of Medicine and Surgery* 42, no. 7 (August 1892): 200–204.

Sposati, Aldaíza, ed. *Mapa da exclusão/inclusão social da cidade de São Paulo 2000*. São Paulo: PUC/Instituto Pólis/INPE, 2000.

Sposati, Aldaíza, ed. "Mapa exclusão/inclusão social do município de São Paulo—III (2010): Que mundo é este que vivemos, que país é este e que cidade é esta?" Paper presented at the V Fórum Social Sul, October 2013. https://ceapg.fgv.br/sites/ceapg.fgv.br/files/u60/relatorio_-_mapa_da_exclusao_social_-_sposati.pdf.

Sposati, Aldaiza, ed. *Mapa da exclusão/inclusão social da cidade de São Paulo*. São Paulo: EDUC, 1996.

Steffens, Isadora, and Jameson Martins. "Falta um Jorge: A saúde na política para migrantes de São Paulo (SP)." *Lua Nova: Revista de Cultura e Política* 98 (May–August 2016): 275–99. https://doi.org/10.1590/0102-6445275-299/98.

Stepan, Nancy Leys. "Biology and Degeneration: Races and Proper Places." In *Degeneration: The Dark Side of Progress*, edited by J. Edward Chamberlin and Sander L. Gilman, 97–120. New York: Columbia University Press, 1985.

Stepan, Nancy Leys. *Eradication: Ridding the World of Diseases Forever?* Ithaca, NY: Cornell University Press, 2011.

Stepan, Nancy Leys. *"The Hour of Eugenics": Race, Gender, and Nation in Latin America*. Ithaca, NY: Cornell University Press, 1991.

Stewart, Danielle J. "Framing the City: Photography and the Construction of São Paulo, 1930–1955." PhD diss., CUNY Graduate Center, 2019.

Sugayama, Soraya. "Ferréz: Produção material e cultural na quebrada." PhD diss., Universidade Tecnológica Federal do Paraná, 2019. https://repositorio.utfpr .edu.br/jspui/bitstream/1/4660/2/CT_PPGTE_D_Sugayama%2C_Soraya _2019.pdf.

Taunay, Afonso d'Escragnolle. *História da cidade de São Paulo*. 1953. Brasília: Senado Federal, Conselho Editorial, 2004. https://www2.senado.leg.br/bdsf /bitstream/handle/id/1085/690133.pdf?sequence=4&isAllowed=y-.

Taylor, Diana. "Performing the 'Thing': Teatro da Vertigem's Bom Retiro 958 metros." *Afterall: A Journal of Art Context and Enquiry* 35 no. 35 (March 2014): 60–71.

Teixeira, Luiz Antonio, and Marta de Almeida. "Os primórdios da vacina antivariólica em São Paulo: Uma história pouco conhecida." *Manguinhos* 10, suppl. 2 (2003): 475–98. https://www.scielo.br/j/hcsm/a/63pwhBVBZMDRdwKX3SWrRYb/.

Teixeira, Rosane Siqueira. "Sob a perspectiva de uma política expansionista: Hospedarias de imigrantes de Pernambuco, 1889–1926." *Clio: Revista de Pesquisa Histórica* 40, no. 2 (July–December 2022): 287–321. https://periodicos .ufpe.br/revistas/revistaclio/article/view/252527/43461.

Telarolli, Rodolpho, Junior. "Imigração e epidemias no estado de São Paulo." *História, Ciências, Saúde—Manguinhos* 3, no. 2 (July–October 1996): 265–83. https:// www.scielo.br/j/hcsm/a/RS8yYKbdSdLjkVpGCtP6Cpw/?format=pdf&lang=pt.

Telles, Edward E. *Race in Another America: The Significance of Skin Color in Brazil*. Princeton, NJ: Princeton University Press, 2004.

Terreros, Abraham. "Saberes y prácticas médicos durante la revolución bacteri-ológica y la ley de inmigración mexicana de 1909." *Historia Mexicana* 73, no. 3 (January–March 2024): 1205–40.

Toledo, Roberto Pompeu de. *A capital da vertigem: Uma história de São Paulo de 1900 a 1954*. São Paulo: Objetiva, 2015.

Toji, Simone. *The Immensity of Being Singular: Approaching Migrant Lives in São Paulo through Resonance*. Chicago: HAU Books, 2023.

Tonini, Sandra Cristina Correia Loureiro. "Saúde da população Síria: Percepções dos profissionais da Atenção Primária à Saúde da Supervisão Técnica de Saúde da Mooca no Município de São Paulo." Master's thesis, Instituto de Saúde— Coordenadoria de Recursos Humanos da Secretaria de Estado da Saúde de São Paulo, 2019. https://docs.bvsalud.org/biblioref/2019/08/1008013/sandra _dissertacao.pdf.

Travassos, Claudia, and David R. Williams. "The Concept and Measurement of Race and Their Relationship to Public Health: A Review Focused on Brazil and the United States." *Cadernos de Saúde Pública* 20, no. 3 (June 2004): 660–78. https://doi.org/10.1590/S0102-311X2004000300003.

Trento, Angelo. "A Itália em guerra: A coletividade imigrada e o Fanfulla de São Paulo durante o primeiro conflito mundial." *Revista Escritos* 9, no. 9 (2015): 97–124. http://escritos.rb.gov.br/numero09/cap_04.pdf.

Truzzi, Oswaldo. "Etnias em convívio: o bairro do Bom Retiro em São Paulo." *Revista Estudos Históricos* 2, no. 28 (February 2001): 143–66. https://periodicos.fgv.br/reh/article/view/2144.

Tsing, Anna Lowenhaupt. *Friction: An Ethnography of Global Connection.* Princeton, NJ: Princeton University Press, 2004.

Turner, Patricia A. *I Heard It through the Grapevine: Rumor in African-American Culture.* Berkeley: University of California Press, 1993.

Udaeta, Rosa Guadalupe Soares. *Nem Brás, nem Flores: Hospedaria de Imigrantes da cidade de São Paulo (1875–1886).* São Paulo: FFLCH/USP, 2016. https://spap.fflch.usp.br/sites/spap.fflch.usp.br/files/PAP-UDAETA_Rosa-15032016-FINAL.pdf.

United Nations, *Population Growth and Policies in Mega-Cities: São Paulo.* New York: United Nations, 1993.

Vanderwood, Paul J. *Disorder and Progress: Bandits, Police, and Mexican Development.* Lincoln: University of Nebraska Press, 1981.

Vann, Michael G. "Of Rats, Rice, and Race: The Great Hanoi Rat Massacre, an Episode in French Colonial History." *French Colonial History* 4 (2003): 191–203. https://doi.org/10.1353/fch.2003.0027.

Vargas, João H. Costa. "When a Favela Dared to Become a Gated Condominium: The Politics of Race and Urban Space in Rio de Janeiro." *Latin American Perspectives* 33, no. 4 (July 2006): 49–81. https://doi.org/10.1177/0094582X06289892.

Vaz, Lilian Fessler. "Dos cortiços às favelas e aos edifícios de apartamentos—a modernização da moradia no Rio de Janeiro." *Análise Social* 39, no. 127 (1994): 581–97. https://www5.pucsp.br/ecopolitica/downloads/art_1994_corticos_favelas_edificios_apartamentos_modernizacao_moradia_Rio_Janeiro.pdf.

Venancio, Giselle Martins. "Lugar de mulher é . . . na fábrica: Estado e trabalho feminino no Brasil (1910–1934)." *História: Questões e Debates (Curitiba)* 34, no. 1 (June 2001): 175–200.

Vertesi, Janet. "Mind the Gap: The London Underground Map and Users' Representations of Urban Space." *Social Studies of Science* 38, no. 1 (February 2008): 7–33.

Vignie, Nicolas, and Olivier Bouchaud. "Travel, Migration, and Emerging Infectious Diseases." *Journal of the International Federation of Clinical Chemistry and Laboratory Medicine* 29, no. 3 (November 2018): 175–79.

Walcott, Susan M. "Overlapping Ethnicities and Negotiated Space: Atlanta's Buford Highway." *Journal of Cultural Geography* 20, no. 1 (2002): 51–75.

Waldman, Eliseu, Luiz da Silva, and Carlos Monteiro. "Trajetória das doenças infecciosas." *Informe Epidemiológico do Sus* 8, no. 3 (September 1999): 5–47.

Walle, Paul. *Au Brésil: L'état de São Paulo*. Paris: E. Guilmoto, 1916.

Weber, Beatriz Teixeira. "Como convencer e curar: a introdução da homeopatia no Rio Grande do Sul." Paper presented at XXIII Simpósio Nacional de História, Londrina, Brazil, 2005. https://anpuh.org.br/uploads/anais-simposios/pdf /2019-01/1548206372_de56ee8cccdfe5c46dd378accdfo445a.pdf.

Weinstein, Barbara. *The Color of Modernity: São Paulo and the Making of Race and Nation in Brazil*. Durham, NC: Duke University Press, 2015.

Wilhelm, Jorge. *São Paulo Metrópole 65: Subsídios para seu plano diretor*. São Paulo: Difusão Européia do Livro, Coleção Corpo e Alma do Brasil, 1965.

Williams, Nathalie E., Arland Thornton, and Linda C. Young-DeMarco. "Migrant Values and Beliefs: How Are They Different and How Do They Change?" *Journal of Ethnic and Migration Studies* 40, no. 5 (January 2014): 796–813.

Williams, Robin B. "The Global Spread of Street Pavement Materials and Technology, 1820-1920." In *The Routledge Handbook of Infrastructure Design: Global Perspectives from Architectural History*, edited by Joseph Heathcott, 211–21. New York: Routledge, 2022.

Willis, Graham Denyer. "Antagonistic Authorities and the Civil Police in São Paulo, Brazil." *Latin American Research Review* 49, no. 1 (2014): 3-22.

Winter, Jay. "History, Memory, and the Flu." In *Re-awakenings: The Forgotten and Unforgotten "Spanish" Flu of 1918–1919*, edited by Guy Beiner, xxv–xxviii. New York: Oxford University Press, 2022.

Wolfe, Joel. *Autos and Progress: The Brazilian Search for Modernity*. New York: Oxford University Press, 2010.

Wolfe, Joel. *Working Women, Working Men: São Paulo and the Rise of Brazil's Industrial Working Class, 1900–1955*. Durham, NC: Duke University Press, 1993.

Wyman, Walter. *The Bubonic Plague*. Washington, DC: Government Printing Office, 1900. https://collections.nlm.nih.gov/catalog/nlm:nlmuid-9803039X18-leaf.

Xun, Zhou, and Sander L. Gilman. *"I Know Who Caused COVID-19": Pandemics and Xenophobia*. London: Reaktion Books, 2021.

Yankelevich, Pablo. "Migración, mestizaje y xenofobia en México (1910-1950)." *Jahrbuch für Geschichte Lateinamerikas Anuario de Historia de América Latina* 54 (2017): 129–56.

Yee, David. "Housing in the Latin American City, 1900–1976." In *Oxford Research Encyclopedia of Latin American History*, article published online May 23, 2019. https://doi.org/10.1093/acrefore/9780199366439.013.787.

Young, Robert J. C. "Postcolonial Remains." *New Literary History* 43, no. 1 (January 2012): 19–42.

Zequini, Anicleide. *O quintal da fábrica: A industrialização pioneira do interior Paulista*. São Paulo: Annablume: FAPESP, 2004.

Zylbersztajn, Decio. *O filho de Osum*. São Paulo: Editora Reformatório, 2019.

INDEX

Page numbers followed by *f* refer to figures; page numbers followed by *m* refer to maps.

vaccination, 28, 35, 38, 145, 161, 196
Vaccine Revolt, 144–45
Vargas, Getúlio, 100–101, 106
vehicles, 74, 112, 113*f*, 123, 149–50, 154, 156–62, 181; collisions with pedestrians, 37; official, 140, 142, 151
verticalization, 73, 90
violence, 1, 14, 34, 37, 73, 85, 99, 103–7, 109, 118, 137–38, 145, 164; bad health and, 129; discussions of, 128; gun, 3, 12, 31, 81; immigrant-on-Black, 72; against immigrants, 176; men and, 120; military dictatorship and, 7; nationality and, 56; obstetric, 27; police, 50; Portuguese, 101; state, 132

waste, 76; food, 87; household, 53; industrial, 49; products, 13; removal, 37, 53, 129, 152
water, 13, 34, 52–53, 83, 133, 154, 165, 184; access to, 38; authority, 119, 124; contaminated, 98; delivery, 86; drinking, 131, 138, 198; iodine, 183; lack of, 52, 137; standing, 27, 29, 37, 51, 53, 76, 131*f*, 135*f*, 136–38, 140–41; tanks, 134, 136*f*, 138–39; wastewater, 109
weapons, 5, 31, 73, 106, 169
white immigrants, 34, 69, 91
whitening, 69, 78, 108, 117, 120, 217n50
women, 41, 68, 87, 108, 120, 127, 206n6; Afro-Brazilian, 232n96; Black, 111, 120; BRPHC and, 24; death rate of, 182; as domésticas, 120, 123; enfranchisement of, 104; health of, 123–24; health jobs and, 140; Hospedaria dos Imigrantes and, 92, 95–96; injuries and, 120; Italian, 33, 100; literacy and, 176; Medical Police and, 107; nonwhite, 116; pregnant, 98; Spanish-speaking, 143; trafficked, 100; white, 79; work of, 36
worker activism, 37, 50
workers, 8, 40, 51, 56, 87, 103, 120, 125, 126, 182, 191; Black, 116; community health, 24, 222n68; domestic, 71, 88, 120, 128, 137; foreign, 83; health, 26, 145, 152, 161–62, 198; health surveillance, 74, 142, 144; housing and, 89, 89–90, 106; immigrant, 14, 35, 49–50, 53; Jardim da Luz and, 54; oficina-residências and, 68, 76; railroad, 98; retail, 195; sex, 9, 93, 100–101, 161; textile, 8–9, 142–43, 197. *See also* health care workers; public health: workers
working classes, 7, 9, 35–36, 42, 84, 86, 88, 110–11, 145; Central Disinfectory and, 154; deratification and, 193; health and, 133; immigrant, 31, 164; mobility and, 96; paternalism toward, 137; prejudices against, 109, 130; prescriptions and, 183; public health officials and, 133, 182, 184; Santa Casa de Misericórdia and, 102; sewers and, 52; Spanish flu and, 165, 181, 191; wages of, 83
working-class immigrants, 34, 36, 39, 41, 56, 61, 112, 129
working-class neighborhoods, 12, 18, 52, 56, 73, 140, 158, 193; in the Americas, 50, 74, 78; built environment in, 23; foreigners in, 168; flu in, 181; geographies in, 78; health outcomes in, 28; immigrant, 190, 195; lack of state intervention in, 86; occupational variation in, 120; rat brokers in, 170; water and, 133
World War II, 67, 74, 133, 138, 142, 162, 236n52; Brás hospedaria and, 95; cortiços and, 82; Japanese immigrants and, 187; Jewish immigrants and, 16

xenophobia, 127, 133, 166, 190, 193

yellow fever, 35, 45, 81–82, 85, 130, 132–34, 149–50, 156, 167
Yiddish, 7, 17*f*, 122, 162, 196
The Year My Parents Went on Vacation (Hamburger), 7, 16

Zika, 29, 134, 136–37, 140–41, 144; mosquito eradication, 145, 146*f*
zombies, 189